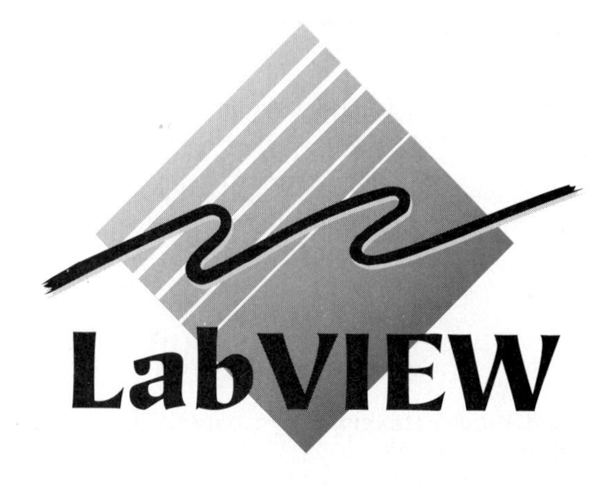

DATA ACQUISITION & ANALYSIS FOR THE MOVEMENT SCIENCES

ANDREW L. MCDONOUGH

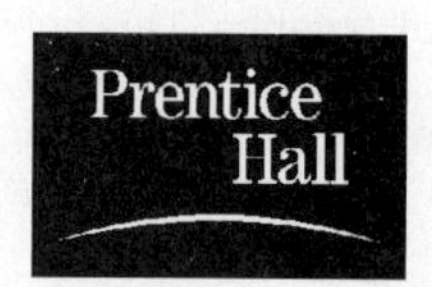

Upper Saddle River, New Jersey

Library of Congress Catologing-in-Publication Data

McDonough, Andrew L.
LabVIEW: data acquisition and analysis for the movement sciences / Andrew L. McDonough.
p. cm.
ISBN 0-13-012847-3
1. Kinesiology–Data processing. 2. LabVIEW. 3. Scientific apparatus and instruments–Computer simulation. 4. Computer graphics. I. Title

QP303 .M357 2001
612.7'6'0285–dc21 00-037491

Publisher: *Julie Alexander*
Acquisitions Editor: *Mark Cohen*
Director of Production and Manufacturing: *Bruce Johnson*
Managing Production Editor: *Patrick Walsh*
Senior Production Manager: *Ilene Sanford*
Production Liaison: *Julie Boddorf*
Production Editor: *Amy Gehl*
Creative Director: *Marianne Frasco*
Cover Design Coordinator: *Maria Guglielmo*
Cover Designer: *Joe Sengotta*
Interior Designer: *Carlisle Graphics Services*
Director of Marketing: *Leslie Cavaliere*
Marketing Coordinator: *Cindy Frederick*
Editorial Assistant: *Melissa Kerian*
Composition: *Carlisle Communications*
Printing and Binding: *R.R. Donnelley & Sons*

Prentice-Hall International (UK) Limited, *London*
Prentice-Hall of Australia Pty. Limited, *Sydney*
Prentice-Hall Canada Inc., *Toronto*
Prentice-Hall Hispanoamericana, S.A., *Mexico*
Prentice-Hall of India Private Limited, *New Delhi*
Prentice-Hall of Japan, Inc., *Tokyo*
Prentice-Hall Singapore Pte. Ltd.
Editora Prentice-Hall do Brasil, Ltda., *Rio de Janeiro*

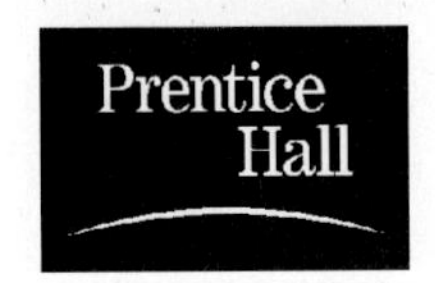

10 9 8 7 6 5 4 3 2 1
ISBN 0-13-012847-3

For Nancy

You've always been my source of inspiration and interest
for any project I've undertaken.

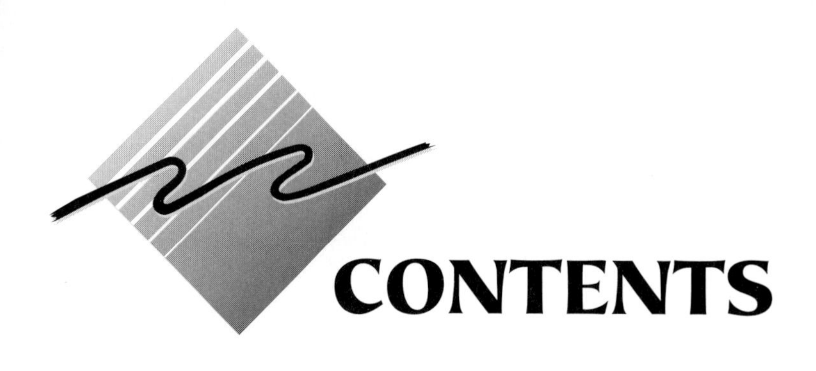

CONTENTS

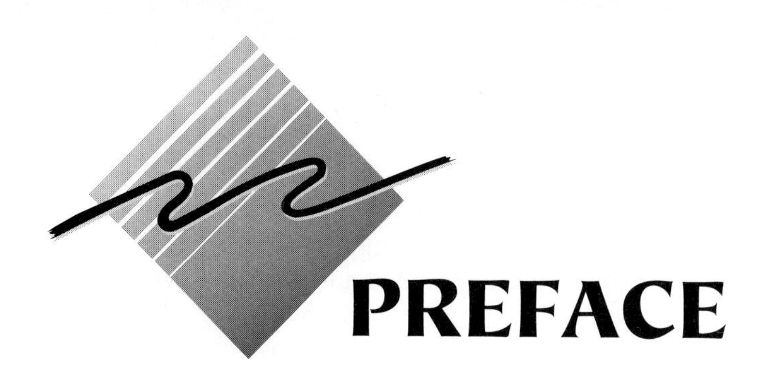

PREFACE

I was first introduced to the LabVIEW programming language when I was in graduate school pursuing my doctorate. Immediately after learning how powerful and flexible this graphical software was for acquiring and analyzing data, I introduced LabVIEW to our Human Performance Laboratory in the Department of Physical Therapy at New York University. For the past 5 years, I have been encouraging my colleagues and graduate students to use LabVIEW as the front end for many of the instruments we use to measure and study kinematic and kinetic aspects of movement science. Our laboratory focuses on the study of normal and pathological gait, posture control and balance, reaching and grasping, and other motor control and motor learning topics. To this end, I have been teaching a graduate course that focuses on the use of LabVIEW to collect signals from electromyographs, dynamometers, electrogoniometers, and force transducers, to name a few. The course emphasizes hands-on training in basic programming and data collection techniques that are routinely employed by researchers in physical therapy, applied physiology, physical education, motor control, and motor learning laboratories, among others. Early on, I developed an in-house laboratory manual that takes students step-by-step through writing and using simple and rather complex LabVIEW programs over an 8-week period. Toward the end of the course, students learn about the power and ease-of-use of graphical programming, and they incorporate this newly learned skill directly into their thesis or dissertation research. The original manual for this course has served as the substrate of the current text and retains many of the hands-on elements I first introduced several years ago.

To learn about LabVIEW and keep current with the newest information and features of this evolving software, I have participated in a number of courses, workshops, and seminars offered by National Instruments Corporation of Austin, Texas, the makers of LabVIEW. It has been my experience that few, if any, of the participants at these meetings are involved in the study and measurement of human performance issues. Most attendees come from the ranks of engineering, manufacturing, or process control in industry. Accordingly, most texts written over the past few years tend to focus on applications that address industrial and commercial uses of LabVIEW. And while I am personally aware of researchers who use LabVIEW, some of whom are colleagues and former mentors, few textbooks or manuals relate directly to the use of LabVIEW to study human motion. This manual attempts to fill this niche, offering the user a practical and direct way to learn, write, and use programs for the purpose of collecting and analyzing human performance data. It is not, however, intended to be a complete overview of LabVIEW. A number of good books currently on the market delve into virtually every aspect of this graphical programming environment; to have included this detail would have been redundant. This manual provides the user with an understanding of the essentials needed to become a LabVIEW programmer specifically to get the user up and running writing programs that apply directly to the study of movement science.

Andrew L. McDonough
Department of Physical Therapy
New York University

About the Author

Andrew McDonough is an Associate Professor of Physical Therapy at New York University. He has been a member of the NYU faculty since 1977 and served as department chairman from 1989 through 1997. Dr. McDonough received his doctorate in Motor Learning from Teachers College—Columbia University, where he was first introduced to LabVIEW. He teaches a master's and doctoral-level course at NYU entitled "Measurement and Evaluation III" that focuses on a "hands-on" approach to LabVIEW programming. In developing this course, he wrote an in-house laboratory manual that has served as the substrate for the current book. Most of his current research involving the measurement of manually applied forces with transducers and the elicitation of H-reflexes using electromyography uses LabVIEW VIs. He also teaches anatomy and kinesiology in the entry-level Doctor of Physical Therapy program as well as research methods to advanced master's students.

Dr. McDonough is the co-author with David Saidoff, a former student, of *Critical Pathways in Therapeutic Intervention: Upper Extremity*, published by Mosby. A second, expanded volume entitled, *Critical Pathways in Differential Diagnosis: Strategies for Therapeutic Intervention*, is in press and scheduled for release in 2000.

Dr. McDonough may be contacted via email at
alm3@is2.nyu.edu

His Web Site is at
http://www.nyu.edu/classes/mcdonough

Acknowledgments

Several of the VIs involving spectral analysis, and others, were a collaborative effort between myself and Dr. Joseph P. Weir, a colleague and friend. I'd like to acknowledge Joe's contribution to this book and thank him for his valuable input.

Second, I'd like to thank Mark Cohen, Acquisitions Editor, of Prentice Hall/Pearson Education, for his support and interest in this project.

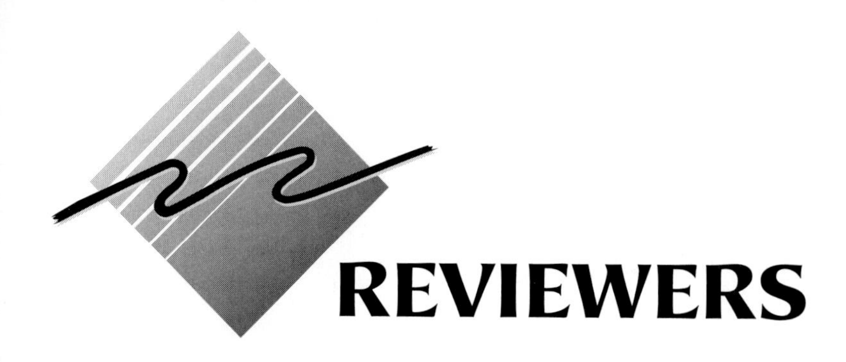

REVIEWERS

Joan Edelstein, MA, PT
Associate Professor of Clinical Physical Therapy
Director, Program in Physical Therapy
Columbia University
New York, New York

Joseph P. Weir, Ph.D.
Assistant Professor
Program in Physical Therapy
University of Osteopathic Medicine
Des Moines, Iowa

Nabil Dajani, Ph.D.
Research Assistant/Teaching Assistant
Bioengineering Department
University of Chicago
Chicago, Illinois

Charles S. Lessard, Ph.D.
Associate Professor
Biomedical Engineering
Industrial Engineering Department
Texas A&M University
College Station, Texas

Dr. Eng. Sherif Hussein
Research Assistant
Bioengineering Unit
University of Strathclyde
Glasgow, United Kingdom

S.D. Filip To, Ph.D., P.E.
Associate Professor
Agricultural and Biological Engineering
Mississippi State University
Mississippi State, Mississippi

1

GETTING STARTED

OBJECTIVES

- ❖ Distinguish between graphical and text-based computer languages.
- ❖ Use LabVIEW to measure aspects of human performance.
- ❖ Understand the text structure and conventions for this book.

WHAT IS LabVIEW?

LabVIEW is a graphical programming language, sometimes known as G, developed by Jeff Kodosky in the mid-1980s for the National Instruments Corporation based in Austin, Texas. Programs written in LabVIEW, known as *virtual instruments* (VIs) simulate hardware devices that acquire and analyze electrical signals. In some ways, LabVIEW may be likened to a sophisticated voltmeter. Analog electrical signals output from measuring devices, and sensors are interfaced with a computer via various input devices (e.g., analog-to-digital [A-to-D] converter boards) and fed to LabVIEW programs. Signals from virtually any device that emits a direct-current analog signal (± 10 volts) may be acquired and analyzed by LabVIEW VIs. With known conversion and calibration factors, the digitized electrical signal is configured in the appropriate units of measure (e.g., degrees, Newtons, foot-pounds, meters/second, etc.). LabVIEW is used in industry to run and monitor assembly lines; for process control; by engineers to develop and test sophisticated electromechanical devices; and by computer programmers, educators, and scientists of every persuasion. LabVIEW's strength is its generalizability to many uses over a broad range of commercial and scientific applications.

The ease with which even complicated and sophisticated programs can be written is due to LabVIEW's graphical interface. Compared with traditional text-based programming code, VIs written in LabVIEW can be up and running very quickly. Students taking my graduate course are amazed that simple VIs can be structured and run, without errors, literally in a matter of a few minutes, whereas a program written in conventional text-based code could take hours and sometimes days, to write, debug, and run. A simple analogy may be useful to describe LabVIEW's graphical interface. As Windows is to DOS, LabVIEW is to a conventional text-based language such as BASIC or C+. That is, programming in LabVIEW is handled by the manipulation and connection of icons (i.e.,"wiring" VIs and subVIs [subroutines] together), which establish a logical flow of information to acquire signals, do calculations, do analyses, or drive electronic or mechanical devices. A single icon may represent tens or even hundreds of lines of conventional text-based code.

Beyond the ease of operation issues, the benefits of using LabVIEW become immediately obvious. Flexible and adaptable graphical software can be used as a front-end replacement for expensive, dedicated hardware devices. Thus, as conditions change, objectives are reoriented, and the need for additional processing power becomes apparent, LabVIEW VIs are easily modified to meet those needs. The focus of this text is the use of LabVIEW to acquire and analyze physiological and mechanical signals that measure various aspects of normal and pathological human performance. Examples of commonly used measurement devices in the movement sciences include electromyographs to measure electrical output of contracting muscles, dynamometers to analyze torque and angular velocity of joints, and transducers and other strain gauges to measure the amplitude of forces applied to human tissues. Traditionally, electrophysiological testing devices are expensive, become obsolete quickly, and are subject to wear-and-tear, eventually breaking down and requiring frequent replacement or upgrades. Today, many of these devices are operated by proprietary software that requires a steep learning curve and frequent upgrades and that sometimes has or develops bugs causing programs to crash or operate unpredictably. When intervention is required, unless the user has a knowledge of traditional computer programming, it's an expensive and time-consuming proposition to ask the manufacturer to repair or modify proprietary software. Going outside the company and hiring your own programmer is likewise a major chore and expense. Since LabVIEW VIs are written specifically to monitor measuring devices, often by the user him- or herself, changes and troubleshooting problems can be handled locally, inexpensively, and with substantially less downtime.

Who Uses LabVIEW Software?

This book evolved originally from an in-house laboratory manual I developed in conjunction with a graduate course I teach in the Department of Physical Therapy at New York University. The course focuses on the use of LabVIEW for the acquisition and analysis of measures of human performance in the movement sciences. The course and accompanying manual are intended to give participants—the majority of whom are graduate students in my and other departments in the university—hands-on experience in programming specific VIs to collect and analyze biomechanical and kinesiological data. The current text continues along these lines and provides not only basic information concerning the LabVIEW environment but also specific opportunities to apply LabVIEW programming directly to measurement of normal and pathological human movement.

Thus, faculty who teach courses similar to mine may find this text useful in organizing a practical programming experience using LabVIEW for their students. This text may also be useful in advanced biomechanics or kinesiology courses in which students are directly involved in data acquisition. In my experience, learning is best facilitated by doing, and given this text's focus on active and practical programming fundamentals, students should find this manual informative and useful.

While originally intended as a course manual, the current text may also be useful to users who are not part of a formal course who want to develop basic skills and proficiencies in LabVIEW programming that specifically apply to parameters of human performance. Specific areas of focus include physical and occupational therapy, basic and applied physiology, physical education, biomechanics, kinesiology, motor learning, and motor control. One of the advantages of LabVIEW VIs—many of which are included in this text—is that, with some tweaking, these programs will have broad applications and appeal to most, if not all, of the fields described.

Measures of Human Performance: LabVIEW

While not a complete list, the following are areas of human performance analysis and physiological parameters that LabVIEW VIs can measure. LabVIEW programming offers the benefit of taking VIs that measure parameters similar to those noted and easily modifying them to meet the user's specific needs.

LabVIEW Capabilities

- **EMG** measurement including filtering, rectification, normalization, and integration
- **Spectral and power analysis**
- **Dynamometry**—torque and angular velocity measures including peak torque, time-to-peak torque, work, and power
- **Electrogoniometry**—uni- and biaxial devices
- **Force transducers**
- **Biofeedback**
- **Event markers**
- **Timers**

- **Simple oscilloscopes**
- **Data calculations**—percent scores, grading
- **Statistical analysis**—descriptive, ANOVA, correlation, line fitting/regression

Who Should Use This Book?

This text was originally developed for students, educators, and researchers involved in the acquisition and analysis of measures of human motion and physiological function. As such, the text is appropriate for group study and may be used as a course laboratory manual. This book may also have appeal to the individual user who is interested in learning basic LabVIEW programming skills while developing specific VIs to study human motion.

Overview of Text Structure

In addition to the current section, two other sections are presented.

Section 2 presents an overview of measurement theory with a specific focus on the acquisition and analysis of bioelectrical and mechanical-electrical signals generated from sensors and monitors that serve as a substrate for the use of LabVIEW programming.

Section 3 deals with learning and practicing basic and intermediate-level LabVIEW programming skills. The reader is introduced to LabVIEW's organizational structure; the platforms that support LabVIEW and the user interface including menu structures, operating tools, and functions; and the use of help windows. Next, "hands-on" programming concepts are discussed in detail while the user explores the functional capabilities of LabVIEW using specific examples of VIs and subVIs. Instructions are provided as the user starts to build simple VIs incorporating LabVIEW functions of increasing complexity. Basic concepts involving data acquisition are discussed with a practical focus intended to permit the user to explore hardware and software options that facilitate data acquisition and analysis. Instructions are included that enable the user to build a simple generic interface device to acquire analog signals. Finally, a series of VIs and subVIs are provided and discussed that specifically address data acquisition and analysis of various human performance parameters. In addition to appearing in hard copy, all VIs described in this book appear on the accompanying CD-ROM. Also included are sample data files collected with VIs written by the author that may be used to confirm that programs run and function properly. The data files may be especially useful if data acquisition hardware (e.g., an A-to-D converter board) is not available. The specific use of these data files is described elsewhere in this book.

Readers are encouraged to build and use the VIs and subVIs presented in Section 3 for their own data acquisition and analysis purposes and to modify these programs to meet their own specific programming needs.

TEXT CONVENTIONS

The following text conventions are used for this book:

BOLD—USED FOR

- Front panel and block diagram task bar options:

  File Edit Operate Project Windows Help

- Items in pull-down menus associated with the task bar options:

  File/Open or **File/Save**

- Filenames:

  Torque.vi

  Test2.dat

- Tools and control palettes:

  Controls/Numeric (front panel)

  Functions/Structures (block diagram)

  Tools (either front panel or block diagram)

***ITALICS*—USED FOR**

- Functions from **Control, Functions,** or **Tools** palettes:

  Controls/Numeric/*Digital Constant* (front panel)

  Functions/Structures/*Sequence* (block diagram)

  Tools/*hand tool* (either front panel or block diagram)

  Tools palette (descriptions of commonly used tools):

TOOL NAME FOR THIS BOOK	DESCRIPTION FROM LabVIEW
Hand Tool	Operate Value
Arrow Tool	Position/Size/Select
Wiring Tool	Connect Wire

Opened Hand	Scroll Window
Lettering Tool	Edit Text
Paint Brush Tool	Set Color

BOLD ITALIC **USED FOR *EMPHASIS***

"QUOTES" USED FOR

- Front panel or block diagram "labels"
- Numbers or strings inserted into controls and indicators

HOW TO USE THIS BOOK

Experience has shown that the layered pop-up and pull-down menu structure that LabVIEW uses, while not difficult to use, is complex, and first-time programmers are sometimes frustrated by their inability to locate needed VIs and other functions. Therefore, VI and subVI locator pages are shown opposite each figure in which a program is described. Locator pages specifically identify in which palette and menu (and submenu) programming functions may be found. The spiral-bound format for this book was intentionally selected so that the pages being studied can "lay flat" in front of the computer monitor or on an easel for easy viewing. Within a few programming sessions, users begin to recall the location of often-used functions, and toward the end of their programming experience, users tend to rely on these locators less and less, if at all.

As noted previously, a companion CD-ROM is provided with this book. All VIs and subVIs described in Section 3 are provided. A description of how the disk is organized and instructions for copying the contents of the CD-ROM to your hard drive are described in Section 3. Although I recommend that all VIs presented be written by the programmer, if time does not permit or if a particular VI is too complex, the user can call up the VI from the CD-ROM for review.

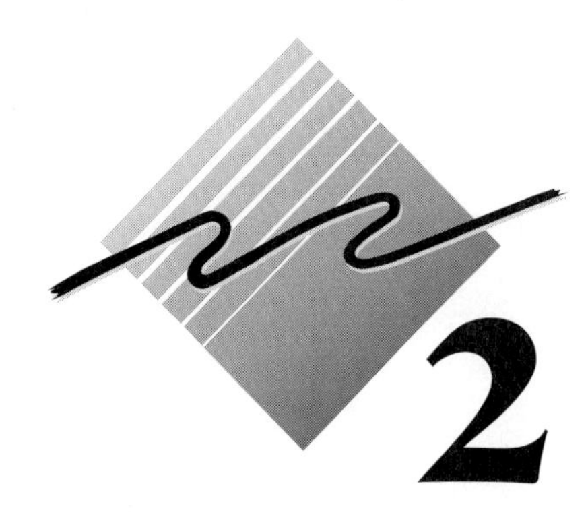

2

MEASUREMENT

OBJECTIVES

- ❖ Review and understand basic concepts of signal measurement.

MEASUREMENTS REPRESENTED AS VOLTAGES

Many electrophysiologial measurement tools output their results as ***voltages*** that are linearly proportionate to units of measure (e.g., Newtons with a force transducer or foot-pounds with an isokinetic dynamometer). A programming language like LabVIEW is written in binary format that allows signals to be processed ***digitally.*** In many ways, LabVIEW might be thought of as a sophisticated and very sensitive ***voltmeter*** that measures electrical output from an instrument. Thus, the initial ***analog signal*** must be converted to ***digital format*** by an ***analog-to-digital (A-to-D) converter*** connected to a computer, before it can be used by LabVIEW.

ANALOG-TO-DIGITAL CONVERSION

A typical A-to-D converter is a card that sits in a slot in a computer's motherboard and is connected to the signal source with cables. In some cases, the A-to-D converter may be a stand-alone piece of hardware. In Section 3-13, "Data Acquisition," basic elements of signal collection are discussed, with some practical examples for configuring an A-to-D converter board and building a simple interface device for acquiring analog signals.

Once the signal has been converted to digital format, it's ready to be used by software programs using data acquisition subroutines to communicate directly with the computer's A-to-D board. At this point, the acquired digital signal may be manipulated (e.g., filtered, tabulated, graphed, etc.) to meet specific data collection and processing needs.

SAMPLING RATE

As the name implies, the ***sampling rate*** is the number of data points acquired and converted to digital format per unit of time (typically per second). An adequate sampling rate ensures that an acquired analog signal is accurately represented in digital format and thus properly processed by LabVIEW. A sampling rate that is ***too low*** for the signal being acquired will cause ***data points to be missed.*** An ***undersampled signal*** will not be truly representative of the signal source, leading to calculation errors. One of the key parameters of an A-to-D board is the total number of samples that may be converted by all channels acquired by the board. A board with an underrated sampling capacity will likewise lead to signal errors. The sampling rate therefore must be matched appropriately to the sensor(s) being used for measurements.

A generally accepted rule is to always sample data ***at least twice*** the anticipated rate at which the data are generated. This will ensure adequate data collection and provide a sufficient margin for error, especially when the signal source demonstrates high variability. For example, the potentials measured from Type II (i.e., phasic) motor units in contracting muscle have a top firing frequency of approximately 250 Hertz (Hz) (i.e., 250 cycles per second). Therefore, under most experimental circumstances, a minimally acceptable sampling rate would be 500 Hz (i.e., frequency $\times$ 2). On the other hand, the average gait cycle (i.e., the time it takes between consecutive heel contacts on the same side) is about 1 second. Thus, a sample rate of 2 Hz rounded up to 10 Hz should ensure that no data points will be missed.

While the ***oversampled signal*** will not present problems with respect to the true nature of the signal, the user should understand that collecting more than the required number of samples may tax computer memory (i.e., hard drive) resources. Currently, large-capacity hard drives are relatively inexpensive, so that storage today may not be the issue it was several years ago. Nonetheless, the user should understand that a 1- to 2-gigabyte hard drive could be easily filled if multiple trials are planned in an experiment with a large number of subjects at a sample rating of 1000 Hz. Obviously, pilot work before the actual data are collected should reveal a satisfactory balance between the sample rate and storage capacity.

Another factor that may need to be considered is ***data format*** (i.e., spreadsheet vs. binary), discussed in Sections 3-14, "Writing and Reading Data," and 3-19, "Other Programming Functions and Tools." Data saved in ***binary format,*** although more complicated in terms of programming, is inherently more efficient in data storage. For example, studies looking at fatigue during sustained muscular contraction will, by their nature, consume a large amount of hard drive space. Saving data in binary format will usually ameliorate this problem.

The thoughtful selection of an adequate sampling rate may also assist the user in data interpretation. In Section 3, many of the LabVIEW programs (virtual instruments, or VIs) discuss sample and/or process data at 1000 Hz. Although in many cases this rate exceeds the ***two times rule*** noted earlier, every tic on the ***x-axis*** of a *waveform graph* or *chart* will represent ***1 msec,*** making timing issues easier to manage.

Signal Range

Signal range refers to the ***minimum*** and ***maximal voltages*** an A-to-D board can handle. A typical range is 0 to ± 10 volts. Thus, a signal measured by a sensor of "−12.3" volts would be considered ***out-of-range*** and therefore suspect. Signal range is another important consideration in matching an A-to-D board's data processing capabilities with the anticipated signal sources, sensors, and associated hardware (e.g., amplifiers). Changing the amplifier (and/or preamplifier) ***gain*** and/or selecting a board with a different ***resolution*** may be a way of adjusting the input signal to meet the range specifications of a given A-to-D board.

Resolution

The ability to recognize and measure small detectable changes in voltage is a function of A-to-D board ***resolution.*** A-to-D converters divide analog signals into ***divisions.*** The higher the number of divisions, the greater the board's resolution capability and the greater the ability to differentiate ***small changes in voltage.*** The higher the resolution, the more ***sensitivity.*** Twelve- or 16-bit boards typically offer resolution consistent with the electrophysiological signals described in this book.

Measurement Variables

Variables are used to quantify a set of values for a given measure and take a number of forms consistent with the nature of the measurements being performed. Variables are usually characterized as ***categorical, continuous,*** or ***discrete.***

Categorical variables are used to ***classify*** a phenomenon that is not quantifiable and may be ordered or unordered. ***Ordinal*** variables are classifications that have ***ordered positions.*** For example, some scales that assess pain permit patients to rate their pain from 0 to 10, with 10 being the worst possible pain. ***Nominal*** variables classify information that is ***not ordered*** such as gender or blood type.

Quantifiable variables are either continuous or discrete and from a statistical point of view are handled in a similar manner. ***Continuous*** variables document measures over a period of time, whereas a ***discrete*** variable documents a single point or event in that continuum. In fact, a discrete variable may be selected from a continuous data set.

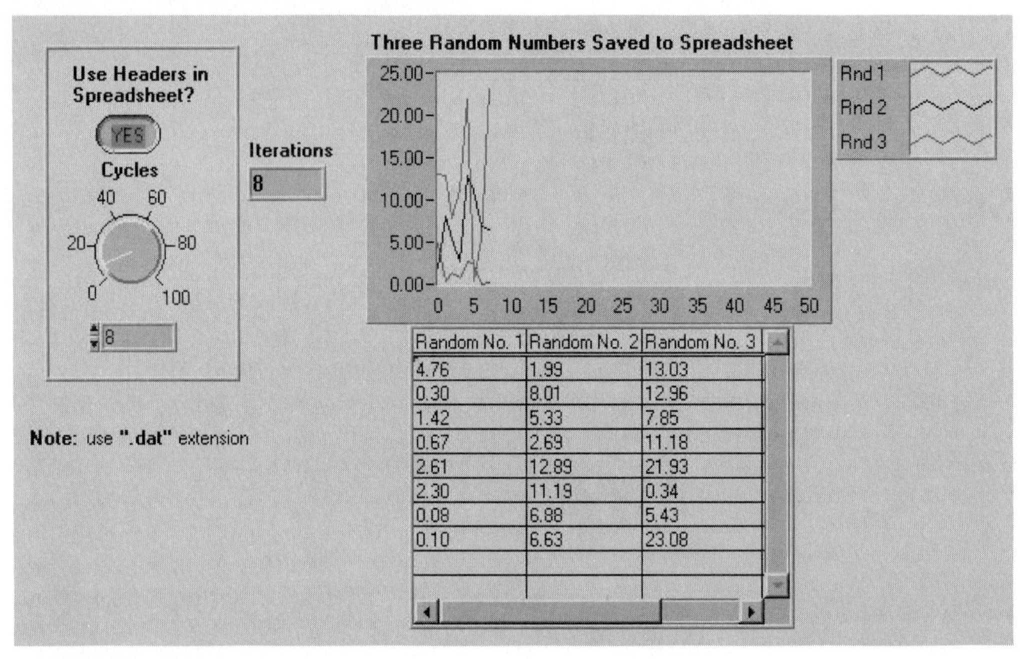

Random No. 1	Random No. 2	Random No. 3
4.76	1.99	13.03
0.30	8.01	12.96
1.42	5.33	7.85
0.67	2.69	11.18
2.61	12.89	21.93
2.30	11.19	0.34
0.08	6.88	5.43
0.10	6.63	23.08

FIGURE 2–1
Front panel of **Gen3col.vi.**

Variables may also be characterized as ***inputs*** or ***controls*** and ***outputs*** or ***indicators.*** LabVIEW and other computer programming languages handle and manipulate variables in either a ***numeric*** or ***string*** (i.e., alphanumeric) format. Thus, control variables may take the form of either numeric or string variables. Likewise, indicator variables may be either numeric or strings.

NUMERIC AND STRING VARIABLES

In LabVIEW, functions that drive programming operations and display data are generically referred to as ***controls*** and ***indicators*** and may be either discrete or continuous variables. In the vernacular of LabVIEW (and other programming languages), continuous variables are described as ***arrays.*** Typically, discrete variables take the form of numeric *Digital Controls* and *Indicators* and physically appear as rectangular boxes on the front panel of a LabVIEW program (for a detailed discussion of LabVIEW front panel functions, see Section 3-2, "Front Panel"). Arrays of continuous data, which may also serve as controls or indicators, usually take the form of *Tables* or *Waveform Graphs.* Figure 2–1 is the front panel of a LabVIEW program called **Gen3col.vi** (see Section 3-12, "Tables," for

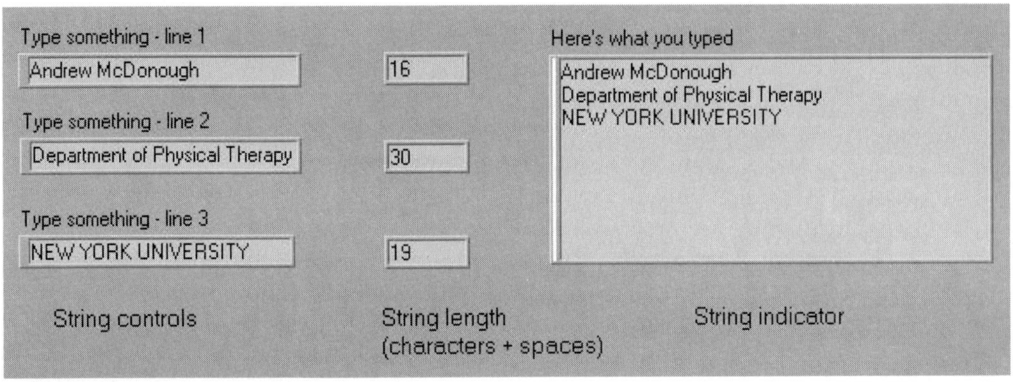

FIGURE 2–2
Front panel of **Strings1.vi.**

a complete description) and demonstrates examples of numeric digital control and indicator variables.

As noted, alphanumeric data are portrayed as ***string variables*** and may also serve as controls or indictors. Figure 2–2 demonstrates commonly used string variables in the front panel of the LabVIEW program called **Strings1.vi** (see Section 3-9, "Strings," for a complete description).

While program functions vary according to their intended design and use, before programs are usually run, control data are first input into their respective variables (numeric or string). In some cases, previously saved data files are called up. After the control variables have been set, the program is run and indicator variables will display the data as numbers, alphanumeric information (e.g., the time and date the data were collected), graphs, or tables.

MEASUREMENT UNITS: CALIBRATION AND UNIT CONVERSION

Raw data acquired by LabVIEW are displayed as ***voltages proportional to the units of measure*** of the sensor being used. Device calibration ensures that the instrument being used is accurate and reliable and provides a valid measure of the variables being studied, while data conversion changes the raw signal into the desired measurement units.

Calibration involves the checking and/or adjustment of the ***gradations*** of an instrument to ensure a ***valid*** and ***accurate*** measure of the variable being studied. Calibration should be done (1) when a new instrument will be used to take measurements and (2) after an instrument has already been used to take repeated measurements. The interval between calibrations varies—between hours, days, or months—depending on the design of the investigation, sensitivity of the instrument, and number of times it's been used.

Calibration usually involves the testing of the instrument against another instrument or set of conditions considered to be a ***gold standard.*** Comparing measurements between the device and gold standard is a means of establishing the instrument's ***validity.*** Calibration also involves the ***zeroing*** of the instrument to the gold standard's zero point. Checking the accuracy of repeated measurements over time and ensuring that measurement error (i.e., variability) is within tolerable limits determine the instrument's ***reliability.***

In Section 3-19, "Other Programming Functions and Tools," a program was written (Figure 3–19.7) that uses a Piezo electric ***force transducer*** and an ***event marker*** that might be used to document the point in time when a criterion force is manually applied to the transducer. As force is applied, a crystal in the transducer deforms and gives off an electric discharge (i.e., voltage) proportional to the amount of force. Before collecting data, the force transducer's ability to provide valid force measurements was checked against a simple validation procedure. Lead shot were placed in containers and measured on a chemist's balance, taking measurements out to the third decimal place. Shot were added or removed to provide precisely measured weights rounded to the nearest 1/2 kg (e.g., 0.500, 1.000, 1.500, 2.000 kg, etc.). These precisely measured weights were considered the gold standard against which the linearity of measurements using the force transducer was tested. In random order, weights were applied to the transducer for a finite period, and the resultant voltages using a LabVIEW program were measured and the data saved to a hard drive. Afterward, the recorded voltages were plotted in ascending order to assess the linearity (i.e., proportionality) of all measurements. A curve that approximated a straight line with minimal variability and that closely matched another line fitted to the curve documented that the transducer was a valid tool for measuring applied forces.

The ***reliability*** of the transducer was checked by applying a single load of known weight to the transducer many times, each time measuring and recording the resultant voltage with LabVIEW. A ***mean voltage*** with a low ***coefficient of variation*** (i.e., an index of variability) showed the transducer to be a reliable means of measuring applied force.

Finally, a ***conversion factor*** was calculated for the transducer by repeatedly measuring the calibration weights and determining the average voltage registered over three trials for each weight. By dividing the ***average weight*** by the ***average voltage*** and creating a proportional ratio to solve for the ***one-volt weight,*** a conversion factor of ***1 volt = 6.25 kg*** was calculated. Note that this conversion factor appears on the front panel of the program named **Readtran.vi** in Figure 3–19.7 and is used in the block diagram (back panel) to calculate a criterion force in kilograms.

ACCURACY AND PRECISION

Accuracy assesses a variable's ability to actually represent what it's supposed to represent. For example, in a game of darts, a dart that lands in the bull's-eye would reflect an ***accurate throw,*** whereas a dart landing in the third concentric circle would be considered ***inaccurate. Precision*** refers to how closely a series of repeated measures approximates one another. Precision and accuracy are not necessarily coupled assessments. If four darts are thrown and all four land in the bull's-eye, this would be considered an accurate and precise performance. However, if all four darts landed in a tightly clustered area in the third concentric circle (i.e., none landed in the bull's-eye), the throws would be considered precise but not accurate. Additionally, if all darts landed randomly in the concentric circles, and none hit the bull's-eye, the performance would be considered not accurate or precise.

With respect to instrumentation, one of the chief ways to improve accuracy is to periodically calibrate an instrument against a known gold standard. This reduces error between measurements, and the error that can't be eliminated will at least be systematically applied across all measurement trials.

Calibration has a similar impact on the precision of measurements. Precision may be further improved statistically through repetition and the averaging of trial data, thus reducing the effect of random error.

The term ***precision*** is also used to describe the number of ***decimal places*** to which a number is taken. Thus, the number "63.45" has a precision of 2. When properly applied, decimal precision serves as an index of the sensitivity of a measurement. A measurement's precision should match an instrument's measurement capabilities. For example, electromyographic electrodes and associated hardware (e.g., preamplifier, amplifier) can identify differences between very small electrical potentials to the second, third, and even fourth decimal place. Conversely, it would not make sense to have ***any*** decimal precision if counting the number of inspirations/expirations of the lungs (i.e., typically "12 to 15" per minute during relaxed breathing). A common mistake in reporting the precision of a number is to use more decimal places than an instrument provides. For example, if a dynamometer measures and calculates torque production to two decimal places, it would be inappropriate to report numbers to three places.

SIGNAL VS. NOISE AND BASELINES

A common problem often encountered in analyzing electrophysiological signals is differentiating ***baseline noise*** from a ***true signal*** (Figure 2–3). In other words, the question arises, "At precisely what point does the true signal rise from the

FIGURE 2–3
Isometric torque curve demonstrating the transition between baseline noise and the true signal.

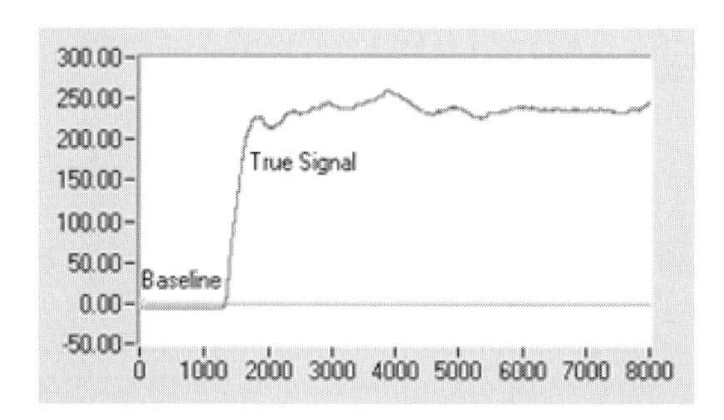

FIGURE 2–4
Subroutine (subVI) in a block diagram used to differentiate baseline noise from the true signal using the *Threshold Peak Detector.vi* function. Note that 0.001 volt has been added to the maximal baseline amplitude, serving as the index point for threshold detection.

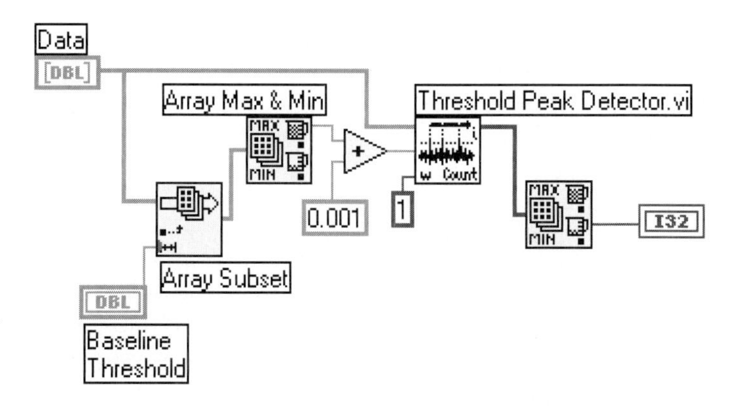

baseline?" This information is often needed to calculate temporal parameters of a signal (e.g., time-to-peak torque during an isometric contraction on a dynamometer). While methods vary somewhat in making this determination, the following procedure is generally applicable to common signal analysis.

After an instrument's baseline has been determined to be stable and its electrical profile has been minimized as much as possible, the mean amplitude and standard deviation of a segment of the baseline preceding the true signal (e.g., 500 to 1000 msec) is calculated. At this point, a program ***subroutine*** capable of documenting when a predetermined threshold is detected is used. The subroutine is configured such that data processing begins at the point in the signal where the average baseline amplitude ***plus 2 standard deviations*** is detected. In this case, programming code often takes the form of ***if . . . then*** statements or their equivalent. This point will in some way be ***indexed*** along the baseline, thereby documenting the point at which true signal may be differentiated from baseline noise.

LabVIEW uses a subroutine (***subVI;*** see Section 3-5, "Creating SubVIs") called *Peak Threshold Detector.vi*, which is used in a number of programs in Section 3 (Figure 2-4). In this case, a 0.001 voltage (vs. 2 standard deviations) is added to the maximal baseline amplitude, thus defining the threshold at which signal processing is triggered. Note that there is a function represented by a small (blue) icon with the label "I32," connected to a terminal on the right side of an *Array Max & Min* function, which, in turn, is connected to a terminal on the *Peak Threshold Detector.vi* icon. This icon corresponds with a front panel (digital) indicator that indexes (i.e., documents) the point along the x-axis where the signal begins to ***rise from the baseline.***

NORMALIZATION

Comparisons made between trials or subjects require that measurement parameters be standardized so that an "apples-to-apples" comparison can be made. Without a standardizing strategy, it may be impossible to determine if differences in measurements are due to an experimental intervention, the normal variability encountered between trials or subjects, or a disparity in some physical or physiological characteristic of the subject or experimental condition. ***Normalization*** has the effect of adjusting for these characteristics so that a meaningful comparison can be made. Normalizing measurements also permits subjects or conditions with different characteristics to participate in the same experiment and thus maximizes the use of a given subject pool. Without normalization, all subjects or conditions would have to have exactly the same physical or physiological characteristics (e.g., height, limb length, pulse, blood pressure, etc.). Stating this problem in the form of a question, one might ask, "Is it valid to directly compare the vertical displacement of the foot while stepping over a 6″-inch-high curb in a subject who is 5′ 2″ tall with someone who is 6′ 2″ tall?" The answer is probably ***no,***and therefore some type of ***adjustment*** or ***normalization*** of measures needs to be made to permit meaningful between subject comparisons.

Normalization usually involves the calculation of a ***ratio*** between a measurement parameter and the standard used to adjust the data. In the example noted above, the vertical displacement of the foot stepping over the curb might be divided by each subject's leg length or total height. The ***derived ratio*** would then serve as the dependent measure on which comparisons or statistical calculations are made.

Meaningful comparison of electromyographic data has historically relied on normalization to correct for between subject variability in the number of motor units found in muscle and/or different patterns of firing frequency. Typically, the ***integrated*** electromyographic signal (see Section 3-15, "Electromyography") is divided by the maximal integral of the muscle being studied during a ***maximal voluntary isometric contraction.*** The derived ratio of integrals then serves as the dependent measure. Historically, this procedure is a well-accepted strategy for assessing ***isometric*** (i.e., when muscle length stays the same) muscle contractions but has been criticized for assessing ***isotonic*** (i.e., when a muscle changes length) contractions. Notwithstanding this criticism, a better method has not emerged, and therefore the procedure, in spite of being a less than perfect solution, is used routinely to normalize electromyographic signals during isotonic contractions. In Section 3-15, "Electromyography," the LabVIEW program called **Normalx2.vi** is discussed as a simple way to normalize two electromyographic signals.

Multiple-Signal Synchronization

Analysis of human performance frequently employs multiple instruments to measure various facets of movement behaviors. When multiple devices are used, to ensure that each instrument starts data collection at precisely the same time, it's necessary to ***synchronize*** each instrument. Historically, in the case of electrophysiological analysis, an ***event marker*** has been used to synchronize multiple channels of data. This usually involves the triggering of a small electrical potential by tripping a switch sometime just before data collection is to begin. This electrical "stamp" along a signal's baseline documents a ***common point in time*** on which all data channels may be synchronized. When instruments function at different sampling rates, the synchronized signals must then be interpolated, usually using the slowest sampling rate as a least common denominator. A higher sampling frequency is thus adjusted as a function of the lower sampling rate.

One of the advantages of using an A-to-D board common to all input channels is that they are ***electronically synchronized,*** thus obviating the need for additional synchronization devices. If LabVIEW is used to acquire each signal, each instrument may be configured to use the same sampling rate, eliminating the need for complicated and sometimes confusing interpolation algorithms.

Summary

Thoughtful attention to basics concepts concerning measurement during hardware and software configuration using LabVIEW will minimize common sources of measurement error and ensure accurate, valid, and reliable data.

3

DEVELOPING LabVIEW PROGRAMMING SKILLS

In Sections 1 and 2, a number of basics concepts concerning measurement were presented. Thoughtful attention to these issues during hardware and software configuration using LabVIEW will minimize common sources of measurement error and ensure accurate, valid, and reliable data.

LabVIEW PROGRAMMING SKILLS AND APPLICATIONS

The third section of this book deals with general programming concepts and the specific application of LabVIEW to ***data acquisition and analysis*** for the movement sciences. Section 3–1 describes basic user information and addresses topics such as operating systems; minimal system requirements; and definitions of LabVIEW structure and terminology including virtual instruments (VIs), front panel and block diagram, pull-down and drop-down menus, and tool and function palettes. Later, functional operations including running and saving VIs, directory structure, and the use of the companion CD ROM, including ***sample data files***, are discussed.

Sections 3–2 and 3–3 provide a comprehensive overview of front panel and block diagram structure for all LabVIEW VIs. Sections 3–4 through 3–12 consider elementary programming concepts that all LabVIEW users should understand, while Sections 3–13 through 3–18 deal with specific data acquisition and analysis applications (e.g., EMG; dynamometry/torque measurements; and feedback devices) for studying human movement. Finally, Section 3–19 describes a variety of programming topics ranging from methods of updating charts and graphs; applications used for statistical analysis; and an introduction to binary programming. Most sections end with ***practice exercises*** that provide the user the opportunity to put into use what is described in the text by either writing recommended VIs or modifying existing programs. A large library of sample data files is included to ensure that each VI works properly.

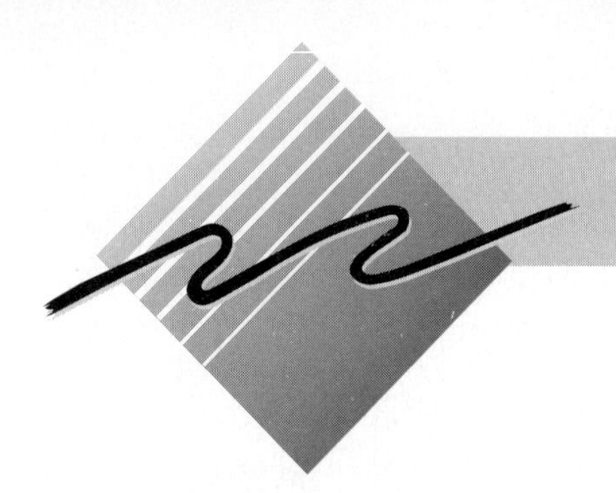

SECTION 3–1

BASICS

OBJECTIVES

- ❖ Compare LabVIEW v5.1 with features from previous versions.
- ❖ Define virtual instruments (VIs) and subroutines (subVIs).
- ❖ Understand and use front panels and block diagrams.
- ❖ Use drop-down and pop-up menus and palettes.
- ❖ Run VIs.
- ❖ Save VIs to directories and subdirectories.
- ❖ Use sample data files in the accompanying CD-ROM disk.

LABVIEW V5.1 AND PREVIOUS VERSIONS

LabVIEW v5.1 is the most current version, released by National Instruments in early 1999. This is the second revision of v5.x since its introduction in February 1998. The previous version was 4.0, which was upgraded to 4.1 in 1997. Version 4.0 marked the first time LabVIEW operated in a 32-bit environment using Windows 95™ or Windows NT™, although it still retains its downward compatibility with the 16-bit environment using Windows 3.1™ and Windows for Workgroups 3.11™. Windows 98™ is now the current version of Windows and imparts new functional capabilities to LabVIEW and other software.

Users always seem to greet software upgrades with some ambivalence. Just after users have spent weeks and months mastering the major features of the current version, the manufacturer releases a new version, sending users back to the drawing board. LabVIEW is no exception. Versions 3.x and 4.x demonstrated significant changes beyond the 16- vs. 32-bit issues. One of the most obvious changes was the reconfiguration of the top task bar on the front panel. In version 4.x, in addition to the ***drop-down layered*** menus that appear when clicking on a menu item,

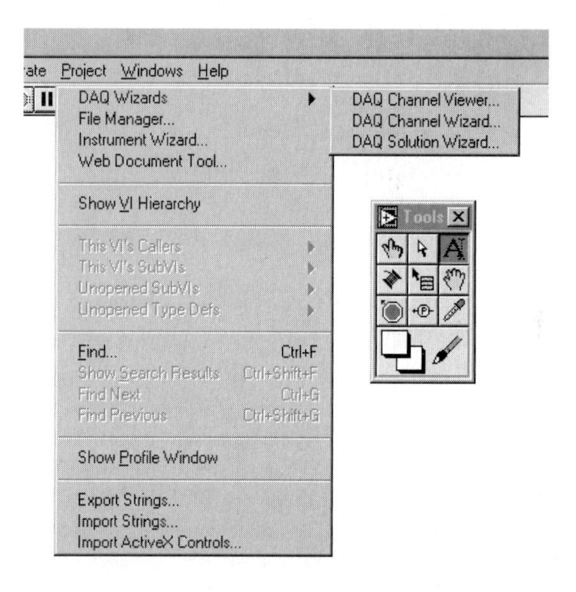

FIGURE 3–1.1
Data Acquisition **(DAQ) Wizards** are located in v5.1 in the **Project** option of the task bar.

two of the most often used palettes—the **Tools** and **Controls** palettes—are now configured as ***pop-up*** menus accessed by right-clicking the mouse. These palettes can be moved about the front panel and block diagram using the Windows ***click-and-drag*** method. Version 4.x also introduced the **DAQ Solution Wizard** (DAQ stands for *data acquisition*), which, along with Windows 95/98's ***plug and play*** capability, makes choosing and configuring hardware input devices (e.g., A-to-D converters) to match data acquisition needs easier. **DAQ Wizards** are located in v5.1 in the **Project** option in the task bar (Figure 3–1.1). Additional "bells and whistles" also appear in version 5.x.

Version 5.x retains many of the original elements of version 4.x and offers a significant number of new features, making the time and money spent upgrading worthwhile. This text is organized from the perspective of v5.1 running on Windows 98™, and many of its most functional aspects will be described. Perhaps some of the more interesting and timely features include Internet connectivity and compatibility with HTML (Hypertext Markup Language), one of the major language formats for the Internet. New print features have also been added, which are significant improvements over previous versions.

As is often the case with software upgrades, LabVIEW will only "read files down." That is, the more recent version is downwardly compatible with files saved using previous versions, but files saved with the current version can't be read ***directly*** by previous versions (i.e., major revisions—4.x vs. 5.x, etc). This can present problems if you use one version at home and another at the office or if a colleague is using a different version. Version 5.1 now allows the user to save VIs and subVIs in v5.0 format using the **Save with Options** selection from **File** in the task bar in the front panel.

WHICH OPERATING SYSTEM SHOULD I USE?

LabVIEW runs on a variety of computer platforms including Mac, Windows 98/95/NT/3.1, Sun work stations, and Hewlett-Packard Model 9000 Series 700 computers, thus providing stand-alone and network capabilities. While Mac historically had an advantage as a graphical operating system, this advantage has largely disappeared. Today, Mac and Windows appear to be quite competitive.

This text presents topics on LabVIEW from the Windows 95/98™ point of view. Regardless of which platform you plan to work on, there are a few basic parameters you should seriously consider. While LabVIEW will function with a 486 PC, you probably won't be happy with its speed and performance. In fact, LabVIEW will even run on a 386 PC with a math coprocessor. As a rule of thumb, to get the most out of LabVIEW, a Pentium™ processor with a minimum clock speed of 133 MHz is recommended. Obviously, the more horsepower, the more speed and relative improvement in performance will be experienced.

MINIMUM SYSTEM REQUIREMENTS

LabVIEW will run on a machine with 8 MB of RAM (random access memory) but coupled with a slow processor, performance will be sluggish at best. Currently, 16 MB of RAM are considered the minimally accepted standard, and in the 32-bit world of Windows 95/98, 32, 64, or 128 MB are better. RAM is a relatively cheap commodity today and shouldn't be a major constraint when configuring a machine to run LabVIEW efficiently.

Hard drive capacity is another important consideration. The rule is, "You can never have enough hard drive space!" Software today, including LabVIEW, is massive, and so it's best to assume that the software and the files you generate with it will require a lot of hard drive memory. Most machines purchased today have a hard drive with a minimum of 4 GB of memory. Like RAM, hard drive memory is currently cheap, so order or expand the computer on which LabVIEW will run with as large a hard drive as possible. Remember, it's unlikely that programs will get smaller in the future, so plan ahead.

LabVIEW may be used on virtually any size VGA color monitor but, remember, while working with a graphical programming language to maximize programming efficiency, consider using a relatively large monitor. A monitor rated nominally at 17 inches will probably cause less eye strain and head, neck, and trunk postural discomfort than the traditional 14- or 15-inch monitor. Also, keep in mind that monitor sizes are usually stated as ***diagonal measures,*** and so the amount of viewable screen area will be slightly less than the nominal size. Graphical programmers tend to "think big," and if a lot of time is spent at the computer, a 19- or 21-inch screen is probably the way to go.

One of the primary input sources for LabVIEW is the mouse. Make sure it's comfortable to use. Be sure that it has at least two control buttons: generally ***point-and-click*** or ***click-and-drag*** techniques require use of the left button (assuming a right-handed user); while pop-up menus and palettes are usually accessed with the right button. A mouse pad will make your work more comfortable. ***Repetitive stress injuries*** such as ***carpal tunnel syndrome*** are quite prevalent today and may be related to prolonged use of a mouse (and keyboard). Certain mice have better ergonomic designs than others. Wrist supports that keep the wrist and hand aligned properly are commercially available. Supports are largely a matter of personal preference, so it's best to try them out before making a purchase.

THE BASIC VS. ADVANCED ANALYSIS PACKAGE

LabVIEW comes packaged in one of two ways. The ***Base Package*** comes with most functions needed to operate LabVIEW. Media are currently provided on a CD-ROM, although a floppy disk version may be ordered. Higher level users, especially those doing data acquisition, will find that the advanced analysis features found in the ***Full Development System*** are a must. While there is, as might be expected, a price differential, exploiting the high-level analytical capabilities of LabVIEW is best achieved and appreciated with the Full Development System. This package also includes new Internet and HTML capabilities now available in v5.x, as well as an extensive number of instrument drivers. A ***student version*** of LabVIEW is also available and is relatively inexpensive.

INSTRUMENT DRIVERS

LabVIEW connects with a vast number of sensors and monitoring devices found in industry, research, and educational settings. For LabVIEW to communicate with these instruments, ***driver*** software is required. For example, an analog-to-digital (A-to-D) converter board that digitizes captured analog signals from a device such as an electromyograph (EMG) amplifier will require a driver, many of which are found in the **NI-DAQ™ 6x Configuration Utility.** This software assigns a device (slot) number and configures system base addresses, DMA channels, and IRQ (interrupt) levels so that LabVIEW virtual instruments (VIs—programs) can properly communicate with the EMG. With the advent of ***plug and play*** technology, much of the drudgery of configuring instruments is now a thing of the past. Plug and play senses and identifies most hardware connected to a computer and automatically configures it to the manufacturer's specifications. In the event that a particular instrument is unknown, the user still can manually configure the equipment.

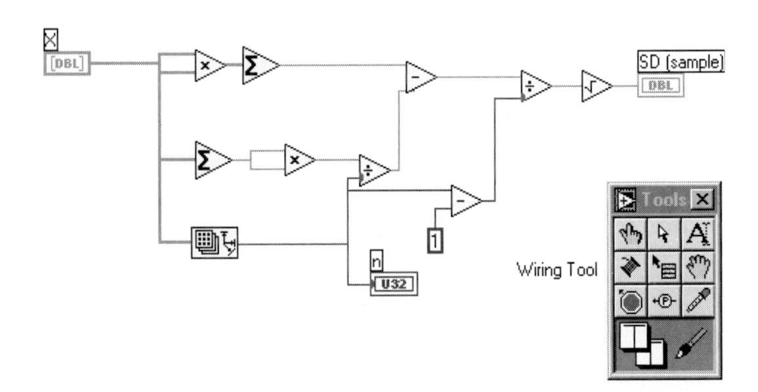

FIGURE 3–1.2
Block diagram of a subVI used to compute the standard deviation of the sample. Note the *Wiring Tool.*

LabVIEW ships with an extensive array of instrument drivers. If a particular instrument is not supported in the software package, most known drivers are available from National Instruments Tech Support Department or may be downloaded from National Instrument's BBS, FTP, or Web site free of charge. An instrument driver library called **INSTRUPEDIA™** is available on a CD-ROM.

WHAT ARE VIS AND SUBVIS?

One of LabVIEW's principle features is the ability to configure software as hardware devices ("the Software is the instrument"). This is accomplished via LabVIEW's graphical user interface with which software programs are written. Icons—representing the equivalent of text-based code (e.g., BASIC or C^{++})—are connected or wired together, creating a computer program called a ***VI,*** or ***virtual instrument.*** An analogy may be drawn with a printed circuit board in electronics. In these devices, components (e.g., microchips, transistors, resistors, capacitors, diodes, etc.) are linked together with solder or other types of connectors, creating a solid-state circuit board. A good example might be the controller board for a hard drive in a computer. The way and order in which each element is connected establish the orderly flow of electrical energy and therefore determine and drive the function of the circuit. In LabVIEW, individual icons (subVIs) with predetermined connection points (terminals) are ***wired*** together using a *Wiring Tool* (a spool of wire) from the **Tools** palette, likewise establishing an orderly flow of information in the VI (Figure 3–1.2).

Repetitive functions in text-based programming known as ***subroutines*** are configured in LabVIEW as ***subVIs.*** Numerous subVIs are included in LabVIEW's menu structure. In the event that a subVI does not exist, users may create and save their own. For example, in Figure 3–1.3, a subVI called **SDsam.vi** calculates the

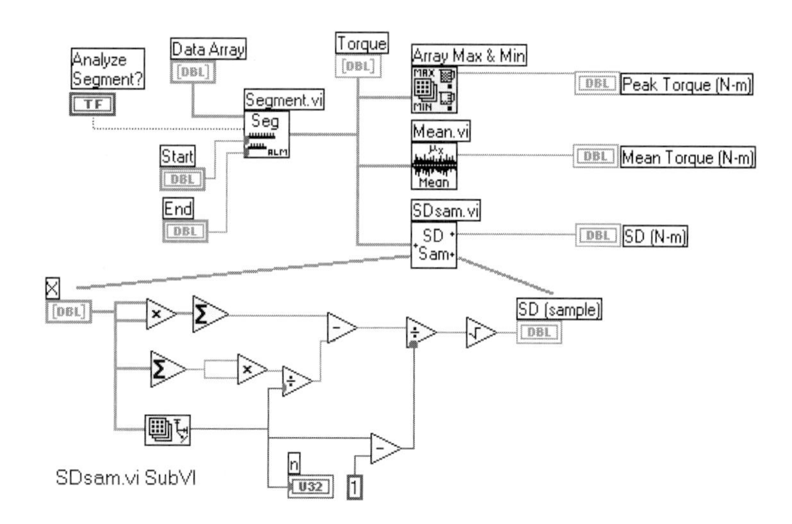

FIGURE 3–1.3
Block diagram with the **SDsam.vi** subVI used to compute the standard deviation of the sample. Double-clicking on the icon will reveal the code used to write this subVI. See the exploded view below the **SDsam.vi** icon.

standard deviation of the sample from an array of values. Rather than creating this code each time a VI requires this function, a subVI may be written and saved and later inserted into subsequent VIs when needed. While this is a simple example, subVIs can be complex, and the benefits of using a subVI vs. reinventing the wheel each time should be immediately obvious. The user also can create a subVI icon face that helps the programmer or user more easily identify a particular subroutine's function in the context of a large VI. The subVI may also be personalized to give credit to the original developer. A subVI editor permits making changes either to the icon face or to the terminals that link the subVI to the rest of the VI. SubVIs will be discussed in greater detail in Sections 3–5, "Creating SubVIs," and 3–6, "More SubVIs."

LabVIEW Structure

Front Panel and Block Diagram

When LabVIEW is started, the user is immediately brought to two blank overlapping panels, which represent the fundamental structure of a VI. The panels may be toggled between in the usual way by placing the cursor on any part of the panel and left-clicking the mouse. Similarly, each panel's size may be changed by left-clicking the corner of the window (a corner bracket tool appears) and dragging the panel larger or smaller. Toggling is also possible using the **Windows** menu and clicking on **Show Diagram** if you're working on the front panel and **Show Panel** from the block diagram. Both panels may be tiled horizontally or vertically by selecting the

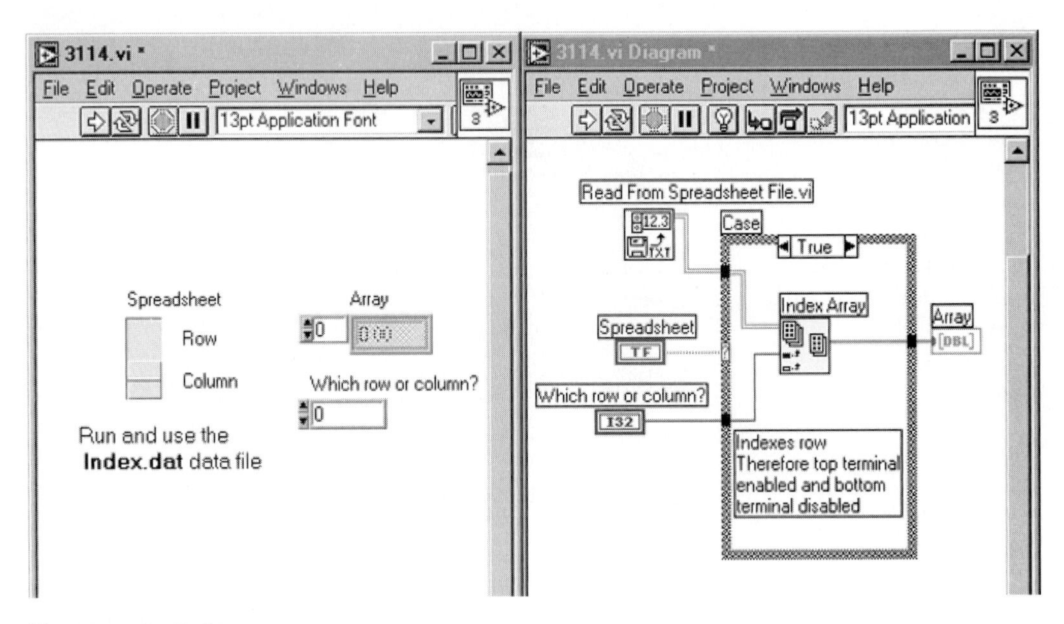

FIGURE 3–1.4
The front panel and block diagram may be displayed simultaneously using the **Windows/Tile Left and Right** menu option. Tiling can also be done vertically.

appropriate option from **Windows** in the task bar. In fact, this is an excellent way to visualize what's going on in the two panels while building a VI (Figure 3–1.4).

The ***front panel*** is the user interface from which the VI is operated. It consists of various types of controls (e.g., knobs, dials, slides, etc.) gauges, graphs, and tables laid out and positioned by the user. The front panel is built and controlled by selecting menu items from the task bar across the top of the screen. Most of the items have ***drop-down*** or ***pull-down*** menus and operate in the usual Windows fashion. Note that, each time an element is accessed and placed on the front panel, an ***icon,*** a subVI, will appear on the block diagram (see Figure 3–1.4).

The ***block diagram*** includes the actual "program" being written and might be likened to a wiring diagram on a plan to build an electronics device. Each VI has a series of ***terminals*** to which ***wires*** (links) are attached, establishing the flow of information between various functions. Like the front panel, the block diagram is controlled and functions are accessed using the task bar across the top of the screen.

Thus, the user continually toggles back and forth between the front panel and block diagram to write a program—a VI. The VI is therefore the sum-total of all of the graphical elements in the two panels. In Section 3–4, "Build and Run Two Simple VIs," you will construct and run two VIs to become familiar with panel use and other programming functions.

FIGURE 3–1.5
Front panel demonstrating the **Windows** task bar option.

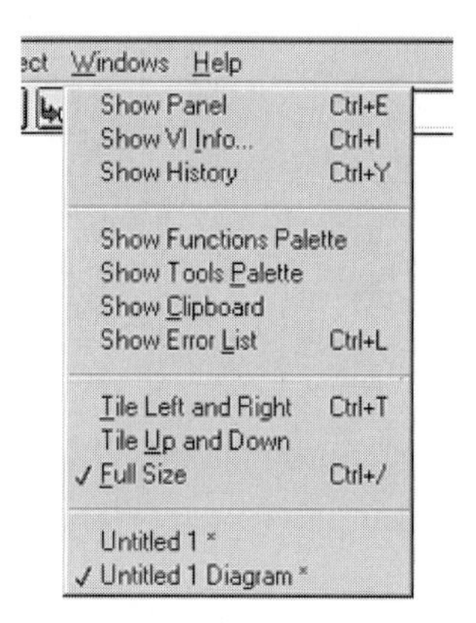

PULL-DOWN AND POP-UP MENUS

Front panel and block diagram functions are accessed and controlled using standard Windows-style ***pull-down*** (from the task bar across the top of the screen) and ***pop-up*** menus. Generally, ***pull-down*** menu items are accessed with the left mouse button, and ***pop-up*** menus (e.g., palettes) are accessed with the right. Certain key combinations using either the ***Control*** or ***Alt*** keys also permit access, but using the mouse and cursor will probably be more efficient. For example, begin running LabVIEW, and select **New VI** from the initial dialog box. From the front panel, place the cursor on **Windows** on the task bar across the top of the screen, and left-click the mouse. A pull-down menu like the one in Figure 3–1.5 appears.

On the front panel, right-clicking the mouse pops up the **Controls** palette, while popping up on the block diagram accesses the **Functions** palette. Both of these palettes are layered; thus, submenus may be found by left-clicking the cursor on a submenu item. For example, after popping up the **Functions** palette from the block diagram, left-click on the ***floppy disk image***, and a submenu entitled **File I/O** (i.e., file input/output) will appear, from which may be chosen specific input/output subVIs to save or read data to or from a spreadsheet (Figure 3–1.6).

TOOLS, CONTROLS, AND FUNCTIONS PALETTES

The **Tools, Control,** and **Functions** palettes are the principal tools with which VIs are built and controlled. The **Tools** and **Control** palettes are used for the front panel and block diagram, while the **Functions** palette appears only in the block diagram. The **Tools** palette will automatically appear each time **New VI** or **Open VI** is selected from the LabVIEW start-up dialog window. The **Tools** palette may also be toggled on or off by selecting the **Show Tools Palette** item from the **Windows** pull-down menu (see Figure 3–1.5). The **Controls** palette may also be accessed by either right-clicking anywhere on the screen or from the **Windows** pull-down menu. All palettes may be repositioned using the *Arrow Tool* and "tacked"

FIGURE 3–1.6
Right-clicking anywhere on the block diagram will bring up the **Functions** palette. By default, the **Tools** palette will appear in the block diagram. Both palettes may be toggled on and off by left-clicking on the **Windows** task bar option and selecting a **Show** option.

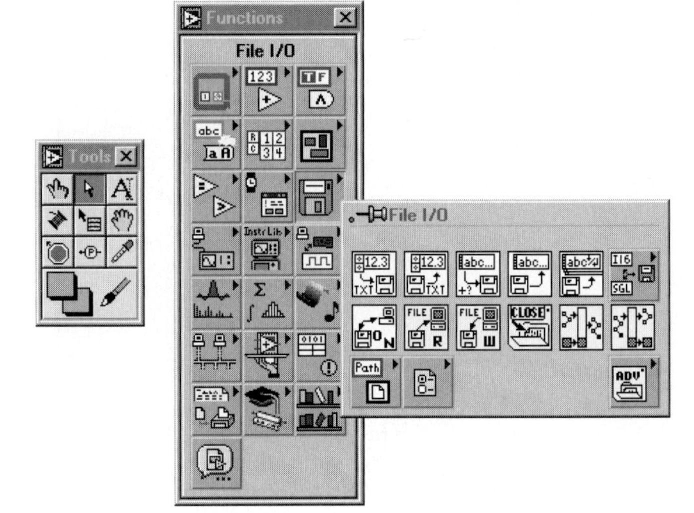

FIGURE 3–1.7
The **Tools** palette.

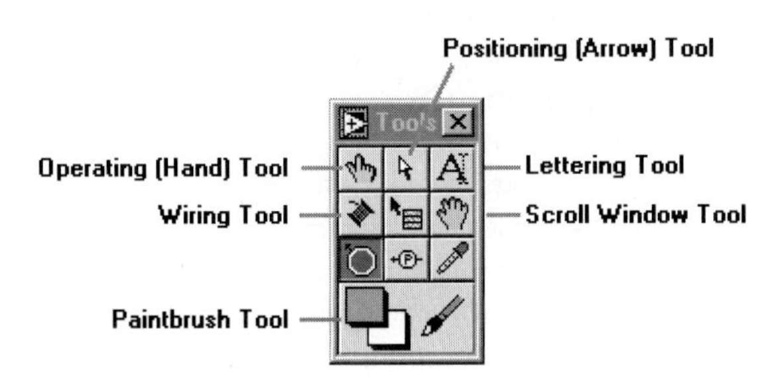

into place. In the block diagram, the **Functions** palette is accessed the same way as the **Controls** palette.

The **Tools** palette (Figure 3–1.7) provides operational and navigational tools to lay out and organize the front panel and block diagram. Some of the tools include a *Positioning Tool* (arrow), *Operating Tool* (hand), *Wiring Tool* (spool), *Lettering Tool* (A) and *Color Tool* (paintbrush). The *Positioning Tool* is the main cursor and permits selection, movement, and resizing of objects. The *Operating Tool* runs various devices requiring manipulation such as control dials; cursor-controlled indicators; or the **Run** button, which executes the VI. The *Wiring Tool* is used in the block diagram to connect subVIs and other programming functions. The *Lettering Tool* allows for labels to be placed on either panel. Font control (e.g., type, size, style, etc.) is achieved by left-clicking on the pull-down **Application Font** menu located beneath the **Project** menu at the top of the screen. The color of objects is controlled with the *Paintbrush Tool.* The *Paintbrush Tool* is placed on the object to be colored. Right-

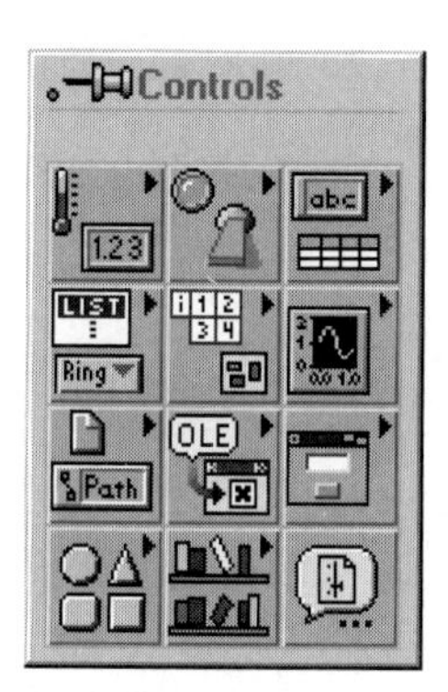

FIGURE 3–1.8
Right-clicking anywhere on the front panel will bring up the **Controls** palette. The palette may be toggled on or off by left-clicking on the **Windows** task bar option and selecting the **Show** option.

TABLE 3–1.1 Submenus available from the **Controls** palette.

SUBMENU	FUNCTIONS INCLUDED
Numeric	Digital Indicators and Controls; Knobs, Dials, and Slides
Boolean	Boolean (true/false) Switches, Buttons, Lights, and LED's
String & Table	String Indicator and Controls; Table Set-up
List & Ring	List and Ring Menu Controls
Array & Cluster	Array and Cluster
Graph	Waveform Charts and Graphs; X–Y Graphs; Intensity Graphs
Path & Refnum	Path Indicators and Controls
ActiveX	Container, OLE Variant
Dialog	Dialog Numeric and String Controls, Dialog Ring
Decorations	Shapes and Patterns for the Front Panel
User Controls	Access to Directories
Select a Control	Access to Directories

clicking pops up a color palette from which a color is selected by left-clicking the appropriate color tile. Left-click to exit the palette. Touching the object to be colored with the *Paintbrush Tool* and left-clicking turns the object the desired color.

The **Controls** palette (Figure 3–1.8) includes a series of submenus for front panel objects that determine the overall layout and function of the VI. Variables and other controls are selected using the *Arrow Tool.* Left-click on a submenu from the **Controls** palette, and an additional submenu appears showing various choices. Left-click the choice, and drag the object to the desired location on the front panel. Then, left-click to paste the object to the front panel. The position and size of the object may be fine-tuned using the *Arrow Tool.*

The submenus shown in Table 3–1.1 are available from the **Controls** palette.

Structures and subVIs from the **Functions** palette (Figure 3–1.6) are chosen and located on the block diagram in the same way as with **Control** palette objects and are described in Table 3–1.2.

TABLE 3–1.2 Submenus available from the **Functions** palette.

SUBMENU	FUNCTIONS INCLUDED
Structures	Sequence, Case, For Loop, While Loop, Formula Node, Global and Local Variables
Numeric	Plus, Minus, Divide, Multiply, Square Root, etc., Numeric Constant
Boolean	And, Or, Not, etc.
String	Length, Subset, Concatenate Strings, etc., String Constant
Array	Size, Index, Subset, Reshape, Build, Reverse 1D Array, Transpose 2D array
Cluster	Unbundle, Bundle, Build Cluster Array, etc.
Comparison	Equal, Less Than, Greater Than, Min/Max, Range, etc.
Time & Dialog	Tick Count, Wait, Wait Until Next ms Multiple.vi, Get Date/Time String, 1-Button Dialog, 2-Button Dialog
File I/O	Write Spreadsheet File.vi, Read Spreadsheet File. vi, Open/Create/Replace File.vi, Read File, Write File, Close File, etc.
Instrument I/O	VISA, GPIB, GPIB 488.2, Serial
Instrument Drivers	
Data Acquisition	Analog Input and Output, Digital I/O, Counter, Calibration and Configuration, Signal Conditioning
Signal Processing	Signal Generation, Time Domain, Frequency Domain, Measurement, Filters, Windows
Mathematics	Formula, 1D and 2D Evaluations, Calculus, Probability and Statistics, Curve Fitting, Linear Algebra, Optimization, Zeroes, Numeric Functions
Graphics & Sound	3D Graphics, Picture Plots, Picture Functions, Graphics Formats, Sound
Communications	Active X, DataSocket, HiQ, DDE, TCP, UDP, System Exec.vi
Application Controls	Open Application Reference, Open VI Reference, Close Application or VI Reference, Call By Referencing Node, Property Node, Invoke Node, Call Chain, Print Panel.vi, Stop, Quit LabVIEW, Menu, Help
Advanced	Call Library Functions, Code Interface Node, Data Manipulation, Synchronization, Memory
Report Generation	Easy Text Report.vi, New Report.vi, Set Report Font.vi, Print Report.vi, Dispose Report.vi. Report Layout, Append Report Text.vi, Append Numeric Table to Report.vi, Append Text Table to Report.vi, Append File to Report.vi, Advanced Reports
Tutorial	Demo Voltage Read.vi. Digital Thermometer.vi, Generate Waveform.vi
User Libraries	Access to Directories
Select a VI . . .	Access to Directories

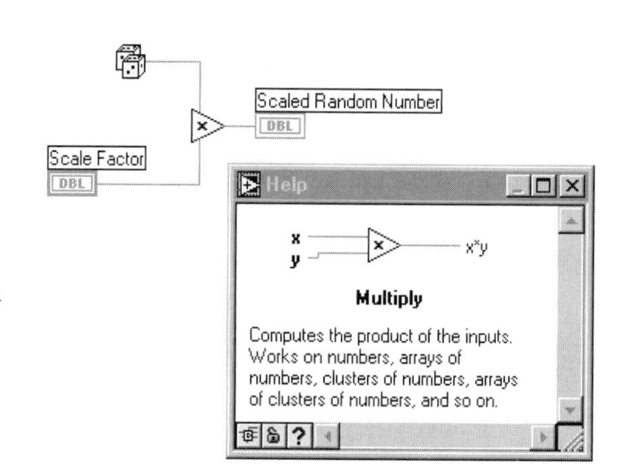

FIGURE 3–1.9
The **Help** window is toggled on and off by left-clicking on the **Help** task bar option in either the front panel or block diagram and selecting the **Show** option. Each time an icon or function is touched with the cursor, a description appears in the Help window.

HELP WINDOW

The Help window (Figure 3–1.9) may be accessed from either the front panel or block diagram by left-clicking on **Help** in the task bar at the top of the screen. The window is resizable and movable using the *Arrow Tool.* In the block diagram, touch a subVI with the cursor (there is no need to click either mouse button), and note that a ***help message*** is displayed in the window describing the function of the subVI and wiring terminals. Now, get the *Wiring Tool* from the **Tools** palette, and touch the tip on any wiring terminal on a subVI. Note that in the **Help** window, the terminal area on the icon face begins to ***pulsate*** and ***terminals pop out*** from the icon, helping to further distinguish the terminals. SubVIs frequently have multiple, closely spaced terminals, sometimes making identification difficult. Using the **Help** window makes distinguishing one terminal from another easier. It's a good idea to leave the **Help** window on, especially when building a complicated VI with multiple subVIs. This will also be useful when troubleshooting a bad or improperly wired terminal.

RUNNING A VI

To activate a text-based program in BASIC, the user types the word "Run" and presses the Enter key on the keyboard. This sets the program into motion until the last line of code is executed. To execute a LabVIEW VI, the user left-clicks the **Run** button (white arrow pointing to the right) located beneath **File** and **Edit** on the task bar at the top of the screen (Figure 3–1.10). The user does not need to change the cursor when clicking the **Run** button. As soon as whatever cursor being used is placed over the **Run** button, it automatically changes to the *Hand Tool.*

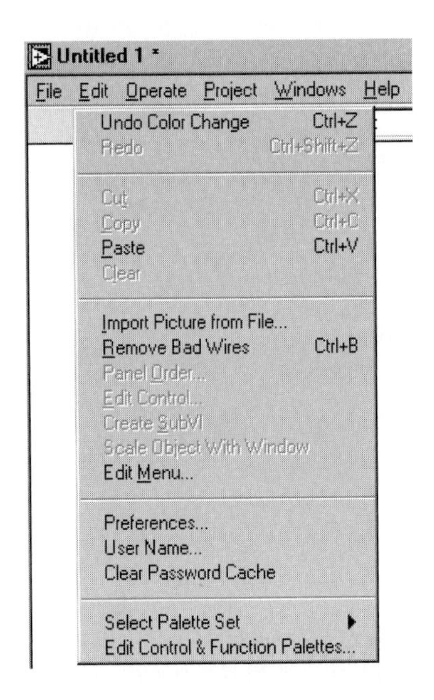

FIGURE 3–1.10
Edit option of the task bar with pull-down menu.

Note that, when the VI executes properly, the **Run** arrow changes from white to black, signaling all is well with the VI. To stop the VI, the user left-clicks the **Stop** button (looks like a ***Stop*** sign) beneath **Edit** and **Operate.** Stopping a program may also be accomplished by installing a *Boolean* switch associated with a *While Loop* on the block diagram (see Section 3–7, "Loops and Structures," for more information on this function). Some VIs are programmed to cycle through a specified number of iterations, at which time the VI stops automatically.

Bad terminal connections, broken wires, or logic errors in a VI will cause the program to abort when the **Run** button is clicked. When this happens, the **Run** arrow will ***turn gray and appear broken.*** At the same time, a ***dialog box*** will be displayed, describing any errors that have been identified. For example, if a terminal on a subVI was not wired or was wired incorrectly, an error message such as, "unwired terminal or bad wire" will be returned. Left double-clicking on the error message will bring the user to the block diagram, and the specific area in the VI where the problem occurred will be highlighted. ***Bad wires*** will appear as ***broken lines*** and are a common mistake if terminals aren't properly wired. In some cases, the terminal is incompatible with another terminal from another subVI. Bad wires may be removed by left-clicking and highlighting the wire and pressing the delete key. If numerous bad wires are present, left-clicking on the **Edit** menu and clicking on the **Remove Bad Wires** option will delete them all at once (Figure 3–1.10).

Immediately to the right of the **Run** arrow is the **Continuous Run** arrow (two white curved arrows tracing a circular path (see Figure 3–1.11). Some VIs that are intended to execute for a single iteration may be made to run repetitively by

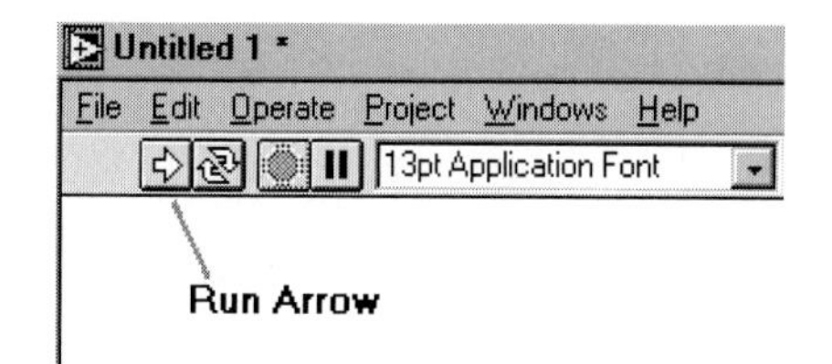

FIGURE 3–1.11
The **Run** arrow is located on the left side of the task bar in the front panel and block diagram. Left-clicking on the **Run** arrow executes a VI.

left-clicking the **Continuous Run** arrow. Note that the color changes from ***white*** to ***black*** while in continuous mode. The **Run** arrow will also change to black. Pushing the **Stop** button will halt execution of the VI.

SAVING VIS, DIRECTORIES, AND LIBRARIES

VIs are saved using conventional Windows 95/98 procedures by left-clicking the **File** menu and choosing the **Save** or **Save As . . .** option. Clicking either option will bring the user to a dialog window where a prompt to ***choose*** or ***create*** a directory will appear. Windows 95/98 permits the use of ***long filenames*** rather than being constrained by the original DOS/Window's v3.x 8 + 3 format. Unless another extension is appended, VIs will automatically be given the ***.vi* extension.** It's a good idea to use this convention, which will make VIs more obvious if they are stored in directories where LabVIEW files are mixed with executable files (e.g., files with the extension ***.exe*** or ***.com***).

LabVIEW offers the option of saving files in ***libraries.*** Libraries permit multiple files to be stored under a single file name. The dialog box that appears after **Save** or **Save As . . .** is clicked, providing the option to ***create a library*** by clicking on the **New VI Library** button. The ***.llb*** extension automatically will be appended to the library name.

Libraries are a handy place to store related VIs. A disadvantage is that damage to a library file may result in ***all files*** saved being damaged or unrecoverable.

NATIONAL INSTRUMENTS EXAMPLE VIS

National Instruments includes with LabVIEW an extensive number of prewritten VIs and subVIs, providing a wide variety of data acquisition and analysis capabilities. Many of these VIs may be adapted for specific programming needs by editing and resaving. It's best to save the VI using another filename and store it in a new directory. Otherwise, the edited version will be overwritten and the original version will no longer be available. **Example VIs** are stored in libraries (**.llb**) in the **LabVIEW/Examples** directory.

CD ROM DISK AND SAMPLE DATA FILES

Included in this book is an accompanying **CD ROM disk.** This disk contains all VIs and subVIs described in succeeding pages. Note also that ***modified*** or ***other types*** of VIs that are suggested as ***Practice Exercises*** in some chapters are contained on this disk. Presaved ***data files,*** used to confirm that data processing and analysis VIs are running properly, are also included. After doing a ***Practice Exercise,*** you may want to call up and/or print out a VI from the disk to compare the version just written with a version of the VI on the **CD ROM disk.**

To optimize performance during programming, I recommend that you copy the contents of the **CD ROM disk** to a convenient directory on the computer's hard drive. Instructions for this transfer are described in the first ***Practice Exercise.*** From this point forward, the phrase **"CD ROM disk directory"** refers to the VIs and data files that have been copied ***from*** the original **CD ROM disk *to*** a directory in the hard drive. The **CD ROM disk directory,** referenced by section number and filename, including sample data files, is shown in Appendix A.

SUMMARY

Current and past versions of LabVIEW were discussed including overall structure of VIs and subVIs using front panels and block diagrams. VIs and subVIs are run from the task bar at the top of the screen and saved using options from the **File** menu. Most VIs and subVIs and data files are included on a companion CD-ROM.

PRACTICE EXERCISES

Copy the contents of the **CD ROM disk** included with this book to the computer's hard drive using the following procedure: Put the **CD ROM disk** in the CD-ROM drive. Using ***Windows Explorer*** or other ***file manager*** software, find the ***drive letter*** of the CD ROM drive. Left-click on the CD ROM drive folder on the left side of the screen, and note that the contents of the disk, referenced by section number (e.g., 3–1, "Basics"), appear on the right side of the screen. Left-click, hold, and drag the **CD ROM Disk *folder*** to the ***C: prompt*** near the top of the listing on the left side of the ***Explorer.*** This assumes that the ***main directory*** is in the ***C:*** hard drive. If it is not, or if another hard drive is to be used, select the appropriate hard drive letter (e.g., D:). When the cursor (with the **CD ROM disk** folder) is over the ***C: prompt,*** release the mouse button; then the files, in their original folders and order, will be copied to the hard drive. Depending on the processor and clock speed, this may take several minutes. From this point forward, when you are asked to open a VI or subVI, use the VI and subVI just copied for all programming.

To become acquainted with using the contents of the **CD ROM disk** files just copied to the hard drive, open LabVIEW. At the opening dialog window, left-click on the "Open VI" button. At the prompt, navigate through the hard drive directories until you locate the **CD ROM disk** folder. Left-click and highlight the folder, and then press the **Open** button. Scroll through the directory until the Section 3–16, "Torque and Velocity Measurements," folder is found. Left-click and highlight the folder, and again press the **Open** button. Left-click and highlight on the VI icon (disk) called **Torque.vi,** and press the **Open** button, and the file will be called up. The first time you open the VI or any other VI from the **CD ROM disk directory,** you may be prompted to identify the location of one or more subVIs (these will be described in detail in Sections 3–5, "Creating SubVIs," and 3–6, "More SubVIs"). Scroll through the directory for Section 3–5, and select, highlight, and open the subVI(s) being requested. Note that ***resaving*** **Torque.vi** back to its original directory location will "teach" LabVIEW where subVIs are located. The next time **Torque.vi** is opened, LabVIEW will "remember" where the subVIs are located. That is, you ***won't*** be prompted to identify subVI files again.

When **Torque.vi** is opened, several controls, indicators, and two graphs appear on the screen (front panel). This VI is intended to measure ***isometric torque signals*** from an ***isokinetic dynamometer.*** (**Torque.vi** will be discussed in detail in Section 3–16, "Torque and Velocity Measurements".) For now, to practice using a sample data file from the **CD ROM disk directory,** do the following: Left-click the **Run arrow.** As soon as the VI begins to run, a dialog window appears, prompting you to "Choose (a) file to read." Scroll through the directories until you find a folder called **Sample Data Files.** Left-click and highlight the folder, and press the **Open** button. Find the data file called **Torq2.dat,** and open it using the same procedure. This is a data file recorded during a ***maximal isometric contraction*** of the quadriceps during knee extension on a dynamometer. Note that two graphs appear, and values for some of the indicators for torque measurements are displayed in a framed panel toward the bottom of the screen. The main graph and three of the indicators with measurements will look like Figure 3–1.12. To confirm that the correct data file was selected, check the "Data File" path indicator above the graph. The filename should read "Torq2.dat." Compare the overall shape of the graph in Figure 3–1.12 with the one on the screen. Also check to see that three indicators below the graph display the following values: "Peak Torque" should be "230.29 Newton-meters," "Peak Torque Index" should be "2263 msec," and "Start of Rise from Baseline" should be "1039 msec." In Section 3–16, "Torque and Velocity Measurements," you will build **Torque.vi,** and you will learn to interpret other measurements and select a ***segment*** of the torque signal for further analysis and display.

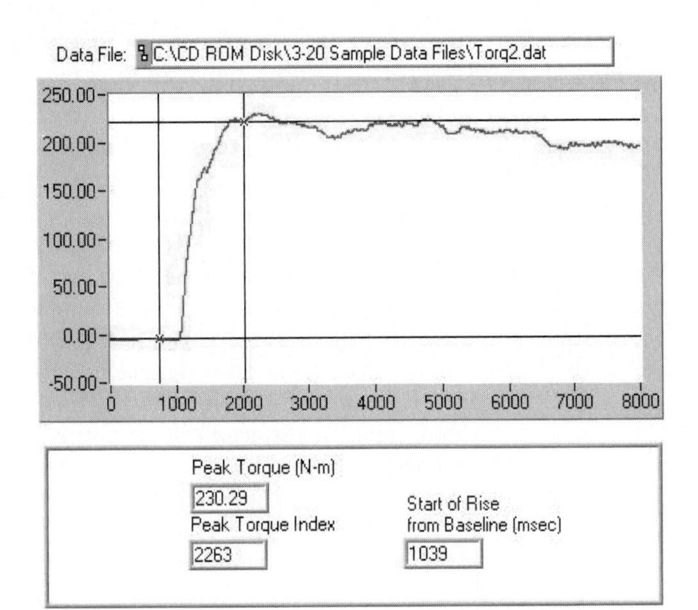

FIGURE 3–1.12
Waveform Graph displaying an isometric torque curve and three *Digital Indicators*.

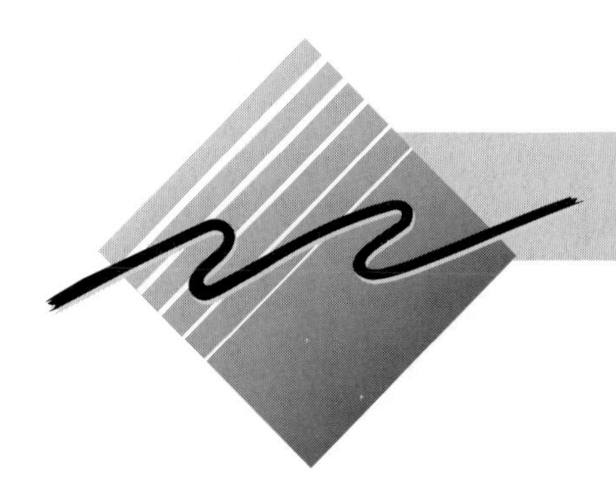

FRONT PANEL

OBJECTIVES

- ❖ Review and understand basic front panel programming functions.
- ❖ Practice basic front panel programming functions.

INTRODUCTION

As noted in Section 3–1, "Basics," LabVIEW VIs consist of a ***front panel*** and ***block diagram.*** The front panel represents the user interface for the VI where various controls and indicators are found. Usually, the VI is run from the front panel. The block diagram is the area where the actual programming occurs. Here, icons representing a wide variety of data collection and processing and analysis functions are wired together to establish a logical flow of information. This and the next section build on programming concepts introduced in Section 3–1, "Basics." What follows is a discussion of basic front panel functions focusing on the **Controls** and **Tools** palettes.

LAYOUT

Precisely how the user organizes and lays out front panel elements is largely a matter of preference; however, a few conventions may make programming and use of the VI easier. The first issue to resolve is to identify who will be the ultimate user of the VI. If the programmer and user are the same individual, front panel organization and appearance may be of less concern, since the location and functions of front panel elements are known and understood. In this case, less polish and attention to details may be tolerated. On the other hand, if the VI is intended to be used by someone other than the programmer, then efforts should be made to make running and understanding the VI as ***user friendly*** as possible. A number of programming tips may facilitate this goal. Using a ***left-to-right input/output*** convention, organizing controls and indicators in ***groups,*** and using ***colors*** to distinguish categories of controls should make the VI more understandable to the user and easier to run and operate.

While a ***left-to-right input/output*** convention is probably easier to adhere to in the block diagram, using this idea in the front panel is advisable whenever possible. This convention involves locating controls (e.g., *Digital Controls, Dials, Knobs, Slides,* etc.) toward either the ***left*** or ***top*** of the front panel. Indicators (e.g., *Digital Indicators, Graphs, Meters,* etc.) should be located to the right or bottom of the panel. Since the eyes are comfortable with a left-to-right visual scan, as in reading a sentence or page of text, a front panel laid out this way may be easier to interpret.

Complicated VI front panels do not always lend themselves to putting all controls to the left and all indicators to the right. Another strategy that may help to orient the user is to group elements that have similar functions. For example, if *Dials, Buttons, Slides,* or other types of control devices need to be preset before the VI is run, it may be helpful to organize them in the same geographic location on the front panel, labeling them with an appropriate heading. For example, in Figure 3–2.1, controls used to operate a segment analyzer, filters, and rectification options are located in the upper left corner of the screen. This VI displays force transducer and event marker signals on two *Waveform Graphs,* indexing force output at the point where an event marker is triggered. Note also that "Transducer" and "Event Marker" channels are selected using two *Digital Controls* underneath the "Rectification" control. To the center and right of the controls are two *Waveform Graphs* and several *Digital Indicators* that display the data in various units of measurement. Another strategy that may help to group controls and indicators in a logical way is to ***group*** them in ***frames*** or other figures (e.g., boxes or triangles). Not only will this strategy physically cause a separation between front panel elements, but it gives the VI a finished look that approximates that of a piece of hardware. *Raised Frames* from the **Decorations** menu in the **Controls** palette have been used in Figure 3–2.1 to group and separate controls from indicators. The **Decorations** (Figure 3–2.2) menu is found in the lower left corner of the **Controls** palette. After popping up the menu, use the *Arrow Tool* to select the appropriate frame or shape by left-clicking the mouse. The palette disappears, and the cursor changes to the *Scroll Tool* (open hand), to which is attached a ***highlighted box.*** Position the box in the approximate place where the figure is to be located, and left-click again. Note that a small version of the figure is first laid down. ***Resize*** the figure using the *Arrow Tool* by ***clicking and dragging*** any of the corners of the figure.

Finally, ***colors*** may be used to further distinguish front panel elements and may complement or be used in place of frames. Call up the **Readtran.vi** VI from

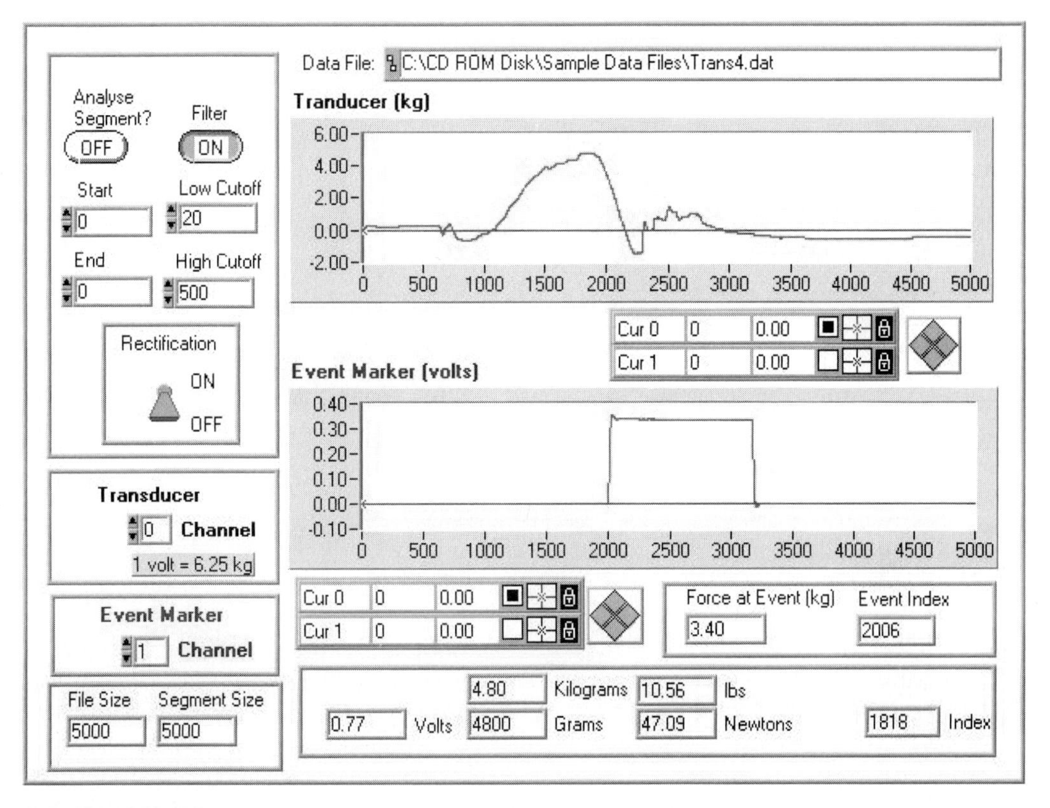

FIGURE 3–2.1
Front panel of **Readtran.vi.**

the **CD ROM disk directory** (Section 3–19, "Other Programming Functions and Tools"). Note that a ***light purple*** color was selected to highlight the "ON/OFF" button and *Digital Controls* for "Start" and "End" values for the segment analyzer in the upper left corner of the front panel. A ***salmon*** color was used to identify the "Filter" control. At the bottom of the screen are a series of *Digital Indicators* used to display force transducer output that are colored ***yellow.***

Changing the color of front panel elements is done with the *Paint Brush Tool* in the **Tools** palette. Using any cursor, left-click on the bottom of the palette, and note that the cursor changes to a small ***paint brush*** as it's dragged away. Position the *Paint Brush Tool* over the front panel element to be colored, and right-click. Note that a ***color palette*** pops up. Select a color by left-clicking the mouse, and note that the object's color changes. Obviously, color selection is a matter of personal preference, but try to pick colors that are easy on the eyes, especially if it's anticipated the user will spend a lot of time in front of the monitor.

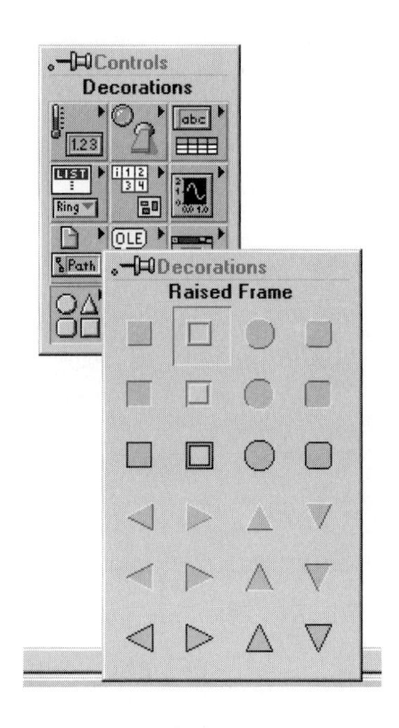

FIGURE 3–2.2
The **Decorations** menu is selected by left-clicking on the *Decorations* option of the **Controls** palette in the front panel.

NUMERIC AND STRING VARIABLES

As with all computer programming languages, ***variables*** are handled as either ***numbers*** or ***strings*** and may function either as ***controls*** or ***indicators.*** Strings are groups of ***alphanumeric*** characters. A string therefore, may be ***all letters*** (e.g., abc) or a ***group*** of ***letters and numbers*** (e.g., abc123). A good example might be someone's street address, which usually includes a house number as well as the name of the street the house is on. Numeric and string variables essentially drive a program and make it operate. Usually, before the VI is run, numeric or string variable data are placed into controls that define the limit of operation of the program. Variables may be fixed and held constant or may be frequently updated to reflect changes in data processing needs. After the program is run, indicators will display the processed data in various formats.

CONTROLS AND INDICATORS

Numeric and string variables may be configured as either ***controls*** or ***indicators*** and are accessed in the front panel from the **Controls** palette (Figure 3–2.3). Moving the *Arrow Tool* over the **Numeric** menu (Figure 3–2.3A) in the upper left corner of the palette causes a series functions to appear, including *Digital Controls* and *Indicators, Vertical,* and *Horizontal Slides, Knobs, Dials,* and *Meters.* Moving the cursor over the **String & Table** menu (Figure 3–2.3B) will similarly display ***string*** *Controls* and *Indicators.*

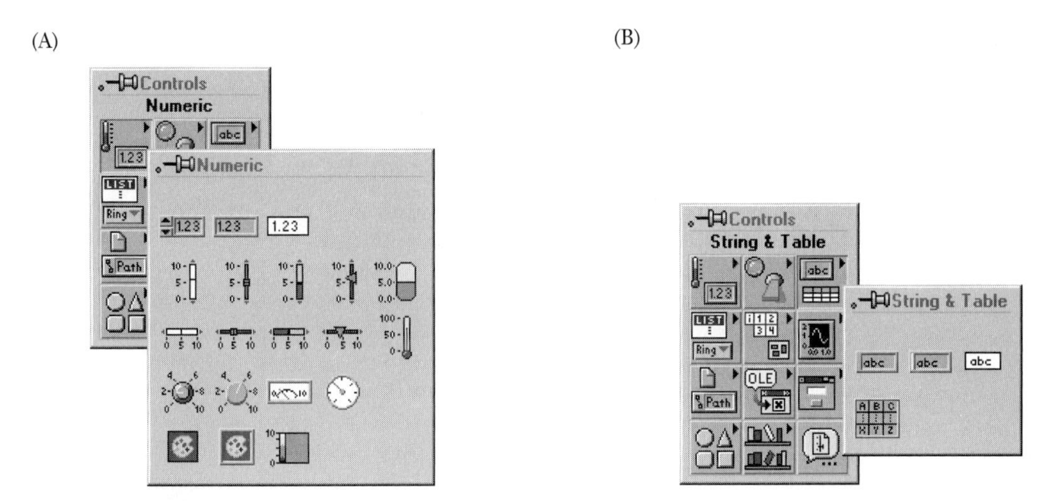

FIGURE 3–2.3
(A) The **Numeric** Menu is selected by left-clicking on the **Numeric** option of the **Controls** palette in the front panel. (B) String variables are located in the **String & Table** menu.

NUMERIC DATA PRECISION AND REPRESENTATION

In LabVIEW, when controls or indicators are used to display numeric data, the level of ***decimal precision*** defaults to ***two decimal places*** (i.e., Double Precision). Decimal precision is changed by right-clicking on a control or indicator from which is chosen the **Format & Precision** option from the pop-up menu. A left-click causes a **Format & Precision** dialog window to be displayed. Toward the center of the dialog window is a "Digits of Precision" control (default = 2), which may be changed. Pushing the OK button returns the user back to the front panel with the new level of precision now registered.

Numeric data *Representation* (e.g., single or double precision, integers) may also be changed in a similar way. For example, to change a *Numeric Control* from the default ***double precision*** case to an ***integer***, right-click on the control and move the cursor over the *Representation* option (Figure 3–2.4). Note that a secondary menu appears with 12 data representation choices. Select "I32 (Long)," and left-click the mouse. After the menu disappears, the control is reconfigured as an integer (i.e., no units of precision).

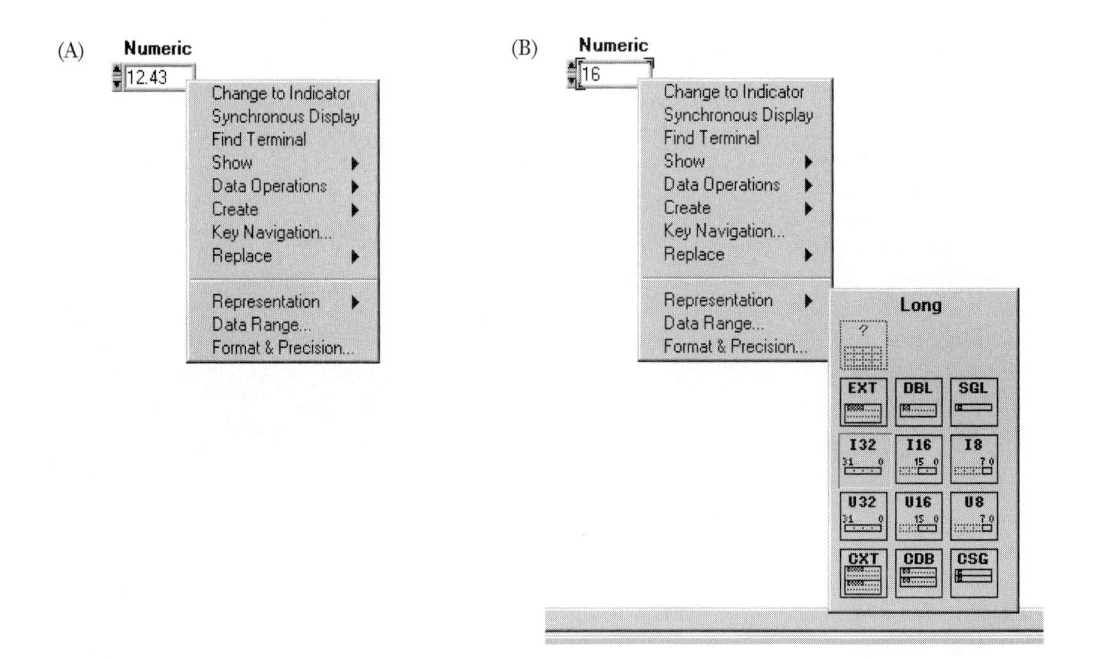

FIGURE 3–2.4
(A) Right-clicking on a *Digital Control* pops up a menu. (B) Touching the cursor on the **Representation** option pops up a second menu.

BOOLEANS

Boolean variables are ***either–or*** conditions and usually take the form of ***true/false*** or ***on/off*** statements. For example, a toggle switch (Figure 3–2.5) is essentially a Boolean control that provides the user with two options. The default condition for the switch (e.g., off) may be changed by flipping the switch to the alternate condition (e.g., on). In Section 3–7, "Loops and Structures," *While Loops* will be discussed. *While Loops* are used to afford ***on/off control*** to a VI. All functions placed in the loop will execute when the *While Loop* operates in the ***true*** (i.e., on) condition. Choosing the opposite ***false*** (i.e., off) condition will stop the VI. Boolean functions in LabVIEW take a variety of forms including switches, buttons, and light-emitting diodes (LEDS).

To select a Boolean function, place the *Arrow Tool* over the **Boolean** menu in the **Controls** palette. Note that a large secondary menu will pop up (Figure 3–2.5). After left-clicking on the object, the menus disappear and the object may be located and resized.

FIGURE 3–2.5
The **Boolean** menu is selected by left-clicking on the **Boolean** option of the **Controls** palette in the front panel. Note the *Vertical Toggle Switch* to the left.

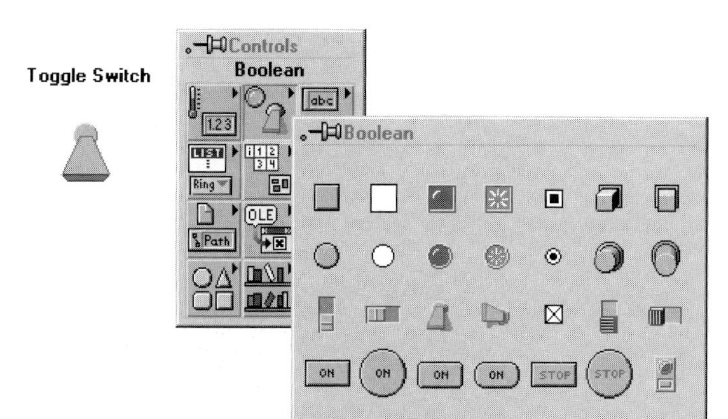

GRAPHS AND GRAPHING OPTIONS

Front panel data display is often achieved using various forms of ***graphs.*** Note that LabVIEW distinguishes between ***graphs*** and ***charts.*** Both are configured and display data in a comparable way. *Waveform Graphs* are used to display data that have been ***previously saved,*** whereas *Waveform Charts* display data in ***real-time*** as, for example, when a signal is acquired from an A-to-D board using an oscilloscope VI. Several other formats are offered including *XY Graphs*, *Intensity Charts*, *Intensity Graphs*, and several forms of *3D Graphs*.

Graphs are selected from the **Graph** menu in the **Controls** palette (Figure 3–2.6) in the usual manner. After the graph has been positioned on the front panel, it may be resized using the ***click-and-drag*** method. By default, the *Waveform Graph* will appear with a gray border, a black background with green horizontal and vertical grids, a legend, and label, all of which may be changed. *Waveform Charts* are essentially the same; however, the grids are absent. Graphs and charts may display single or multiple data plots, the details of which will be handled in several VIs presented in later sections. Figure 3–2.1 uses two *Waveform Graphs.* The ***top*** graph displays ***transducer force*** data and the ***lower*** one an ***event marker.*** Note that both graphs have been reconfigured so that the legend and grid patterns have been removed. In the actual VI found in the **CD ROM disk directory,** the border and background colors also have been changed.

Graphing options are accessed by placing the *Arrow Tool* anywhere on the graph and by popping up a menu by right-clicking the mouse (Figure 3–2.7). To change most graph parameters, select the **Show** option and then the parameter of interest with a left-click. The menus disappear and the graph is updated. Note that X and Y axis ***scaling*** may be changed using the method just described or by using the **X** and **Y Scale** options from the bottom of the first menu.

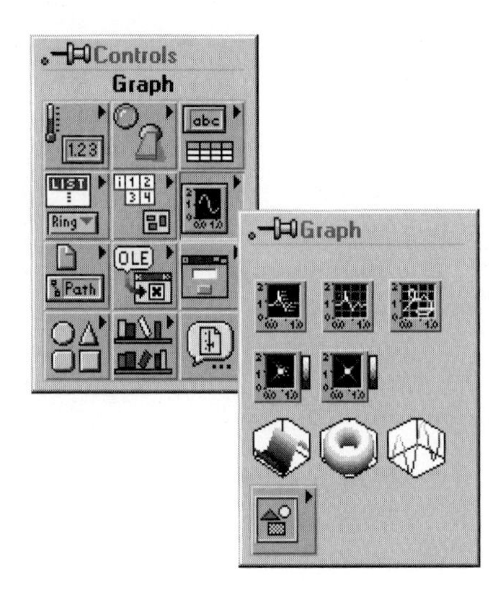

FIGURE 3–2.6
Various graphing functions are found in the **Graph** option of the **Controls** palette in the front panel.

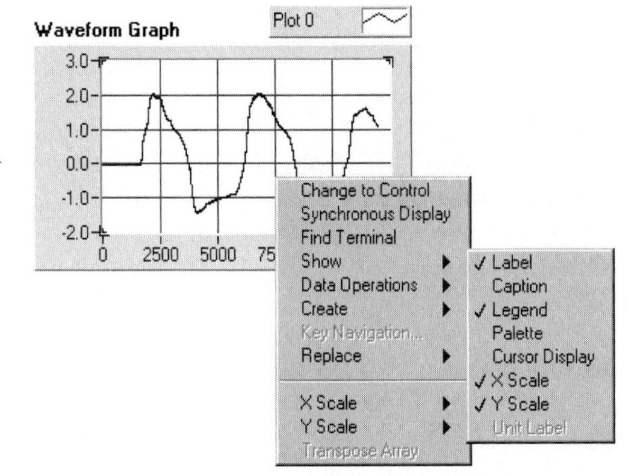

FIGURE 3–2.7
Graphing options are selected by left-clicking anywhere on a graph in the front panel and selecting an option from the pop-up menu using the **Show** option.

ARRAYS

Data that are grouped together as lists (e.g., as in a column of spreadsheet data) are known as ***arrays.*** A ***single*** column of tabular data constitutes a ***one-dimensional (1D)*** array, while ***multiple columns*** provide a ***two-dimensional (2D) array.*** Arrays of data may be used as ***controls*** or ***indicators*** and may be numbers or strings. Figure 3–2.8 is the front panel of the **Index.vi** VI found in the **CD ROM disk directory** and described in Section 3–10, "Indexing." Note that this 1D array contains 21 cells.

FIGURE 3–2.8
An *Indicator Array* in the front panel of **Index.vi.** By default, *Arrays* are single celled. To expand the *Array* to expose multiple cells, left-click and drag one of the lower corners with the **Arrow Tool.**

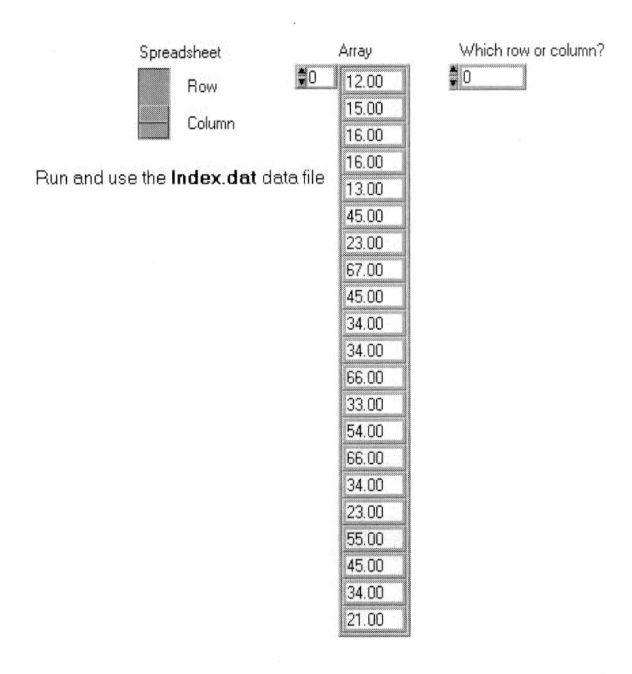

FIGURE 3–2.9
The *Array* (shell) is selected by left-clicking on the **Array & Cluster** menu of the **Controls** palette. *Arrays* are configured as either indicators or controls by inserting the appropriate variable. In this case, the *Array* is configured as an *Indicator Array* with a *Digital Indicator.*

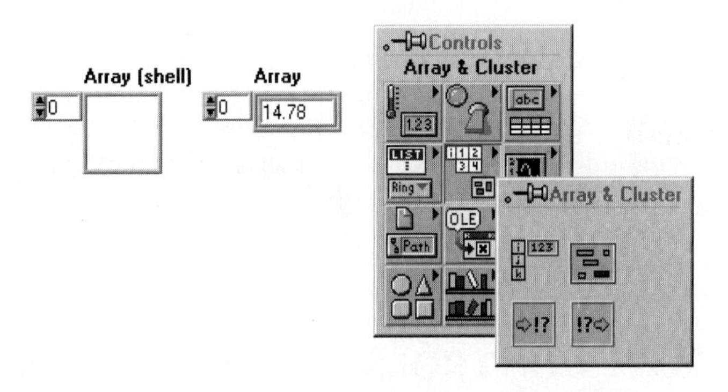

Building arrays is a two-step process. To build a 1D indicator array, first select an *Array* (shell) from the **Array & Cluster** menu in the **Controls** palette, and place it on the front panel in the usual manner (Figure 3–2.9). In its current configuration, the array shell is ***empty*** and may be configured in the next step as either a ***control*** or ***indicator*** array. Next, place the *Arrow Tool* anywhere over the empty array shell, and right-click the mouse to pop up the **Controls** palette. Another copy of this palette may also be located somewhere on the front panel. Select the

FIGURE 3–2.10
Ring structures are selected from the **List & Ring** menu of the **Controls** palette in the front panel.

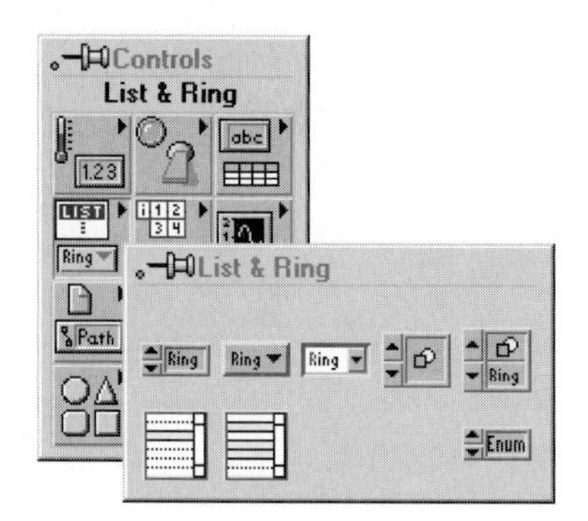

Numeric menu and, from that, a *Digital Indicator* by left-clicking the mouse. Now, loosely position the cursor over the *Array* shell, and left-click again. The *Digital Indicator* is seated into the *Array*. Note that the *Array* is initially configured so that a ***single cell*** shows. To expand the *Array* as in Figure 3–2.8, ***click and drag*** a lower corner of the cell downward.

RINGS

Rings are ***multiple-option string control*** variables that permit the user to choose from a list of actions rather than having to input them separately each time a VI is run. Two common ring controls include *Text* and *Menu Rings*, which are accessed from the **List & Ring** menu in the **Controls** palette (Figure 3–2.10). A description of how rings are used is provided in Section 3–19, "Other Programming Functions and Tools," using the **Rings.vi** VI as an example.

PATH CONTROLS AND INDICATORS

Path functions indicate the ***file path*** and ***filename*** of a data file (Figure 3–2.11). Path functions may be configured as either ***controls*** or ***indicators.*** When path functions are used as a control, the user will be prompted to identify the ***file path directory*** and ***filename*** of a data file needed for analysis. A path ***indictor*** indicates the ***file path directory*** and ***data filename*** used by the VI. In Figure 3–15.6, note that a *File Path Indicator* has been inserted into the top of both *Waveform Graphs*, which, in this example, display the power spectra of two electromyogram (EMG) data files. Confirm that the top graph, *File Path Indicator*, reads "C:\CD ROM Disk\3-20 Sample Data Files\Powspec1.dat". Path functions are accessed from the **Path & Refnum** menu in the **Controls** palette.

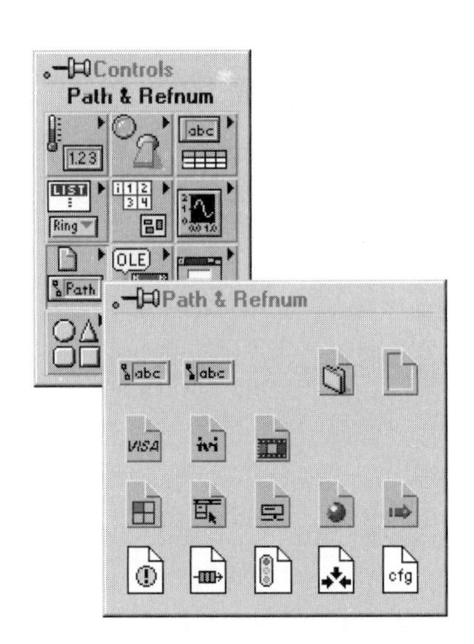

FIGURE 3–2.11
File Path Controls and *Indicators* are selected from the **Path & Refnum** menu of the **Controls** palette in the front panel.

MOVING AND RESIZING OBJECTS

Most front panel objects are easily ***moved*** and ***resized.*** To move an object, left-click the *Arrow Tool* anywhere on the structure. A ***pulsating broken line*** appears around the object. Next, left-click and drag the object to the desired location.

Groups of front panel (and block diagram) objects may also be moved en masse. Using the *Arrow Tool,* hold the left mouse button down, and ***draw a box*** around the elements to be moved. Release the button, and each object is surrounded by a ***pulsating line.*** Left-click and hold on any one of the highlighted objects, and drag the ***entire group*** to a new location.

To ***resize*** most front panel elements, use the *Arrow Tool,* and advance it toward any corner of the highlight line until the cursor changes to an ***angle bracket.*** At that point, left-click and drag the corner until the desired size is achieved, and release the mouse button. This procedure will ***not*** work for numeric and string controls and indicators. To change the size of these elements, click the *Lettering Tool* onto the control or indicator. Move to the **Text Settings** of the task bar at the top of the screen, and left-click on the ***menu ring.*** A long menu with various font parameters drops down (Figure 3–2.12). Select the **Size** option, and then left-click on the desired ***font size.*** When the cursor is released, the control or indicator resizes itself consistent with the font size selected. A ***shortcut*** to ***change*** font size involves holding the Control (Ctrl) key on the keyboard down while simultaneously pressing the "+" (increase) or "−" (decrease) keys.

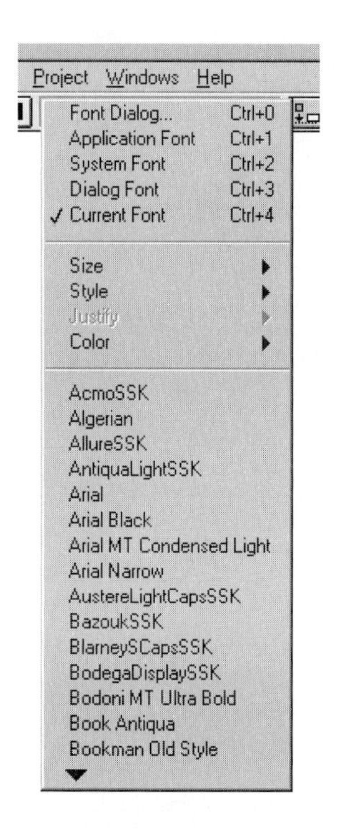

FIGURE 3–2.12
Font style, color, and size may be changed by left-clicking on the **Text Settings** option of the task bar in either the front panel or block diagram and making a choice from the drop-down menu.

LABELS

Labels are used to name and describe front panel objects and identify corresponding icons in the block diagram. The latter function is especially helpful when the block diagram is complicated and has multiple icons. In fact, it's good programming practice to ***label*** front panel objects as soon as they are called up from their menus precisely for this reason.

There are two options for labeling front panel objects. First, as objects are called up from menus and positioned (i.e., when the left mouse button is released), the ***label area*** is ***highlighted*** with white type and a black background, displaying a generic name. For example, after calling up a *Digital Control* from the **Numeric** menu of the **Controls** palette, the label name "Numeric" appears. To change the label, type the desired name, and press the Enter key; note that the label is "stamped" in place, the black background disappears, and the text turns black. Labels may also be typed in ***after*** objects are in place using the *Lettering Tool.* Left-click the cursor onto any part of the label, or swipe across it entirely. This causes the label area to be highlighted again, but this time the background turns white while the text remains black. If the ***click-on*** method was used, use the backspace key to remove some or all of the original characters and retype a name. For the ***swipe across*** method, just begin typing and press the Enter key when finished.

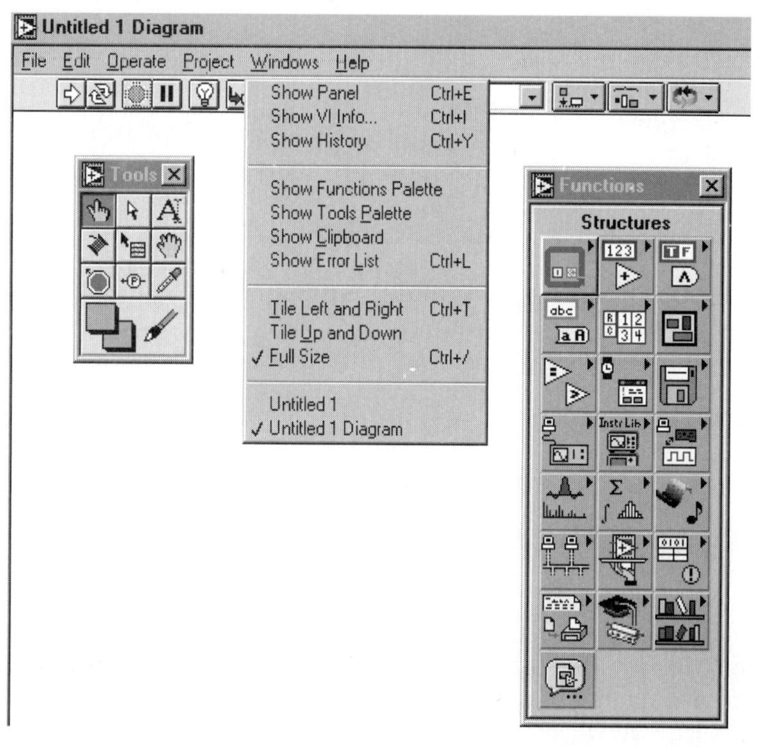

FIGURE 3–3.1
The **Functions** palette is popped up by right-clicking anywhere in the block diagram. By default, the **Tools** palette will appear in the block diagram. Both palettes may be toggled on and off by left-clicking on the **Windows** task bar option and selecting a **Show** option.

THE TOOLS AND FUNCTIONS PALETTES

The **Tools** palette (Figure 3–3.1) described in the previous section is common to both the front panel and block diagram. When the "New VI" button is pushed in the LabVIEW start-up dialog window, the **Tools** palette automatically appears in the front panel. When the user switches to the block diagram, this palette appears in the same relative position, and just as in the front panel, it may be moved to any new location using a ***click-and-drag*** technique with the *Arrow Tool.* This palette is toggled on and off by selecting the **Show Tools Palette** option in the **Windows** drop-down menu from the task bar (Figure 3–3.1).

Just as the **Controls** palette served as the central focus for programming in the front panel, the **Functions** palette (Figure 3–3.1) in the block diagram represents a

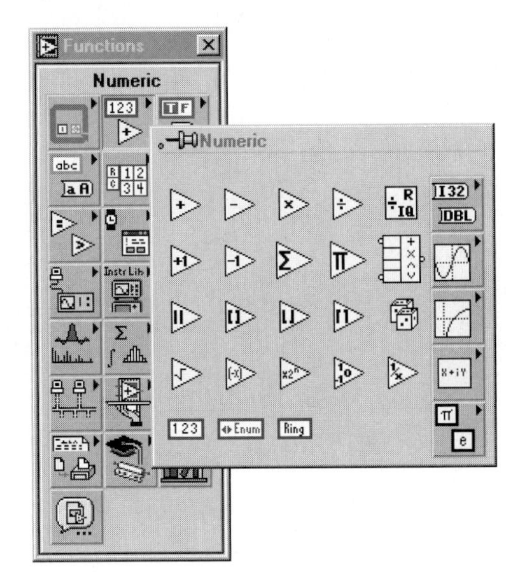

FIGURE 3–3.2
Mathematical functions are selected from the **Numeric** menu of the **Functions** palette in the block diagram.

series of menus and layered submenus from which programming functions and operations may be selected. Functions are chosen the same way as with the **Controls** palette in the front panel. Using the *Arrow Tool,* left-click a menu item on the **Functions** palette, and then navigate through the pop-up submenu(s) to select a function by left-clicking again. In Figure 3–3.2, left-clicking on the **Numeric** menu option in the **Functions** palette causes a layered submenu to appear with common mathematical functions (e.g., add, divide, square root, etc.). Releasing the button causes the menu to disappear and the cursor changes to the *Scroll Window Tool* (open hand) with the outline of the function selected attached. Move the *Scroll Window Tool* to the desired location, and left-click again, stamping the icon in place.

The **Functions** palette includes 22 submenu options that represent an almost unlimited number of programming functions ranging from simple operations to advanced mathematics and signal generation. In succeeding sections, many of these basic functions are explored and described in building simple and more complex VIs.

TERMINAL CONNECTIONS AND WIRING VIS

Block diagram elements are connected together with ***wires*** at ***terminal sites*** on each icon. Wires are the way block diagram functions communicate and establish an orderly flow of information to and from icons. An analogy may be drawn with a printed electronic circuit board. A circuit board contains various electronic components in the form of diodes, capacitors, relays, and so on, that define the board's

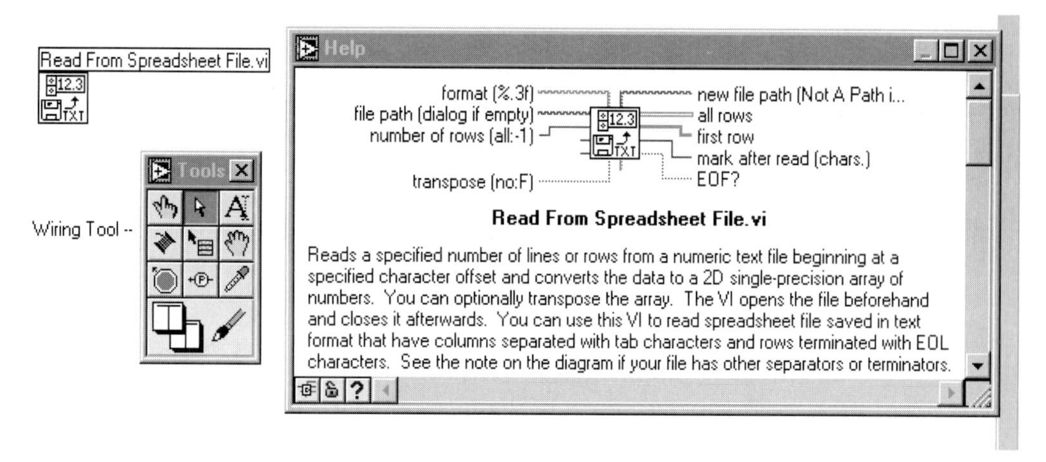

FIGURE 3–3.3
With the **Help** window turned on, touching the *Wiring Tool* to a terminal on the *Read From Spreadsheet File.vi* subVI will cause that terminal to blink in the Help window to help identify its location on the icon.

functional capabilities. Each component is linked to the next with a soldered connection. In a LabVIEW VI, think of the block diagram as a ***circuit board*** with icons being analogous to electronic components. Wires connect icon terminals in the same way that solder connections link electronic components.

Turning on the **Help** window in the task bar and touching the cursor on a block diagram icon will help you to visualize terminal connections, especially when multiple terminals are present. In Figure 3–3.3, the *Read From Spreadsheet File.vi* subVI from the *File I/O* menu of the **Functions** palette has been positioned on the block diagram with the **Help** window turned on. Note that all terminal connections, with their labels, appear and define each terminal's function. When the user selects the *Wiring Tool* cursor from the **Tools** palette and moves it over an icon terminal, each terminal begins to ***blink*** in the **Help** window. It's often a good idea to turn the **Help** window on when wiring icons, especially when multiple terminals are present.

As described in Section 3–5, "Creating SubVIs," a ***left-to-right input/out*** convention for subVI construction is used whenever possible. Terminals on the ***left side*** of a subVI icon are usually ***input*** terminals, and ***right-sided*** connections are ***outputs.*** Note that in Figure 3–3.3, many terminal connections are present and that the top and bottom of the icon have also been used for connection sites.

As noted, terminal wiring is accomplished with the *Wiring Tool*, which looks like a ***spool of wire*** or ***solder.*** The ***tip*** of one end of the wire extends to the left and is used to make the actual connection with icon terminals. To make a connection between two terminals, first locate the tip of the *Wiring Tool* over the icon (turn on

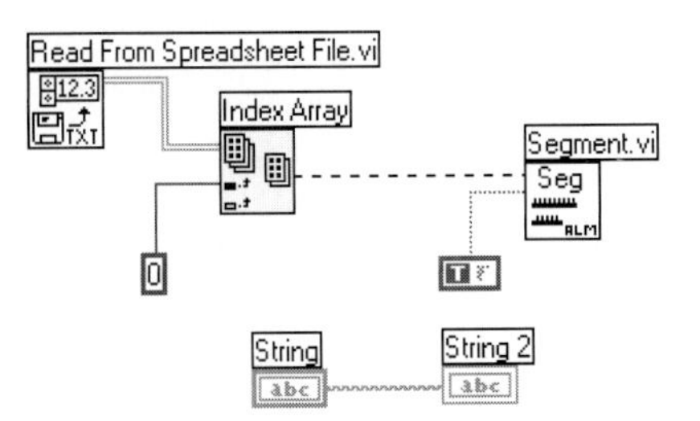

FIGURE 3–3.4
A bad wire (dotted line) is located between the terminals of the *Index Array* function and **Segment.vi** subVI.

the **Help** window to visualize this process). Note that as soon as the cursor touches the icon all associated terminals ***pop out*** from the icon, identifying them as potential wiring sites. Select the terminal of interest, and ***left-click, hold, and drag*** a wire from this terminal to the downstream terminal of another icon to which a connection will be made. Once the *Wiring Tool* is positioned over the next terminal, release the left mouse button, and the connection is completed. The wire just connected takes on the color and wire shape and size (see later) consistent with the terminals' predetermined function. In Figure 3–3.4, the "all rows" ***output terminal*** of the *Read From Spreadsheet File.vi* function has been wired to the "n-dimension array" ***input terminal*** of the *Index Array* function. One **90° turn** (i.e., a change in direction) is automatically provided during wiring. To make a turn, hold the left mouse button down, and turn either to the right or left. Pressing the space bar on the keyboard will have the same effect. To make multiple changes in direction, release the left mouse button, and then immediately push it again as many times as are required, dragging the wire to its downstream connection terminal.

To ***disconnect*** a wire, use the *Arrow Tool,* and left-click and highlight the wire (it will begin to pulsate). Next, either push the Delete (Del) key on the keyboard, or select the **Cut** option from the **Edit** drop-down menu in the task bar at the top of the screen.

If terminal connections are ***incomplete*** during the wiring process or if terminals are ***incompatible*** (e.g., making an output terminal connection with another output terminal), when the left mouse button is released, a ***bad wire*** results and appears as a ***broken dashed line.*** In Figure 3–3.4, a bad wire is seen between the "element or subarray" terminal of *Index Array* and the "Input Array" terminal of the **Segment.vi** subVI. To ***remove*** the bad wire, highlight and delete it as described previously, or select the **Remove Bad Wires** option from the **Edit** drop-down menu. Single or multiple bad wires may be deleted using the latter method.

WIRE COLOR, SHAPE, AND SIZE

In LabVIEW, wire color, shape, and size (cross-section caliber) have specific meanings and uses. Wires that are ***orange*** (or ***blue***), ***green,*** or ***purple*** are associated with functions that deal with or operate on ***numbers, Boolean,*** or ***string functions,***

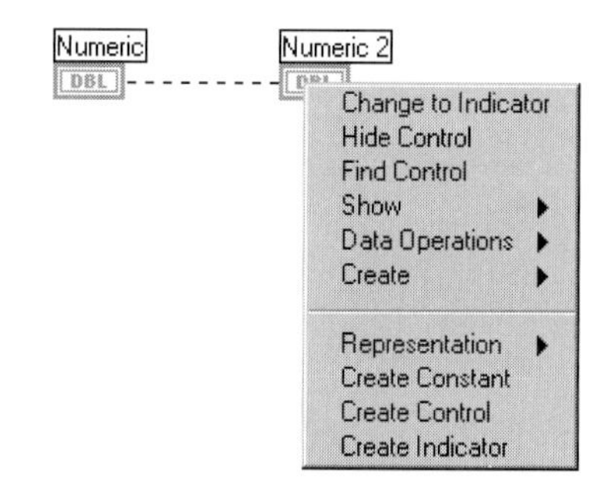

FIGURE 3–3.5
To change a control or indicator into the opposite form, right-click on the object with the *Arrow Tool* and select the **Change** option from the pop-up menu. In this case, a numeric control ("Numeric 2") will be changed to an indicator.

respectively. For numbers, an orange wire represents a ***floating point*** (i.e., multiple decimal point) function, while a ***blue*** wire indicates an ***integer.*** A bad wire will occur if wiring is attempted between mismatched terminals.

Wires that are ***solid*** (orange or blue color) are associated with ***numbers. Dotted green*** wires connect *Boolean* functions, while ***curled purple*** wires are used for ***strings.*** A ***thin*** wire ports a ***scalar*** (single) data signal. ***Intermediate***-thickness wires convey a ***single-dimension (1D) array*** of data, while the ***thickest (double)*** wires are associated with ***2D-array*** functions.

In Figure 3–3.4, an ***orange 2D-array*** wire connects an output terminal of the *Read From File Spreadsheet.vi* function with an input in *Index Array.* The upper indexing terminal (lower left corner) of *Index Array* is wired with a ***thin blue*** wire indicating an ***integer.*** A *Boolean* constant ("True" condition) is wired with a ***thin green*** wire to the "Analyze segment" input terminal of the **Segment.vi** subVI. Finally, an ***intermediate-thickness purple*** wire connects a *String Control* ("String") with a *String Indicator* ("String 2").

ICON SHAPE

Similar to the way that color and size of block diagram icons differentiate various functions and operations, the **shape** of control and indicators icons imparts different functions as well. In Figure 3–3.4, note that the two icons associated with front panel string functions appear ***different.*** The icon to the left is a *String Control* and has a ***thick outer border,*** while the *String Indicator* to the right has a ***thin border.*** *Numeric Controls* and *Indicators* have the same shape border appearance.

A common programming error is to attempt to wire ***mismatched*** functions. For example, attempting to connect ***two controls*** together results in a bad wire due to the functions' incompatibility. In other words, a control (output) only connects with an indicator (input). To ***change*** to the opposite function, right-click on the icon, and from the pop-up menu, select the **Change to Indicator (or Control)** option (Figure 3–3.5). This operation will also work in the front panel.

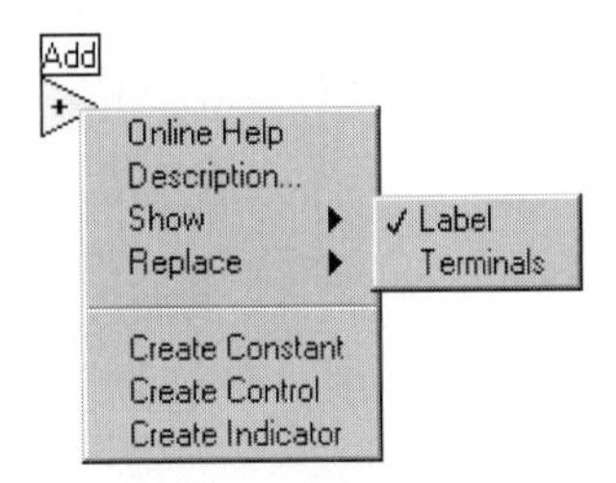

FIGURE 3–3.6
Labels for block diagram objects are toggled on and off by selecting the **Show** option from the pop-up menu.

LABELS

In many cases, block diagram functions have a ***label*** already associated with them. After a function or operation is selected from the **Functions** palette and stamped into position, the user has the option of ***displaying a label*** by right-clicking on the icon and selecting the **Show** and **Label** options from two submenus in the pop-up menu (Figure 3–3.6). When a function does not have an associated label, the user has the option of typing one in when a blank label placeholder pops up.

SUMMARY

The block diagram of a VI represents the place where actual programming occurs, establishing the way information is processed. Icons representing front panel objects and other block diagram programming functions are wired together at icon terminal connector sites to create an orderly flow of information from one function to the next. Many block diagram functions are accessed from the **Functions** palette containing multiple menus and submenus of programming, data acquisition, and signal processing functions.

PRACTICE EXERCISE

To practice basic block diagram layout and wiring techniques, call up the VI named **Block.vi** from the **CD ROM disk directory.** This simple VI uses several mathematical functions to calculate a numerical value. All of the necessary functions have been called up and laid out in their approximate locations necessary to make a calculation. A *Digital Control* (to input a number) labeled "Starting Number" and *Digital Indicator* labeled "Calculated Number" are the only front panel objects. ***None of the functions have been wired.*** After reviewing the overall layout of the block diagram and the information provided above, wire the icons together according to the description below. When finished, call up the VI named **Block2.vi** from the **CD ROM disk directory,** and compare the version of the VI just wired with it. Finally, ***run the VI*** several times from the front panel. Use the following chart to input a number in the *Digital Control* and observe the result in the *Digital Indicator*. Note that the first number ("94.56") has already been inserted into the *Digital Control.*

"STARTING NUMBER"	"CALCULATED NUMBER"
94.56	15.45
78.30	13.78
56.21	11.12
88.88	14.89
11.86	5.19

DESCRIPTION OF THE VI

This VI will **start** with the number input into the "Starting Number" *Digital Control* on the front panel, ***subtract 15*** from it, ***multiply*** that difference by ***3,*** and take the ***square root*** of that quotient. The result will be read in the "Calculated Number" *Digital Indicator* on the front panel.

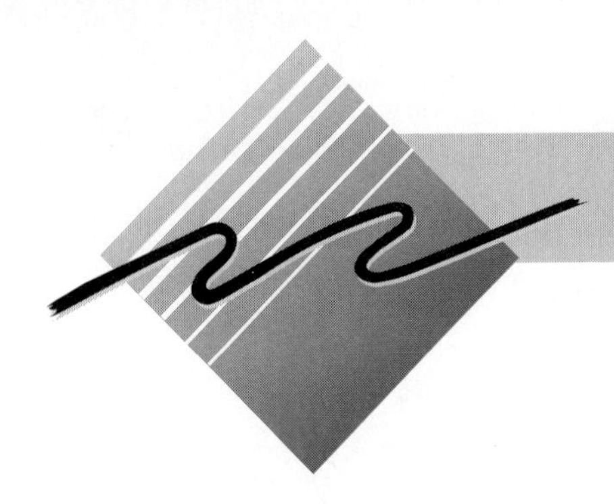

SECTION 3-4

Build and Run Two Simple VIs

Objectives

- Build, run, and save two simple VIs using basic LabVIEW functions.
- Run VIs one time or "on-the-fly."
- Modify basic VI functions.

Introduction

This section provides your first "hands-on" programming experience using LabVIEW. You will build two simple VIs to demonstrate basic front panel and block diagram functions. Before starting, review Sections 3–1 to 3–3 to review programming conventions and the location of **Tools** and **Functions** palettes. Before beginning each VI, it might be helpful to practice popping up palettes and selecting a function from it. Recall there are two ways to access palettes. From the front panel, left-click on the **Windows** option on the task bar. A pull-down menu appears from which is selected the **Show Controls** or **Show Tools** palette options. The same procedure in the block diagram yields the **Show Functions** palette. Palettes pop up on the screen and may be moved around using the *Arrow Tool* or fixed in place while programming. The second method for popping up a palette involves right-clicking anywhere on the screen. The **Controls** palette appears on the front panel, and the **Functions** palette appears on the block diagram. After a palette is accessed, move the *Arrow Tool* over each menu item, and note that a listing of all functions appears. Left-click on the desired function. The palette disappears, and the *Scroll Window Tool* (opened hand) appears with an outlined box (containing the function) attached. Position the cursor wherever the function is needed, and left-click again. The function is placed on the screen ready for use. Note also that after touch-down, an option to label the function is given immediately.

CALCULATE A PERCENTAGE SCORE

The first VI in this chapter is a simple program that calculates a ***percentage score*** based on a total score and the number missed as, for example, when calculating an exam grade (Figure 3–4.1). While programming style will evolve and become more efficient with practice, to get started, it may be a good idea to first locate and then place all VI elements out on the front panel and block diagram ***before*** wiring. Be sure to label each function on the front panel to keep track and identify terminals on the block diagram. Use the **Object/Function or SubVI Locator** tables (e.g., facing Figure 3–4.1) to find each function. Next, using the *Arrow Tool,* place each function in its approximate location. It's good programming etiquette to place ***control functions on the left side*** of the block diagram and ***indicators on the right side.*** This suggests a logical flow of information from ***left to right.*** Layout on the front panel depends more on how the VI will be used. In this case, since there are only three front panel elements, the same ***left-to-right*** (controls-to-indicator) convention has been used. Once the layout has been determined, wire the block diagram terminals using the *Wiring Tool,* as indicated in Figure 3–4.1. Note that on the front panel instructions have been included to orient the user as to how this VI should be used. This is often a good idea, especially if the user is not the programmer. Text may be added using the *Labeling Tool.*

To run the VI, insert a "Total Score" value (e.g., "95") and the "No. Missed" (e.g., "6"), and run the VI by left-clicking on the **Run** arrow on the task bar. In this example, a "Percent" score of 94 is returned in the *Digital Indicator.* This VI may also be run "on-the-fly." Click on the **Continuous Run** arrow, and with the *Hand Tool,* increase or decrease either the "Total Score" or "No. Missed" or both; note that the "Percent Score" is automatically updated. Clicking on the **Stop** button (Abort Execution) turns the VI off. After the VI is functioning properly and the front panel and block diagram have been laid out appropriately, **Save** the VI using a convenient filename and subdirectory. This VI is available in the **CD ROM disk directory** to compare the version of the VI just built to that in Figure 3–4.1.

GENERATE AND PLOT RANDOM NUMBERS

This VI generates a series of ***scaled random numbers*** and displays the current number in a *Digital Indicator* and on a *Waveform Chart* (Figure 3–4.2). The *Random Number* function, by default, provides numbers from 0 to 1. In this example, random

OBJECT/FUNCTION OR SUBVI LOCATOR
PERCENT.VI

Panel	Object/Function or SubVI	Palette/Menu or Directory
Front	*Digital Control* × 2	**Controls/Numeric**
	Digital Indicator	**Controls/Numeric**
Diagram	*Subtract*	**Functions/Numeric**
	Divide	**Functions/Numeric**
	Multiply	**Functions/Numeric**
	Numeric Constant	**Functions/Numeric**

numbers may be ***scaled*** by a ***factor*** of up to "10" using a *Dial.* Note that, when the *Dial* is initially brought up to the front panel, it defaults to a maximum of 10 as a ***double precision*** (i.e., two decimal places) number. Since a scale factor by its nature may be thought of as an integer, the format is changed by left-clicking the center of the *Dial* using the *Arrow Tool* and popping up a menu. Select the **Representation** option, and click on "I32." This sets the scale factor as an ***integer.*** In this example, the *Digital Indicator* labeled "Random No. x Scale Factor" has been similarly configured as an integer. To configure this number as a real number with ***.xx*** units of ***precision,*** bring up the **Representation** menu, and choose the desired configuration.

When the *Waveform Chart* is first displayed on the front panel, it is small. To resize the chart, left-click on any corner with the *Arrow Tool* (note angle bracket), and drag the chart to its desired size. Note also that by default the chart is displayed with a *Legend* (upper right corner). If this option is not needed, right-click anywhere on the chart, and select the **Show** option. Note that ***a check mark*** (✓) lies next to *Legend* and *Palette.* Selecting each checked item will turn it off.

Layout and build this VI using the Object/Function or SubVI Locator. To see how the VI works, click on the **Continuous Run** arrow, and note that scaled random numbers are generated and displayed on the chart and *Digital Indicator* until the **Stop** button is clicked. **Save** the VI using a convenient filename and subdirectory. This VI is available in the **CD ROM disk directory** to compare the version just created with that in Figure 3–4.2.

SUMMARY

To become familiar with basic LabVIEW programming functions, two simple VIs were constructed using commonly used ***controls*** and ***indicators.*** Both VIs can run "on-the-fly," giving the user the best picture as to how these VIs operate. Subsequent sections will build on these basic programming techniques.

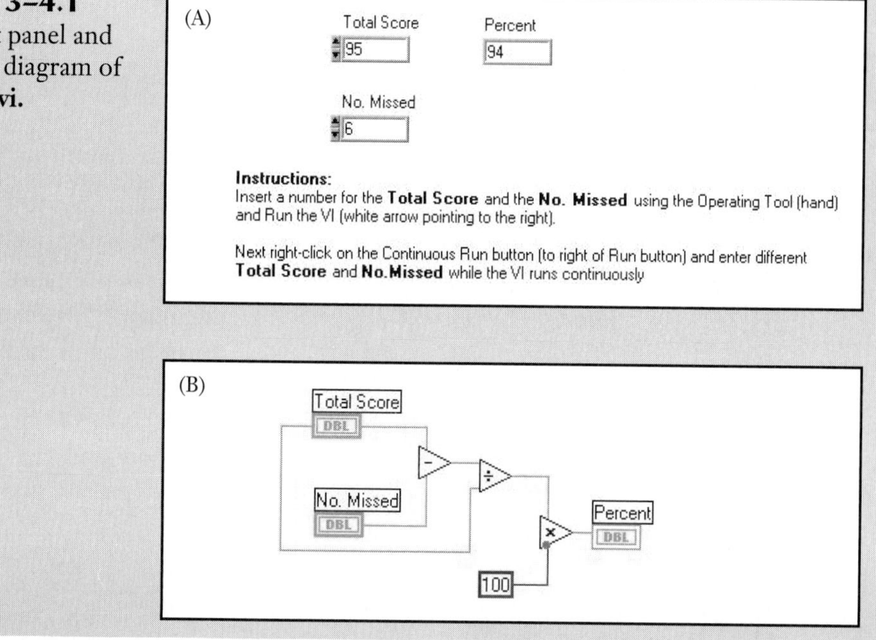

FIGURE 3–4.1
(A) Front panel and (B) block diagram of **Percent.vi.**

PRACTICE EXERCISES

For **Percent.vi,** practice changing the ***numeric format*** and ***decimal precision*** in the controls and indicators on the front panel using the procedure described here. Next, add a front panel *Digital Indictor* to the front panel, and label it "Raw Score." On the block diagram, wire this terminal in the proper location to return the difference between the "Total Score" and the "No. Missed." Open the VI called **Percent2.vi** in the **CD ROM disk directory,** and/or print it out to compare with the VI just modified.

Practice resizing the *Waveform Chart* and adding chart elements (e.g., a *Legend)* in **Random.vi** using the procedures previously described. Next, change the "Scale Factor" to a maximal value of "100" by swiping over, or clicking on, the number "10" on the *Dial* using the *Lettering Tool* and typing in "100." Now, run the VI continuously with the "Scale Factor" set at 90. Note on the *Waveform Chart* that most of the graphed data have disappeared. This is because most of the numbers being generated are now beyond the range of the chart as initially configured. ***Rescale*** the chart by right-clicking anywhere on the chart and selecting the **Y Scale** menu. Select the **AutoScale** option, and note that the chart automatically rescales the Y axis. All data points should now be visible.

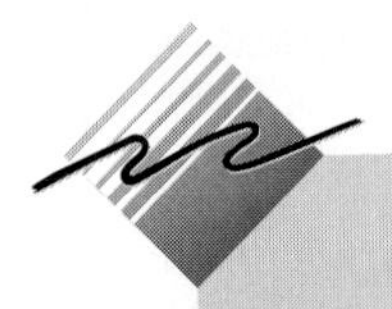

Object/Function or SubVI Locator
Random.vi

Panel	Object/Function or SubVI	Palette/Menu or Directory
Front	*Dial*	**Controls/Numeric**
	Digital Indicator	**Controls/Numeric**
	Waveform Chart	**Controls/Graph**
Diagram	*Random Number (0–1)*	**Functions/Numeric**
	Multiply	**Functions/Numeric**

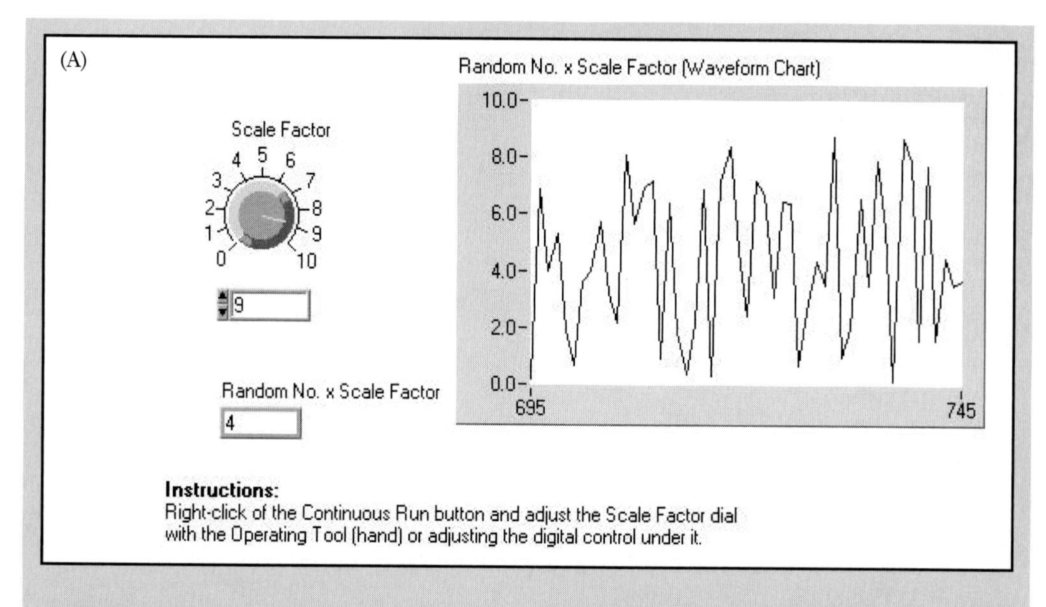

FIGURE 3–4.2
(A) Front panel and (B) block diagram of **Random.vi.**

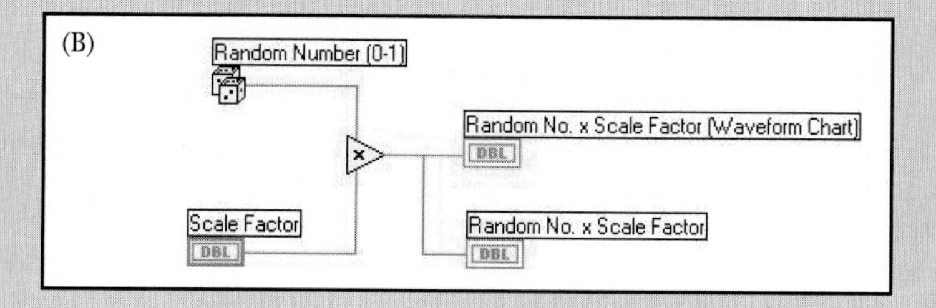

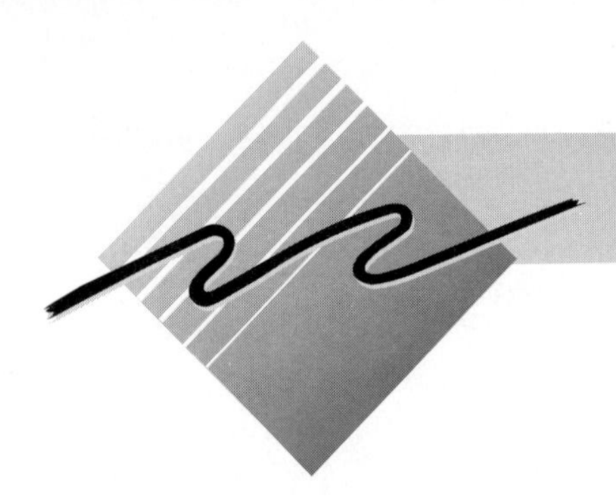

SECTION 3-5

Creating SubVIs

Objectives

- ❖ Understand the use of subVIs as programming subroutines.
- ❖ Write and wire a subVI.
- ❖ Create and edit the subVI face.
- ❖ Save and use a subVI.

What Are SubVIs, and How Are They Useful?

In programming, certain tasks may be used repeatedly. The programmer has two options: write program code each time the task is required, or save chunks of code as a ***subroutine*** and insert it into a program whenever needed. LabVIEW ***subroutines*** are called ***subVIs.*** LabVIEW comes configured with many subVIs, which are found in the **Control** and **Function** palettes in the front panel and block diagram and elsewhere. When unique subVIs are required to meet a programming need, LabVIEW provides the capabilities to create custom subVIs. Once configured, subVIs are available as ***subroutines*** for insertion into subsequent VIs.

Writing and Wiring SubVIs

To demonstrate how subVIs are written and used, a subVI called **Rxscale.vi** (i.e., a random number multiplied by a scale factor) will be constructed. In subsequent activities, the *Random Number* function will be used as a source of sample data to demonstrate LabVIEW programming functions. By default, the *Random Number* generator creates a number from "0 to 1." When larger numbers are required, the programmer must multiply the *Random Number* by a constant or variable ***scale fac-***

tor each time this function is required. Another alternative is to preconfigure the *Random Number* with a ***variable scale factor*** and save this subroutine as a subVI that can then be inserted into a VI whenever larger random numbers are needed.

SubVIs are written in LabVIEW just as any other VI. Figure 3–5.1 demonstrates front panel and block diagram elements needed for this subVI. As an exercise to practice subVI construction, configure each panel as described.

Note that in the upper right-hand corner of the front panel is a ***default icon face*** numbered "1." Right-clicking on the icon causes a menu to pop up with three ***highlighted*** options: ***VI Setup, Edit Icon, and Show Connector.*** Left-click on ***Show Connector,*** and note that the icon face changes and shows two ***wiring terminals*** (i.e., the square face is divided down the middle into two equal-sized boxes). LabVIEW automatically senses how many input and output elements are present on the front panel. In this case, there is one of each: a *Digital Control* (configured as an integer, I32; default = "10") as the ***input*** and a *Digital Indicator* as the ***output.*** If LabVIEW is unsuccessful in recognizing the correct number of inputs or outputs, or if more elements are required later, additional terminals may be added and otherwise manipulated (e.g., rotated, flipped) by going back to the icon face and right-clicking on it again. Also, note that terminals may be wired in any order; however, it's probably a good idea, whenever possible, to treat terminals on the ***left side*** as ***inputs*** and terminals on the ***right*** as ***outputs.*** This may not always be possible with a large number of terminals if the subVI is complex. Choose the *Patterns* menu option to see how many terminal configurations are possible. Since the current example is quite simple and requires only two terminals, the ***left-to-right*** convention described here will be used.

To wire the subVI terminals, use the *Wiring Tool* cursor from the **Tools** palette. Move the cursor to the left terminal on the icon face, and left-click. Note that the terminal turns black or a dark color. Now move the cursor to the *Digital Control* labeled "Scale Factor," and left-click. Note that the control is highlighted and that the right terminal on the icon face has changed color, confirming that this terminal has been wired. Repeat this procedure to wire the right terminal to the *Digital Indicator* labeled "Random No." With both terminals now wired, the subVI has been configured. To rewire the subVI a different way, or if an error was made in connecting terminals, changes are easily made by right-clicking on the icon face and choosing the *Show Connector* option to show the terminal layout plan. Right-click again, and choose *Disconnect All Terminals.* At this point, rewire front panel elements again.

Another method to create subVIs automates the process using the **Create SubVI** option from the **Edit** menu item in the task bar in the block diagram. The *Arrow Tool* is used to surround and "capture" a segment of a VI that is to become a subVI. Invoking the **Create SubVI** option collapses the captured segment into a generic subVI icon, automatically wiring connectors based on LabVIEW's best estimate of the number of inputs and outputs it finds. The subVI face is then ready for editing and saving. See the last Practice Exercise in this section for a more detailed review of automating subVI building.

OBJECT/FUNCTION OR SUBVI LOCATOR
RXSCALE.VI

Panel	Object/Function or SubVI	Palette/Menu or Directory
Front	*Digital Control*	**Controls/Numeric**
	Digital Indicator	**Controls/Numeric**
Diagram	*Random Number (0–1)*	**Functions/Numeric**
	Multiply	**Functions/Numeric**

CREATING AND EDITING THE SUBVI FACE

To give the subVI a unique icon face, right-click and choose *Edit Icon.* The **Icon Editor** (Figure 3–5.2) will open. This is a simple graphics editor used to create an icon face in either black and white or color, working ***pixel by pixel*** with several drawing and lettering tools. Note that by checking the *Show Terminals* box, the user displays the wiring terminals, helping to determine the layout for the icon. In this example, a simple black and white face was chosen with the letters: "RN x SF" (oriented vertically). After editing the face, return to the front panel by clicking the OK button.

SAVING AND USING SUBVIS

With wiring and icon face editing complete, the subVI is ready to be saved. SubVIs are saved just like any other VI into a convenient directory using a unique filename followed by the ***.vi*** extension. Since a library of subVIs is likely to grow quite large with time, it's probably a good idea to create a separate subdirectory to store them so they can be easily retrieved. Note also that, if VIs are moved between different computers that don't have the same menu structure, when a VI is opened for the first time, LabVIEW may prompt for the location of the subVI that's been created. Knowing that all subVIs are stored in the same place will ensure that they are easily found without having to scroll through layers of subdirectories. Subsequently, when the same VI is opened, LabVIEW will "remember" where the subVIs are located.

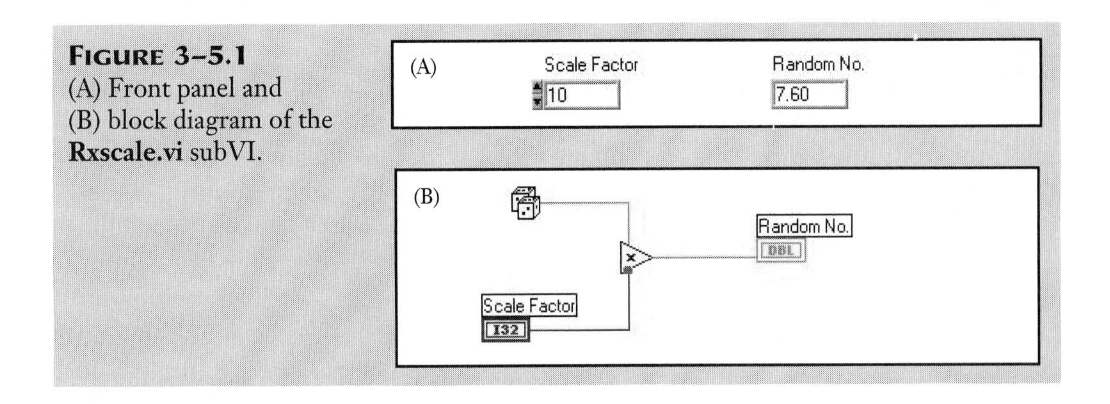

FIGURE 3–5.1
(A) Front panel and (B) block diagram of the **Rxscale.vi** subVI.

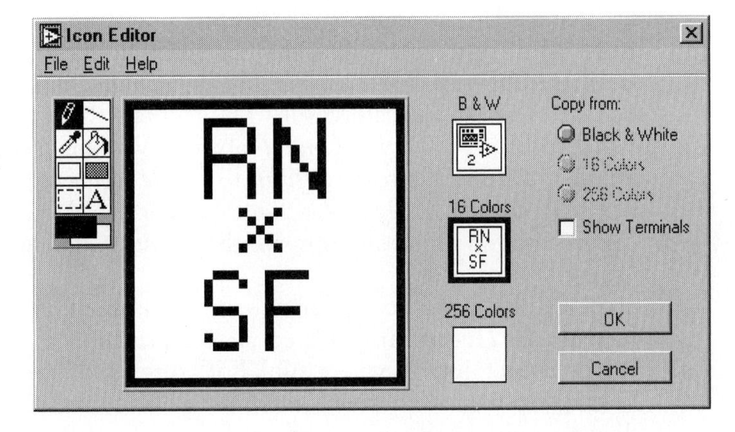

FIGURE 3–5.2
The **Icon Editor** is activated in the front panel by right-clicking on the icon in the upper right corner and selecting the **Edit Icon . . .** option. Editing tools are selected from a menu to the left of the icon.

Using a custom subVI is no different from using subVIs that come preconfigured with LabVIEW. While working in the block diagram, pop up the **Functions** palette, and choose the *Select a VI* . . . option. A dialog window will open to select and open the subVI required. If the subVI is not located in the current directory, scroll through the directories in the usual way until it's found. Highlight the filename, and click on **Open.** The cursor will have "grabbed" the subVI, which may be placed anywhere in block diagram in the usual manner. To wire the subVI, touch the *Wiring Tool* to the approximate site of the terminal being wired, and note that a ***terminal connection*** will pop out from the subVI, indicating its exact location. To "get inside" the subVI, left double-click on the icon face. This opens the front panel of the subVI, and at this point, navigate the front panel or block diagram like any other VI. To exit, click on **File/Close** using the top menu bar. **Save** the subVI in a convenient subdirectory using the **Rxscale.vi** filename. **Rxscale.vi** is also available in the **CD ROM disk directory.**

SUMMARY

SubVIs are ***subroutines*** that are used when repetitive programming functions are required to avoid having to reconstruct the same code over and over again. Once the front panel and block diagram are configured, subVI icons are wired to function terminals. The subVI icon face may be uniquely configured using a simple graphics editor. Once fully set up, the subVI is saved into a convenient subdirectory using a unique filename and is now ready to be inserted into a VI.

PRACTICE EXERCISES

To demonstrate the use of the subVI just constructed, build a VI that will generate ***two*** sets of ***scaled random numbers,*** and display them in two *Digital Indictors* on the front panel. The first set of numbers should be scaled by a factor of "2" and should be generated in the upper part of the block diagram using the *Random Number (0–1)* and *Multiply* functions with a *Numeric Constant* set to "2." Display the random number in the upper part of the front panel in a *Digital Indicator* labeled "Random Number x 2." Use the **Rxscale.vi** subVI to generate the second set of random numbers. Use a front panel *Digital Control* labeled "Variable Control" to scale the random number. Set this control to ***default*** to a ***scale factor*** of "20." Display this number in a *Digital Indicator* labeled "Random Number x ?" When the VI is complete, **Run** in continuous run mode and observe the results. Change the variable *Digital Control* using the *Hand Tool.*

The VI just described may be found in the **CD ROM disk directory.** The filename is: **2Random.vi. Open** and/or print it out, and compare it with the VI just created. Hint: To wire a subVI, it's often useful to turn on the **Help** window. With **Help** turned on, touch the *Wiring Tool* to any part of the subVI. In the window, the subVI will appear with its picture, filename, and terminal layout and descriptors. Touching the *Wiring Tool* to a terminal will cause it to ***blink*** and help specifically identify its location. This is a simple subVI in which terminal identification should not be a problem. In more complex subVIs with multiple terminals, it may be more difficult to differentiate connections.

The second exercise demonstrates an ***automated method*** for creating a subVI. Call up the VI named **Descrip.vi** from the **CD ROM disk directory.** This VI calculates the ***mean*** and ***standard deviation*** for the ***population*** and ***sample*** of an array of data ("X"). The number of array items (i.e., "n") is also calculated. Switch to the block diagram, and note that in the upper part of the diagram LabVIEW functions are used to calculate the mean (*Mean.vi*) and standard deviation (*Standard Deviation.vi*) for the population. In the lower part of the diagram, the ***standard deviation*** for the ***sample*** and the number of array items are calculated using mathematical functions from the **Numeric** palette. In this exercise, this part of the VI is captured and configured as a subVI.

First, break the wire connecting the input array ("X") with the *Mean.vi* and *Standard Deviation.vi* icons. Using the *Arrow Tool,* draw a box around the lower part of the VI including the terminal for the input array ("X"). Release the cursor, and note that the box collapses and highlights all of the surrounded functions. Click on the **Edit** menu item from the task bar, and choose the **Create SubVI** option. This causes most of the enclosed functions to be collapsed into a generic subVI icon. Click on the **Help** window, and confirm that three terminals were automatically configured and wired. On the left side of the icon, a single-input terminal is created, while on the right side, two output terminals are present. Left double-click on the icon to open the subVI front panel. Switch to the block diagram, and confirm that the original functions used to calculate the ***standard deviation*** for the ***sample*** are now captured in the subVI. Switch back to the front panel. At this point, the icon face may be edited using the procedure described previously. Edit the icon face in black and white and using the *Lettering Tool,* and create the following identifier: "SD Sam" (oriented vertically). Close out of the editor, and **Save** the subVI in a convenient subdirectory using the filename **SDsam.vi.** Close out of **Descrip.vi.** When prompted to "Save changes to **Descrip.vi**?" click on **No.** At this point, the subVI is now ready to insert into future VIs. **SDsam.vi** is provided in the **CD ROM disk directory** for comparison with the version just constructed.

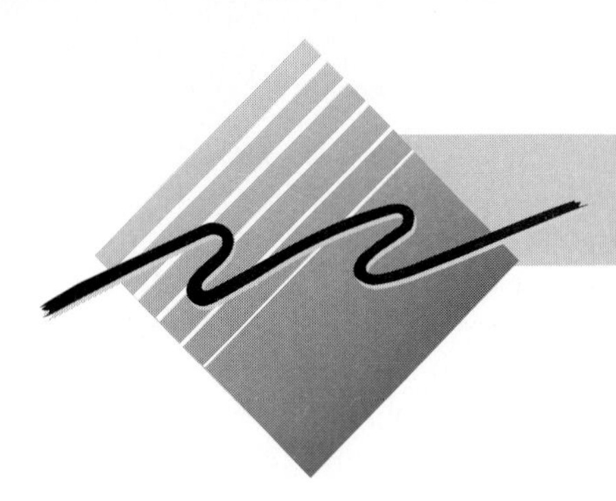

SECTION 3-6

MORE SUBVIS

OBJECTIVES

- ❖ Construct subVIs needed for future programming projects.
- ❖ Practice using a VI with several embedded subVIs.

INTRODUCTION

In Section 3–5, the construction and use of subVIs were introduced using two methods. In subsequent chapters, VIs will be built that require additional subVIs. All the subVIs described next may be found in the **CD ROM disk directory;** however, to understand how each program is written and how it works, I recommend that you build each subVI described in this chapter and save them for future use. After the front panel and block diagram have been laid out and terminals wired, construct an icon face using the subVI editor that uniquely identifies the program to the user. While most subVIs described in this chapter have a specific proprietary function, some may be modified for other programming. Therefore, think of each subVI as a template on which to build other functions.

SAVING SUBVIS

As noted in Section 3–5, "Creating SubVIs," a subVI library is likely to grow rapidly as programming proficiency increases and more applications are generated. It's generally a good idea to save subVIs in a ***separate directory*** labeled **subVIs** or another unique and recognizable name. This will save time when subVIs need to be retrieved by LabVIEW and will avoid the need to scroll through layers of directories and subdirectories.

FIGURE 3–6.1
Block diagram of **Empty.vi.** When a VI is opened and a function cannot be located, a square with a question mark (?) will appear in the block diagram, indicating its position.

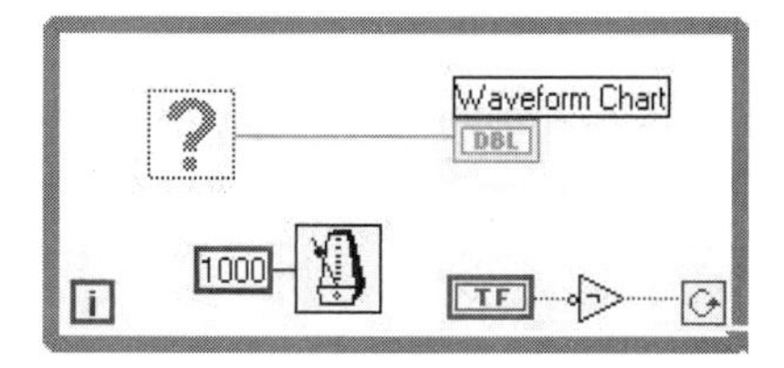

Once each subVI in this section has been constructed and wired, ***save it using the filename specified.*** It's important that ***these filenames*** be used, since later exercises refer to these filenames specifically. If the subVI filename is altered, LabVIEW may have difficulty initially locating the file. If this occurs, a prompt window will open and ask for the subVI location. If the directory or filename is not provided, LabVIEW will retrieve the remainder of the program without the subVI, putting in its place a ***white box with a question mark*** (Figure 3–6.1) in the block diagram. Note also that the **Run** arrow will be ***broken,*** indicating that the VI has an error. To make the VI operational, go into the block diagram, right-click on the subVI placeholder, and select the *Replace* option. Once you have located the subVI, it is inserted into the VI, replacing the question mark. The **Run** arrow reverts to its normal appearance and permits the VI to be executed.

DISVOLTS.VI

Disvolts.vi is used to ***display voltages*** in one of three formats: ***volts, millivolts (mV),*** or ***microvolts (μV)*** (Figure 3–6.2). Physiological signals (e.g., the normal electrical discharge from muscle, as measured by electromyography [EMG]), are by their nature very small. In some ways, LabVIEW may be thought of as a sophisticated ***voltmeter.*** LabVIEW initially reports its data in ***volts.*** In some cases, it may be more useful to display voltages in terms of the magnitudes that are ordinarily encountered.

The heart of this subVI is a *Numeric Case Structure* that's controlled by a three-position *Dial* (configured as an I32 integer) on the front panel that permits switching between three cases (i.e., volts, millivolts, or microvolts). The default setting for the *Dial* is "1" (mV). In the block diagram, for *Case 0,* the voltage is input from an *Input Array* ***unprocessed*** and passed to the *Output Array* in its original form (i.e., volts). *Cases 1* and *2* permit the input voltage to be displayed as millivolts or microvolts, respectively. Note that the subVI has three wiring terminals: two ***input*** terminals (right side) for the *Input Array* and *Dial* and one ***output*** terminal (left) for the *Output Array.* Build and **Save** this subVI into the **subVI directory** using the filename **Disvolts.vi.**

SEGMENT.VI

At times, rather than displaying an entire signal, just a ***segment*** of the signal is required for analysis. Several of the VIs that will be built later will incorporate a ***segment analyzer*** that allows the user to identify the ***start*** and ***ending*** points of the segment to be analyzed. When the VI is rerun, only that part of the signal specified is displayed. For example, Figure 3–6.3 is the front panel of a VI that measures ***torque production*** in an isokinetic dynamometer, in this case, during an isometric contraction. Note that the ***segment analyzer*** ("Analyze segment?") has been turned "ON" by pressing the button. Below the button are two *Digital Controls* into which have been written the "Start" (992) and "End" (2791) point of the segment to be analyzed. The length of the entire data signal is originally "8000 msec." When the VI is rerun with the ***segment analyzer*** turned "ON," a "1799 msec" (i.e., 2791–992) portion of the torque signal is displayed on the two *Waveform Graphs.*

OBJECT/FUNCTION OR SUBVI LOCATOR
DISVOLTS.VI

Panel	Object/Function or SubVI	Palette/Menu or Directory
Front	*Array + Digital Control*	**Controls/Array & Cluster; Numeric**
	Array + Digital Indicator	**Controls/Array & Cluster; Numeric**
	Dial	**Controls/Numeric**
Diagram	*Case Structure*	**Functions/Structures**
	Numeric Constant × 2	**Functions/Numeric**
	Divide × 2	**Functions/Numeric**

Segment.vi (Figure 3–6.4) serves as the ***segment analyzer*** in the current example and will be used in other VIs. This subVI is a *Boolean*-controlled *Case Structure* toggled by a front panel button. In the ***true*** case (i.e., button pressed "ON"), the analyzer uses two *Split 1D Array* functions to partition out a segment of the signal. The ***entire*** data signal is input to the *Case Structure* from an *Input Array,* while a ***segment*** of the signal is fed to an *Output Array.* Two *Digital Controls* are used to establish the beginning ("Start of Read") and ending ("End of Read") points of the segment. Pressing the button to the "OFF" (default) position toggles the *Case Structure* to the ***false*** case, sending the ***entire*** signal to the *Output Array* ***unprocessed.*** Build and **Save** this SubVI into the **subVI directory** using the filename **Segment.vi.**

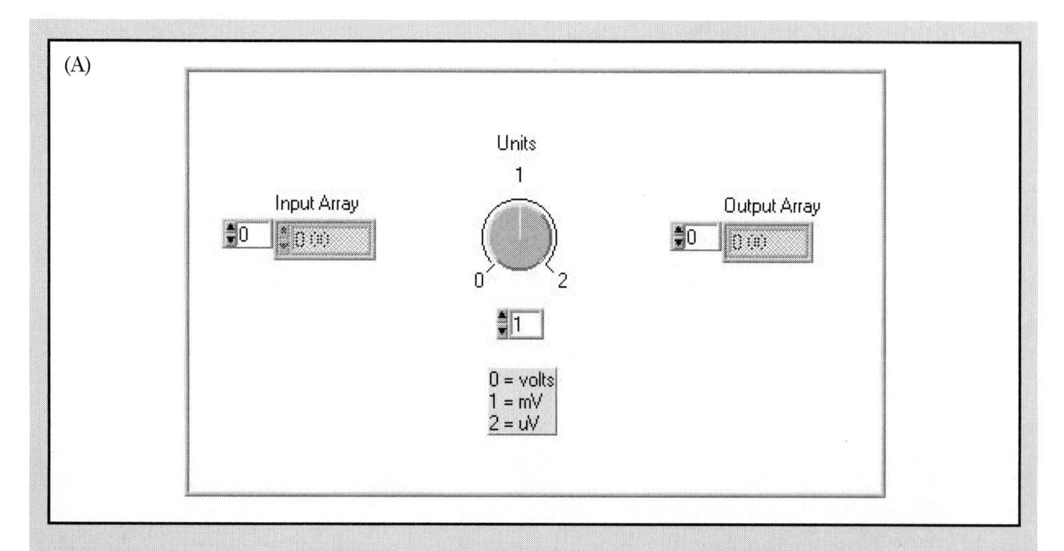

FIGURE 3–6.2
(A) Front panel and (B) block diagram of **Disvolts.vi.** This subVI converts an input voltage to millivolts or microvolts using a numeric *Case Structure*.

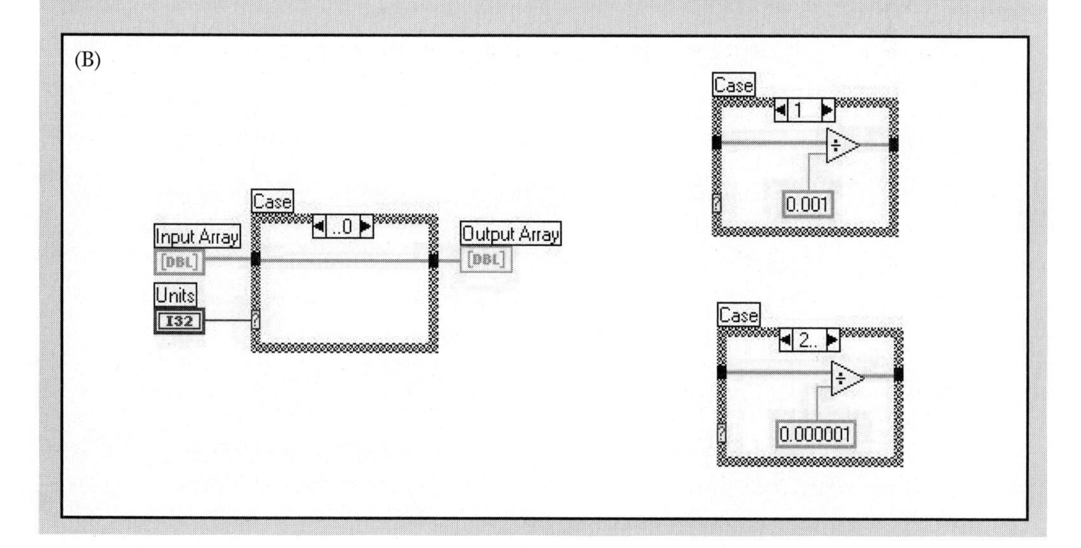

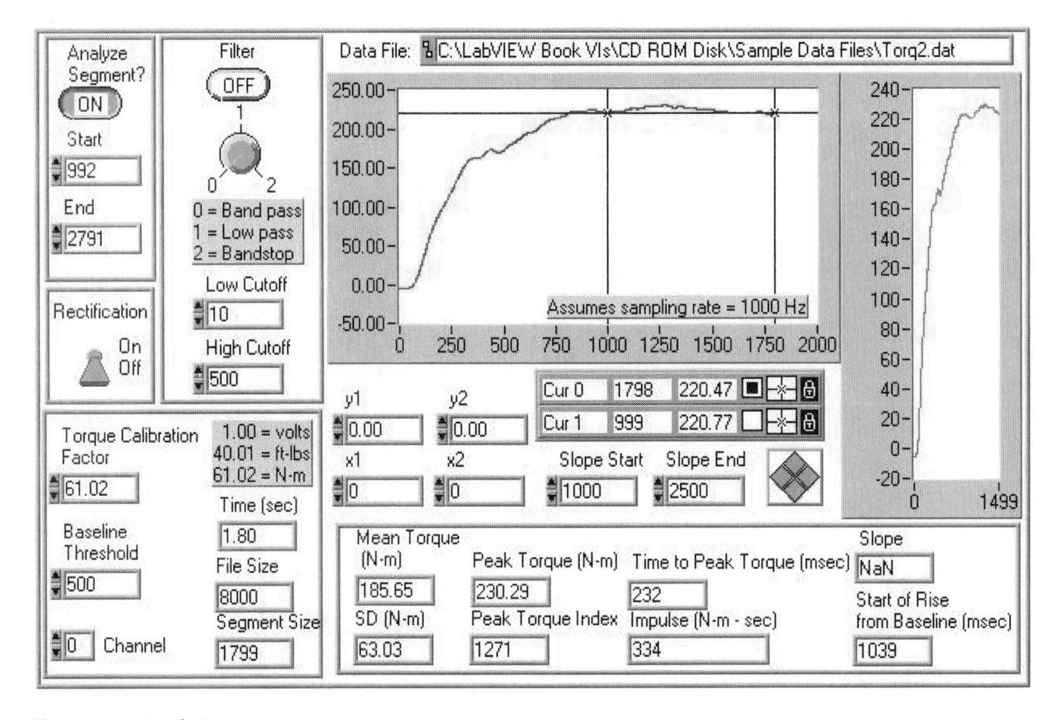

FIGURE 3–6.3
Front panel of **Torque.vi.**

OBJECT/FUNCTION OR SUBVI LOCATOR
SEGMENT.VI

Panel	Object/Function or SubVI	Palette/Menu or Directory
Front	*Array + Digital Control*	**Controls/Array & Cluster; Numeric**
	Array + Digital Indicator	**Controls/Array & Cluster; Numeric**
	Boolean Labeled Oblong Button	**Controls/Boolean**
	Digital Control × 2	**Controls/Numeric**
Diagram	*Case Structure*	**Functions/Structures**
	Split ID Array	**Functions/Array**
	Subtract	**Functions/Numeric**

INTEGRL2.VI

Integration involves the measure of the ***area under a curve*** of graphed data points. Typically, a segment of a curve is selected and subjected to one of several integration algorithms.

Integrl2.vi (Figure 3–6.5) packages LabVIEW's *Integral x(t).vi*—found in the block diagram in the **Functions/Signal Processing/Time Domain** palette—with several *Digital Controls*. The signal is input through an *Input Array* and ported to an *Output Array*. Two *Digital Controls* on the front panel are used to identify the ***start*** ("Initial condition") and ***ending*** ("Final condition") points of the segment to be integrated. A third *Digital Control* specifies the sampling rate ("Sample frequency") set to a default value of 1000. In the block diagram, in the lower left corner of *Integral x(t).vi* is a terminal labeled "dt," which monitors the "sampling interval." In this case, ***one sample will be processed per iteration cycle,*** so the *Reciprocal* function (i.e., 1/1000) is used. An error code is ported to a *Digital Indicator* on the front panel. Build and **Save** this SubVI into the **subVI directory** using the filename **Integrl2.vi.**

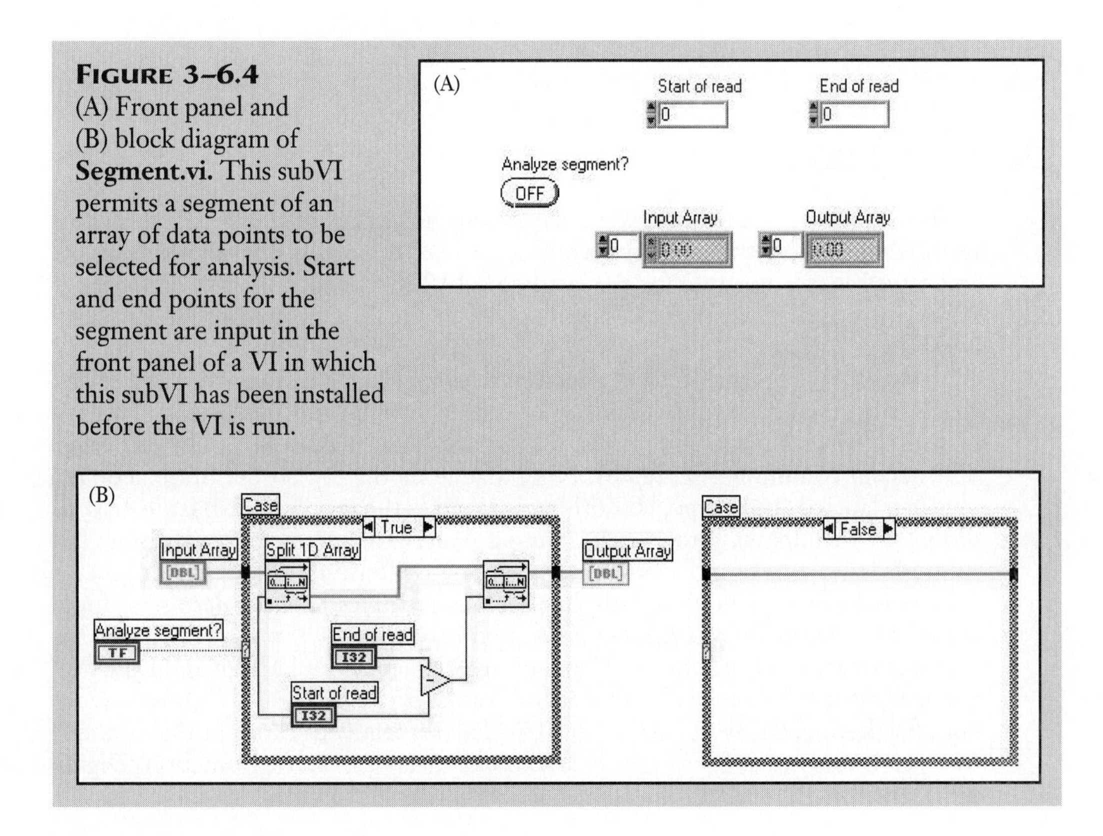

FIGURE 3–6.4
(A) Front panel and (B) block diagram of **Segment.vi.** This subVI permits a segment of an array of data points to be selected for analysis. Start and end points for the segment are input in the front panel of a VI in which this subVI has been installed before the VI is run.

OBJECT/FUNCTION OR SUBVI LOCATOR
INTEGR12.VI

Panel	Object/Function or SubVI	Palette/Menu or Directory
Front	*Array + Digital Control*	Controls/Array & Cluster; Numeric
	Array + Digital Indicator	Controls/Array & Cluster; Numeric
	Digital Control × 3	Controls/Numeric
	Digital Indicator	Controls/Numeric
Diagram	*Integral x(t).vi*	Functions/Signal Processing/Time Domain
	Reciprocal	Functions/Numeric

DIGITAL FILTERS

Filtering smoothes a data curve of extraneous noise (e.g., signal artifact). A Butterworth digital (software) filter is commonly used to process physiological signals and serves as the substrate for the last two subVI in this section. The *Butterworth Filter.vi* is accessed from the block diagram in the **Functions/Signal Processing/Filters** palette.

Bpass.vi (Figure 3–6.6) is a ***bandpass filter*** (i.e., filters above and below a specified frequency range). This subVI centers around the *Butterworth Filter.vi*, providing several filtering options: ***lowpass, highpass, bandpass,*** and ***bandstop.*** The default condition is ***bandpass.*** Note that along the top border of the icon is a terminal labeled "filter type." If nothing is wired to the terminal, it defaults to condition "2" (bandpass). Otherwise, wiring a *Numeric Constant* with a value of "0" through "3" to this terminal will specify alternate filter types (see number scheme below on the front panel). As with the previous examples, the ***raw data set*** is input via an *Input Array*, and the ***filtered data*** are ported to an *Output Array*. Three *Digital Controls* are used to define the "Sampling Frequency" and "High and Low Frequency Cutoffs," respectively. The default values for "Low" and "High Frequency Cutoffs" have been set at "20" and "500 Hz," respectively. Note in this example that ***two*** Butterworth filters are separated by a *Reverse 1D Array* function. Digital

FIGURE 3–6.5
(A) Front panel and (B) block diagram of **Integrl2.vi.** This subVI computes the integral of an array of data points.

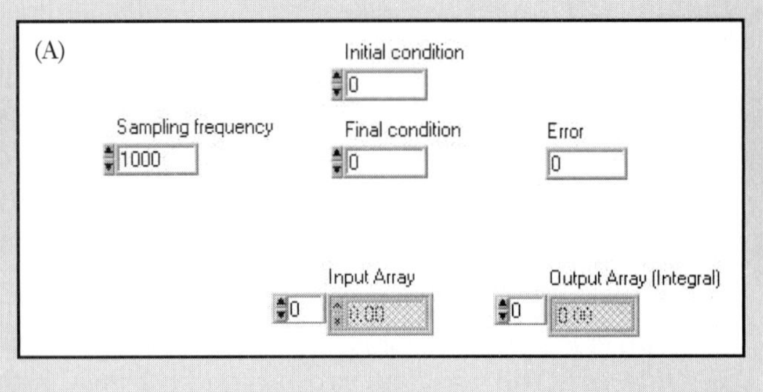

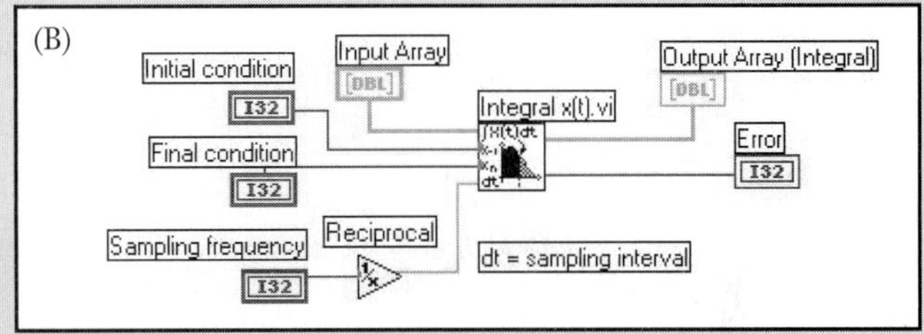

filtering causes a ***phase shift*** (a constant error) and may be corrected by ***reversing polarity*** of the signal using the *Reverse 1D Array* function and passing it through the filter again.

Filters.vi (Figure 3–6.7) gives the user three filtering options: "Bandpass" (default), with "Low" and "High Cutoffs" of "10" and "500 Hz," respectively; "Lowpass"; and "Bandstop." "On/Off" control is provided by a *Boolean Case Structure* toggled by a *Boolean Labeled Oblong Button.* The default case is "Off" (i.e., ***false*** condition). Selection of filter type is handled by a *Numeric Case Structure* with the three cases selected by using a *Dial* on the front panel. Position "0" provides a "Lowpass," "2" provides a "Bandpass," and "3" provides a "Bandstop" filter. In this subVI, the ***sampling frequency*** is fixed at 1000 Hz. A *Digital Control* or other control device could be wired into this terminal and displayed on the front panel to provide variable control of the sampling frequency. Note that this subVI does not correct for the ***phase shift*** problem described in the previous example. Build and save these last two subVIs into the **subVI subdirectory** using the filenames **Bpass.vi and Filters.vi.**

It is a good idea to ***resave*** the subVI called **Rxscale.vi** and **SDsam.vi,** described in Section 3–5, "Creating SubVIs," into the **subVI directory,** as these also will be used in subsequent VIs.

SUMMARY

Several subVIs used in succeeding chapters were described, built, and saved to a **subVI directory.** Locating subVIs in a separate directory makes retrieval easier, especially as the library of subVIs grows.

PRACTICE EXERCISES

To understand how some of the subVIs described previously work, call up the file named **Filtered.vi** from the **CD ROM disk directory.** This VI displays a ***raw*** and ***filtered*** EMG signal on two *Waveform Graphs.* Either a "Bandpass" or "Lowpass"

OBJECT/FUNCTION OR SUBVI LOCATOR
BPASS.VI

Panel	Object/Function or SubVI	Palette/Menu or Directory
Front	*Array + Digital Control*	**Controls/Array & Cluster; Numeric**
	Array + Digital Indicator	**Controls/Array & Cluster; Numeric**
	Digital Control × 4	**Controls/Numeric**
	Digital Indicator	**Controls/Numeric**
Diagram	*Butterworth Filter.vi* × 2	**Functions/Signal Processing/Filters**
	Reverse ID Array × 2	**Functions/Array**
	Numeric Constant	**Functions/Numeric**

filter is activated by toggling the switch on the front panel to the "ON" position. If the switch is left "OFF," the signals displayed will be the same for each graph. "Low" and "High Cutoffs" are preset at "10" and "500 Hz," respectively, and the "Filter Type" defaults to a "Bandpass" filter. To switch to a "Lowpass" filter, set the "Filter Type" to "1" using the *Hand Tool.*

Move to the block diagram, and note that two subVIs described previously were used to build this VI. **Disvolts.vi** allows the signal to be displayed as ***volts, millivolts,*** or ***microvolts.*** A front panel *Digital Control* is used to select a format. **Filters.vi** permits selecting the type of filtering protocol needed. When the **Run** ar-

FIGURE 3–6.6
(A) Front panel and (B) block diagram of **Bpass.vi.** This subVI is a digital bandpass filter with default low- and high-frequency cutoffs of 20 and 500 Hz, respectively. While the default condition is a bandpass filter, lowpass, highpass, and bandstop options are also available.

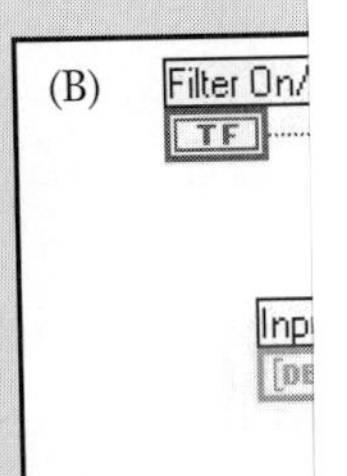

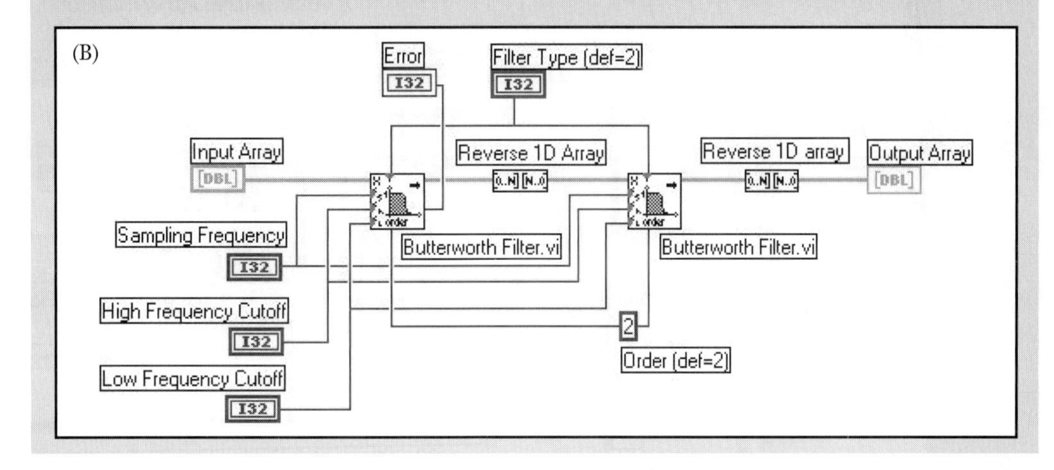

row is pressed, the *Read From Spread File.vi* prompts for a ***data filename.*** When the file is highlighted and the **Open** button is pressed, the *Index Array* function chooses the data channel to display and ports the signal to **Disvolts.vi** and then onto the *Waveform Graphs*, displaying the ***raw*** and ***filtered*** signals.

To become familiar with this VI, practice running it using various combinations of front panel controls. Run the VI, and when prompted, select the data file named **EMGx14.dat** from the **Sample Data File directory** in the **CD ROM disk directory.** This is a single channel of EMG data saved at a ***sampling rate of 1000 Hz*** during an ***isometric contraction*** of the ***biceps brachii*** for ***4 seconds.***

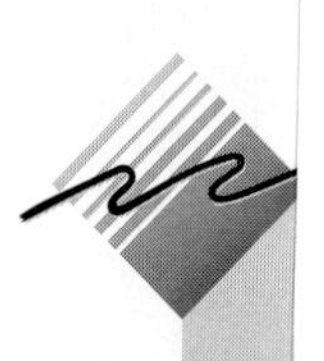

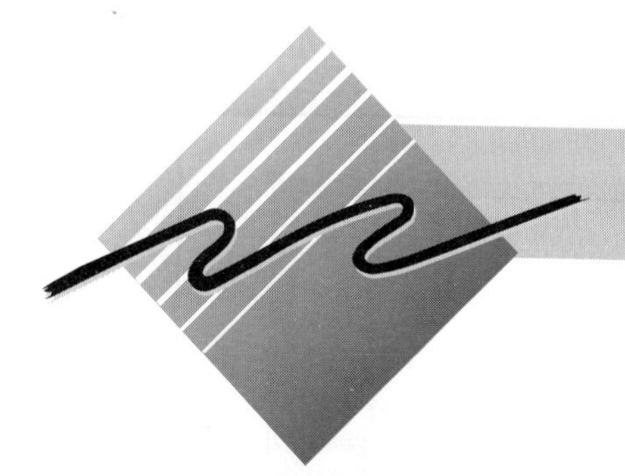

SECTION 3-7

Loops and Structures

Objectives

- ❖ Construct and use a *For Loop.*
- ❖ Construct and use a *While Loop* with *Shift Registers.*
- ❖ Construct and use a *Case Structure* with Boolean and numerical operators.
- ❖ Construct and use a *Sequence Structure* using *Sequence Locals.*

Introduction

Loops and *Structures* are accessed from the block diagram in the **Functions** palette by left-clicking on the **Structures** menu item (Figure 3–7.1). *For Loops* are used to control how many times a VI or subVI will operate. *While Loops* provide ***on/off*** capabilities for VIs. After clicking on the desired function, place the cursor in the approximate location on the block diagram. Note that the cursor changes to a square. Left-click the mouse, and then drag the function to its desired size. To place the loop in its final position, left-click anywhere on its border. Note that a dotted line appears around the loop, highlighting it. Using the *Arrow Tool,* left-click the highlighted loop or structure, and drag it to its desired location. The loop may be resized by left-clicking on any corner of the highlighted loop. The cursor changes to an angle bracket that may be dragged in any direction to resize the loop.

For Loops

For Loops repeat an enclosed VI or subVI a predetermined number of cycles (i.e., iterations). The "**N**" (blue color) in the upper left corner is the "Count Terminal," which is wired with a *Numeric Constant* on the block diagram or a front panel control device (Figure 3–7.1). The *For Loop* repeats the number of cycles specified by the constant or control. The "i" (blue color) in the lower left corner is the "Iteration Terminal" that indicates the number of times (i.e., iterations) the loop has cycled. By default, the first iteration is numbered zero (0).

Shift Registers

Shift Registers are used to transfer a variable of the current iteration of a looping structure to the next iteration. *Shift Registers* may be used with both *While* or *For Loops* and are accessed from the block diagram by placing the cursor on any part of the loop and right-clicking and choosing the *Shift Register* menu option. Note that two terminals pop up: one on the ***right*** (arrow up) and one on the ***left*** (arrow down). New values enter the loop from the right terminal and are then transferred and stored in the left terminal. The left terminal essentially ***remembers*** the previous value after a new value has been entered at the right terminal. If it is necessary to recall past iterations from more than one cycle, ***additional elements*** (i.e., left terminals) may be added by placing the cursor on the left terminal and right-clicking and choosing ***Add Element*** from the pop-up menu.

While Loops

While Loops are located and sized or resized in the same way *For Loops* are handled. On/off control is afforded by the *While Loop* to any enclosed VI or subVI by wiring a *Boolean* control variable (e.g., an "On/Off" switch or button) on the front panel to the *Boolean Condition Terminal* (i.e., incomplete circle with an arrow) in the lower right corner of the loop (see Figure 3–7.1). *Boolean* control variables default to the ***false*** (i.e., off) condition when accessed from the **Controls** palette on the front panel. Thus, flipping a switch or pushing a button reverts to a **true** (i.e., on) condition. When the VI is run, it continues to cycle until the control is turned off (i.e., false condition satisfied). The default condition for *Boolean* controls may be changed by right-clicking on the front panel switch or button and making a choice from a *Mechanical Action* menu item. An "Iteration Terminal" just like the one described for *For Loops* is also provided.

Time Control and While Loops

The rate at which a *While Loop* operates may be controlled by including the *Wait Until Next ms Multiple* function from the **Time & Dialog** menu in the **Functions** palette. Either a *Numeric Constant* in the block diagram or a *Numeric Control* from the **Controls** palette in the front panel may be wired to a terminal on the left side of the *Until Next ms Multiple* function. For example, setting the constant or control to "1000" will cause the VI, when run, to cycle once every second (i.e., 1000 msec). Changing the value to "500" will change the cycle time to once every half of a second, etc.

CASE STRUCTURES

Case Structures are found in the **Functions/Structures** palette in the block diagram (see Figure 3–7.1). *Case Structures* are essentially equivalent to "If/then . . . else" statements and may be accessed using *Boolean* or *Numeric* variables. The default condition is a ***false*** *Boolean Case Structure.* Note the word "False" on the top of the structure. Left-click on the arrows to either side of this label, and note that it changes to "True." On the left side is a terminal appearing as a question mark (?). *Boolean* or *Numeric* variables are wired into the structure here (i.e., at the question mark, which toggles the structure between cases (see Figure 3–7.1). Inside the structure under either the "True" or "False" heading is a function, code, formula

OBJECT/FUNCTION OR SUBVI LOCATOR
FORLOOP.VI

Panel	Object/Function or SubVI	Palette/Menu or Directory
Front	*Array* × 3+ *Digital Control* × 3	**Controls/Array & Cluster; Numeric**
	Digital Indicator × 7	**Controls/Numeric**
	Waveform Graph	**Controls/Graph**
Diagram	*For Loop* × 2	**Functions/Structures**
	Array Size	**Functions/Array**
	Numeric Constant	**Functions/Numeric**
	Multiply	**Functions/Numeric**
	Add	**Functions/Numeric**
	Mean.vi	**Functions/Mathematics/ Probability and Statistics**
	SDsam.vi	**CD ROM/SubVIs**

(node), or special VI. When a condition is ***true,*** anything located inside the structure is activated. When the condition is ***false,*** an opposite or neutral condition is satisfied. If a *Numeric* (vs. a *Boolean)* variable is wired to the structure terminal, the structure will change from a **true/false** conditional structure to a ***numerical*** structure starting with zero (0). Clicking on the arrows to either side of the number advances to the next case (i.e., 1, 2, 3, etc.) To add additional conditions, left-click the cursor on the side of the *Case Structure,* and choose *Add Case.*

Sequence Structures

Sequence Structures—accessed from the **Functions/Structures** palette in the block diagram—are used to run program elements in serial order (see Figure 3–7.1). An analogy might be to frames of a videotape where each part of a VI in the ***first frame*** is executed before the next, etc. *Sequence Structures* are drawn out and sized as you

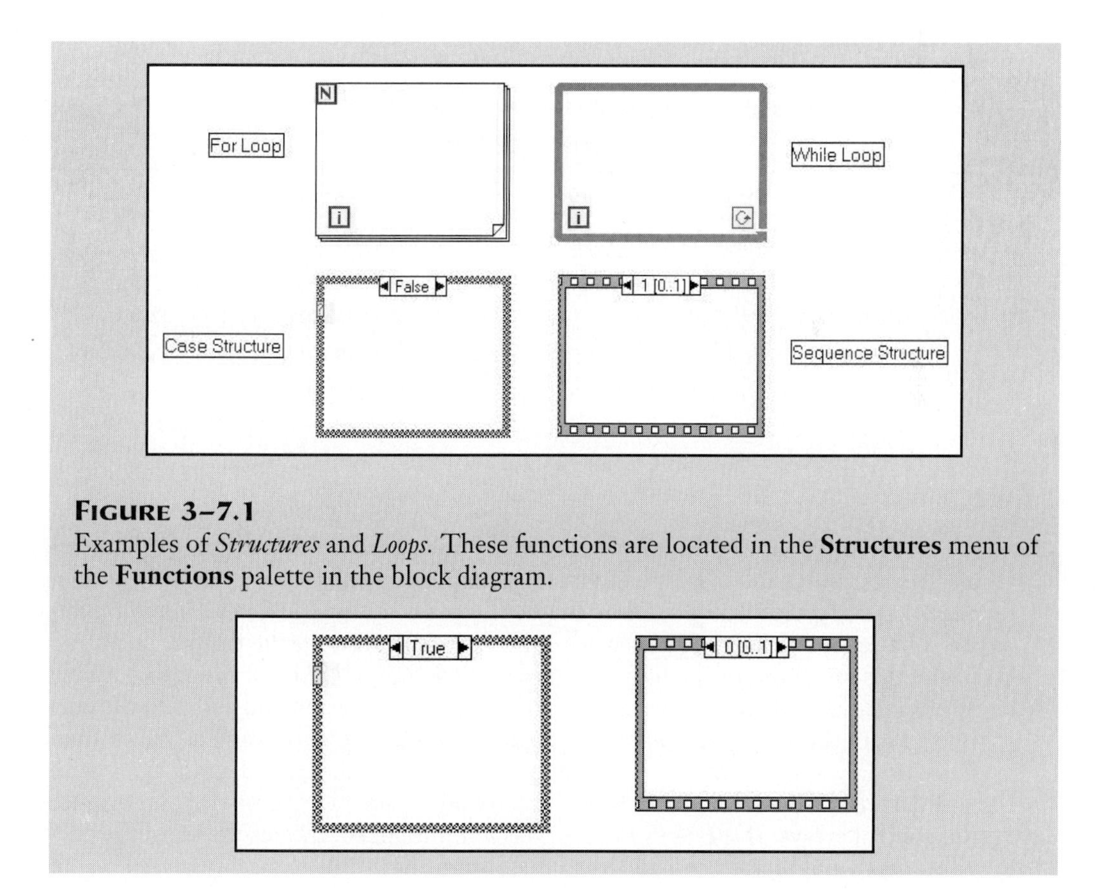

Figure 3–7.1
Examples of *Structures* and *Loops.* These functions are located in the **Structures** menu of the **Functions** palette in the block diagram.

would a *For* or *While Loop.* The first frame is numbered zero (0). To ***add*** additional frames, place the cursor on the border of the structure, pop up a menu using the right mouse button, and choose the *Add Frame After* option. *Sequence Locals* are variables that allow data/information to be passed on from one frame to the next. They are accessed in the same way as adding an additional frame or a *Shift Register.*

SAMPLE VIs

Figure 3–7.2 (**Forloop.vi**) demonstrates the use of *For Loops.* In this VI, two control arrays of numerical data are input by the user in the front panel. When the VI is run, a *For Loop* is used to add first, second, third, and so on, cells of each array together (see block diagram). After the array data are tabulated, the results are passed out of the *For Loop* through a ***tunnel*** and displayed in a third *Indicator Array* on the front panel. In addition, the ***mean*** and ***standard deviation*** for the ***sample*** are calculated and displayed in front panel *Digital Indicators.* The total number of iterations (cycles) completed by the *For Loop* is also displayed in a *Digital Indicator.* The second (lower) *For Loop* adds the five cell values of the output array and passes this result out of the loop to a front panel *Digital Indicator.* Note that a *Shift Register* was used to take the value from the previous iteration and add it to the current cell. In this case, the *Shift Register* was ***initialized*** to ***zero*** using a *Digital Constant.* Initialization ***resets*** the *For Loop* to zero, so that when the VI is run again with new data, the VI will calculate results based only on the new numbers inserted into the control arrays. If the *Shift Register* was ***not*** initialized, the results from the previous data would have been added to the current data.

OBJECT/FUNCTION OR SUBVI LOCATOR
SHIFTREG.VI

Panel	Object/Function or SubVI	Palette/Menu or Directory
Front	*Rectangular Stop Button*	**Controls/Boolean**
	Digital Indicator × 4	**Controls/Numeric**
Diagram	*While Loop*	**Functions/Structures**
	Wait Until Next ms Multiple	**Functions/Time & Dialog**
	Numeric Constant	**Functions/Numeric**
	Not	**Functions/Boolean**

Shiftreg.vi (Figure 3–7.3) demonstrates the use of multiple *Shift Registers* inserted into a *While Loop*. When this VI is run, the value of the first iteration of the *While Loop* (default = zero) is displayed in a front panel *Digital Indicator*. The numbers 1, 2, and 3 are then subtracted from the first iteration value and displayed. As

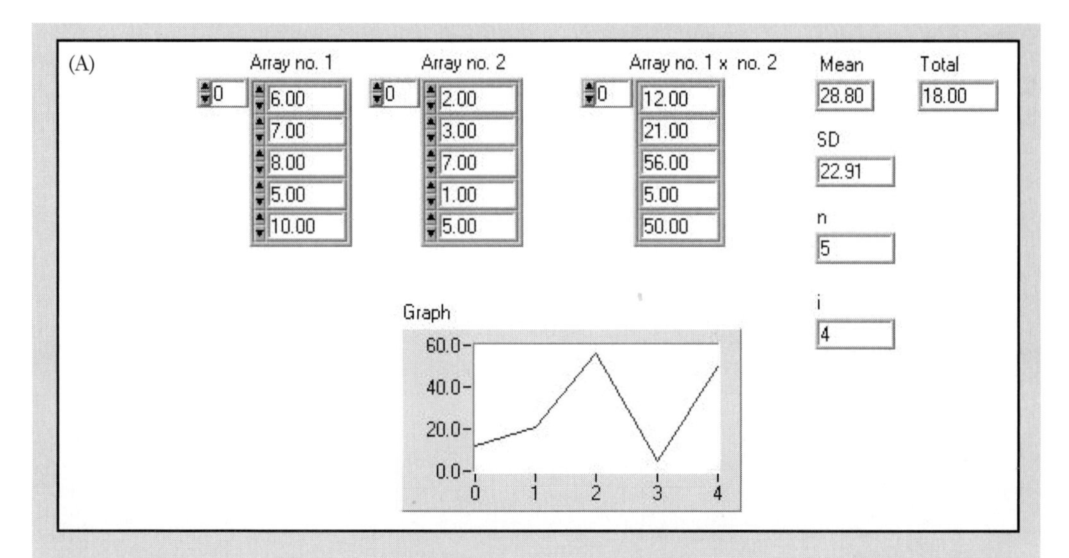

FIGURE 3–7.2
(A) Front panel and (B) block diagram of **Forloop.vi.** This VI demonstrates the use of *For Loops* in the block diagram to process two numeric data arrays.

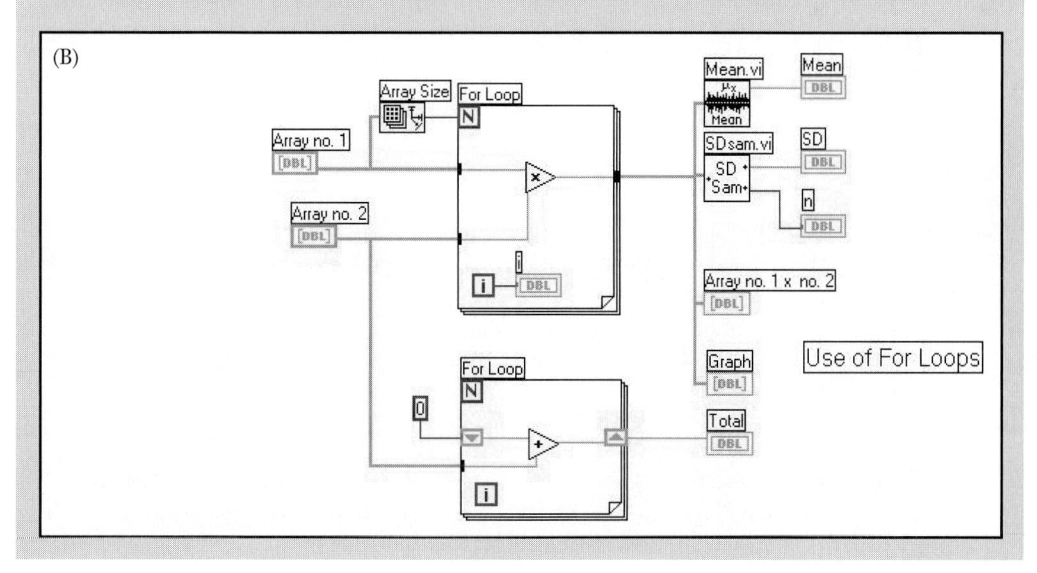

FIGURE 3–7.3
(A) Front panel and (B) block diagram of **Shiftreg.vi.** This VI demonstrates the use of *Shift Registers* used with a *For Loop. Shift Registers* may also be used with a *While Loop.*

(A)

STOP

x (i)
8 Current Value

x (i-1)
7 1 iteration ago

x (i-2)
6 2 iterations ago

x (i-3)
5 3 iterations ago

(B)

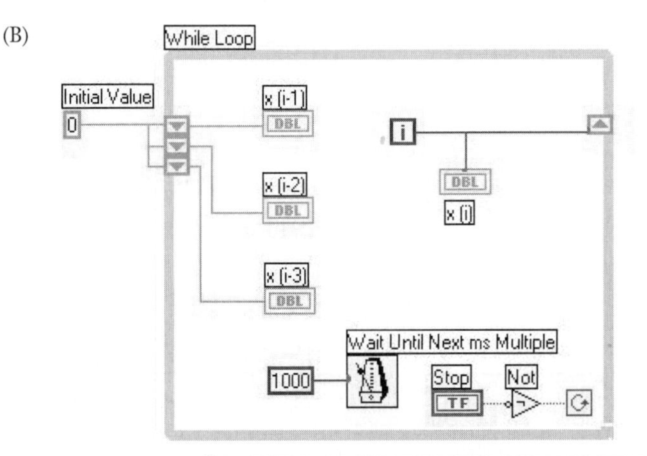

Use the **Execution Highlighting** option (lightbulb) and debugging in continuous run mode to visualize how **Shift Registers** work.

From this panel pop-up a **Probe** (cursor on the wire while the VI is running and right-click and choose probe) on each wire leading from the shift registers elements on the left.

OBJECT/FUNCTION OR SUBVI LOCATOR
CASEBOOL.VI

Panel	Object/Function or SubVI	Palette/Menu or Directory
Front	*Vertical Toggle Switch*	Controls/Boolean
	String Indicator	Controls/String & Table
Diagram	*Case Structure*	Functions/Structures
	String Constant × 2	Functions/String

in the previous example, the *Shift Registers* are initialized to zero when the VI begins to run. The *While Loop* is controlled by a *Boolean Rectangular Stop Button* on the front panel. After the VI begins running, it can be stopped by pressing the "STOP" button. The rate at which values are calculated is controlled by the *Wait Until Next ms Multiple* function wired to a *Numerical Constant* of "1000". In this case, one iteration occurs every second. Variable control of the iteration rate can be achieved by wiring a front panel *Digital Control* (e.g., a knob or slide control) to the *Wait Until Next ms Multiple function.*

Casebool.vi (Figure 3–7.4) and **Casenum.vi** (Figure 3–7.5) demonstrate the use of *Case Structures* with a *Boolean* and *Numeric* control, respectively. In **Casebool.vi,** a *Boolean* switch is used to toggle between two conditions: the "Down" position (false) yields the phrase,"The switch is in the DOWN position" in the *String Indicator* message on the front panel; the "Up" position yields, "The switch is in the UP position." Click on the **Continuous Run** arrow, and toggle the switch using the *Hand Tool.* In **Casenum.vi,** a *Digital Control* has been wired to a *Case Structure,* converting it from the *Boolean* (default) to a numerical condition. Note that three cases are possible. The operator chooses the numbers 0, 1, or 2 and inputs that number into the front panel *Numeric Digital Control.* If case 0 is selected, the quotient of "100" divided by "5" (quotient = 20) is displayed in the *Numerical Digital Indicator* on the front panel, while the phrase "This is twenty" appears in the *String Indicator.* Choosing case 1 returns the number "8" and the phrase "This is eight," while case 2 yields the number "55" and the phrase "This is fifty five." Run the VI in **Continuous Run** mode, toggle the *Numeric Digital Control* between the three cases using the *Hand Tool,* and observe the resultant messages.

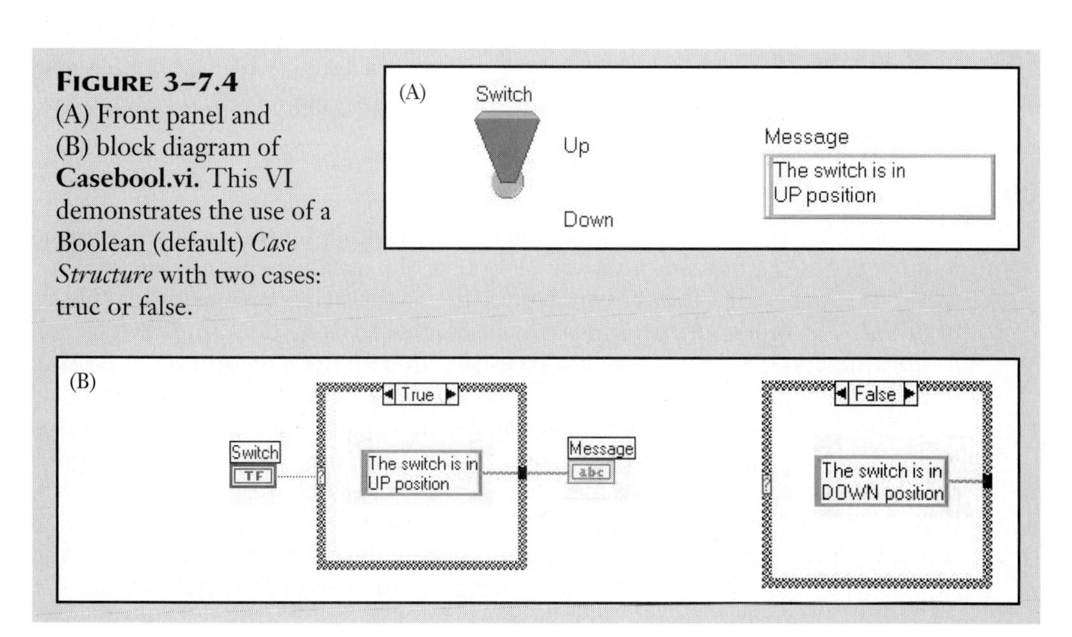

FIGURE 3–7.4
(A) Front panel and (B) block diagram of **Casebool.vi.** This VI demonstrates the use of a Boolean (default) *Case Structure* with two cases: truc or false.

OBJECT/FUNCTION OR SUBVI LOCATOR
CASENUM.VI

Panel	Object/Function or SubVI	Palette/Menu or Directory
Front	*Digital Control*	**Controls/Numeric**
	Digital Indicator	**Controls/Numeric**
	String Indicator	**Controls/String & Table**
Diagram	*Case Structure*	**Functions/Structures**
	Numeric Constant × 4	**Functions/Numeric**
	Divide	**Functions/Numeric**
	String Constant × 3	**Functions/String**

In the final example, **Seqlocal.vi** (Figure 3–7.6) demonstrates the use of *Sequence Structures* using a *Sequence Local.* A number is first inserted in the *Digital Control*, and the VI is run. Three operations are performed on the initial value and displayed in three *Digital Indicators.* In the ***first*** frame (0), the initial value is multiplied by a constant ("100") and then passed on to the ***next*** frame (1) using a *Sequence Local.* Fifty-five is then subtracted from the previous product and passed on to the third and final frame (2), where the value for frame 1 is divided by 2, and that value is displayed as a "Final result" on the front panel in a *Digital Indicator.*

SUMMARY

For Loops are used to ***repeat*** an operation enclosed within the loop a predetermined number of times. Enclosing a VI, subVI, or other operation within a *While Loop* and wiring the loop with a *Boolean* switch gives the operator front panel on/off control of the VI. The timing of operations may be controlled using the *Wait Until Next ms Multiple* function. *Shift Registers* may be used with both *For Loops* and *While Loops* to transfer the value of a variable of the current iteration into the next iteration.

Case Structures permit the ***toggling*** between different conditions enclosed within the case. The default condition is a *Boolean Case Structure*, which gives ***true/false*** control. Wiring the structure with a *Numeric* control permits the addition of multiple cases to be toggled between. *Sequence Structures* permit the serial ordering of programming events. Everything contained within the first frame will be executed before the second frame's contents are operated on, etc. *Sequence Locals* permit the passing of a variable between frames.

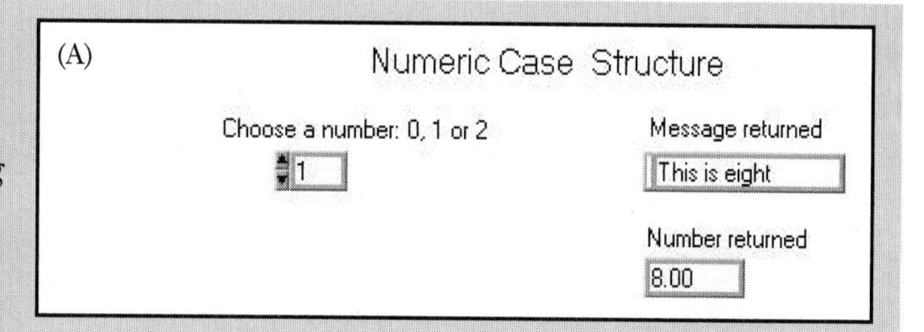

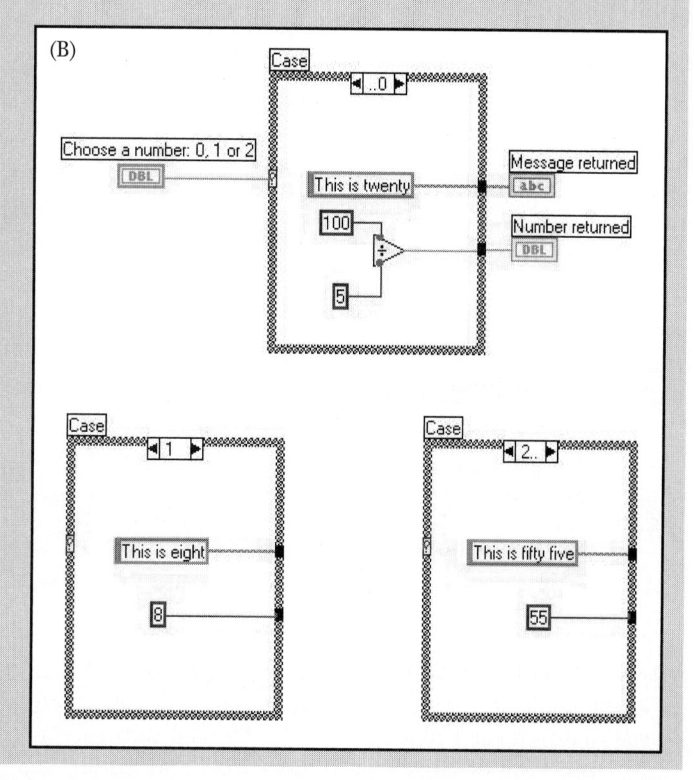

FIGURE 3–7.5 (A) Front panel and (B) block diagram of **Casenum.vi** demonstrating a numeric *Case Structure*. *Case Structures* are by default Boolean structures. Wiring a numeric variable to the input terminal (question mark along left border) will convert the *Case Structure* to a numeric type. While only two cases are possible for a Boolean *Case Structure* (true and false), multiple numeric *Case Structures* may be utilized.

PRACTICE EXERCISES

Following are several additional exercises that build on ideas and concepts just described in this section. Write, or call up from the **CD ROM disk directory,** the VIs just discussed, and modify and **Run** each VI, inserting the following changes/additions. Resave each VI using a unique identifying name in a convenient directory, and/or print out each VI after making changes, and compare the version with the modified version found in the **CD ROM disk directory.** Modified VI versions use the following filenames:

OBJECT/FUNCTION OR SUBVI LOCATOR
SEQLOCAL.VI

Panel	Object/Function or SubVI	Palette/Menu or Directory
Front	*Digital Control*	Controls/Numeric
	Digital Indicator × 3	Controls/Numeric
	Raised Frame × 3	Controls/Decorations
Diagram	*Sequence Structure*	Functions/Structures
	Numeric Constant × 3	Functions/Numeric
	Multiply	Functions/Numeric
	Subtract	Functions/Numeric
	Divide	Functions/Numeric

VI FILENAME	MODIFIED VI FILENAME
Forloop.vi	**Formod.vi**
Shifreg.vi	**Shiftmod.vi**
Casebool.vi	**Casebmod.vi**
Casenum.vi	**Casenmod.vi**
Seqlocal.vi	**Seqmod.vi**

FORLOOP.VI

On the front panel, relabel the *Digital Indicator* called "Total " to "Total Array 2," and add another *Digital Indicator* and label it "Total Array No. 1." Modify the block diagram such that the VI will add the sum total of all cells in Array No. 1 to the sum total of all cells in Array No. 2 and display that total in a *Digital Indicator* labeled "Total Arrays Nos. 1 & 2."

SHIFTREG.VI

Add another *Digital Indicator* on the front panel, and label it "x (I-4)." To the right of the indicator, add the following text: "4 iterations ago." On the block diagram, modify the VI such that the value of the fourth iteration will be displayed in *the Digital Indicator* just added to the front panel. Finally, add a ***control structure*** on the front panel that will permit ***variable control*** of the rate at which the *While Loop* iterates. Note that the original VI is set up such that the *While Loop* always iterates at a rate of ***one cycle per second.***

FIGURE 3–7.6
(A) Front panel and (B) block diagram of **Seqlocal.vi.** This VI demonstrates the use of *Sequence Locals* with a *Sequence Structure. Sequence Locals* pass the value of a variable from one frame to the next.

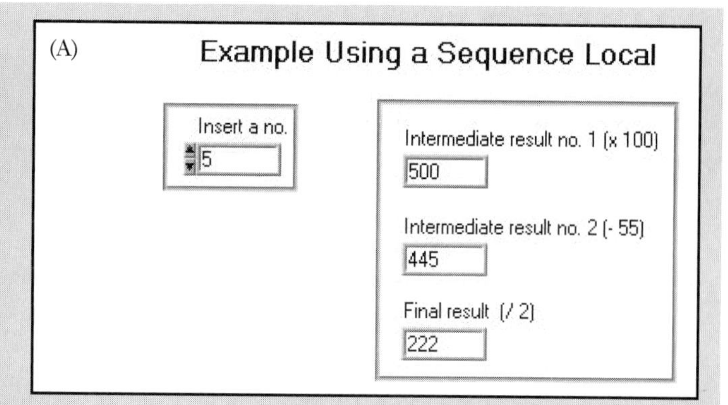

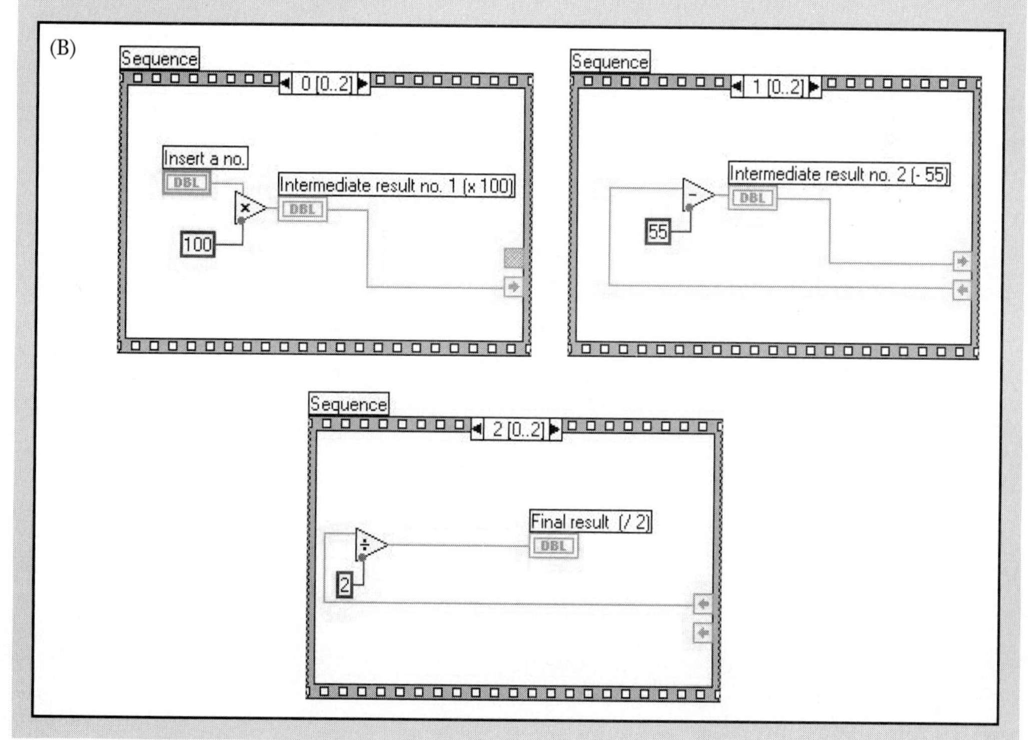

CASEBOOL.VI

On the front panel, relabel the switch position descriptors "Up" and "Down" to "Position 1" and "Position 2," respectively. Modify the block diagram so that moving the switch to ***Position 1*** yields the message "Position 1 returns the True condition," and ***Position 2*** yields "Position 2 returns the False condition."

CASENUM.VI

Add a ***third case*** to the block diagram so that the message displayed on the front panel is, "This is a very big number" and the *Digital Indicator* returns the number, "12345386." You will have to expand the *String* and *Digital Indicators* on the front panel to the right to accommodate the longer message and number.

SEQLOCAL.VI

In the block diagram, add a fourth frame that will take the result of frame 2—the last frame (remember, frame 0 is the first frame, 1 is the second, etc.)—and add "1000" to it. Rewire the front panel *Digital Indicator* labeled "Final result" accordingly.

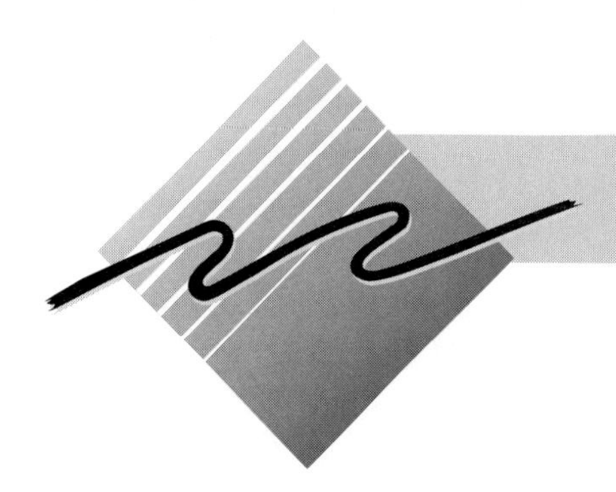

SECTION 3-8

VI PROGRAMMING ERRORS

OBJECTIVES

- ❖ Learn and use error-handling strategies.
- ❖ Learn and use debugging strategies.
- ❖ Learn and use diagnostic probes.

ERROR HANDLING

Programming or logic errors in software are common and can lead to a ***program crash*** or the possibility that it will not run at all. The term ***debugging*** refers to a systematic way of reviewing program code to determine if errors are present. Traditionally, program errors have been referred to as ***bugs.*** LabVIEW bugs generally result in a VI that will not run, which is signaled to the user by a broken **Run** arrow.

A broken **Run** arrow indicates there is a problem with your VI such as a ***bad wire*** or ***mismatched*** numeric control or indicator variable. When the **Run** arrow is clicked in a VI with a programming problem, an **Error List** message will pop up, listing problems in the program. In **Run** mode, left-click on the error, and then click on the **Find** button. The block diagram appears, and the problem area is ***highlighted.*** Clicking on the **Help** window may assist in determining the nature of the problem.

DEBUGGING

Several debugging techniques are available in LabVIEW. Debugging is usually handled in the block diagram. To understand the debugging process, write or call up from the **CD ROM disk directory** a simple VI called **Debug.vi** (Figure 3–8.1).

OBJECT/FUNCTION OR SUBVI LOCATOR
DEBUG.VI

Panel	Object/Function or SubVI	Palette/Menu or Directory
Front	*Array + Digital Indicator*	**Controls/Array & Cluster; Numeric**
	Digital Indicator	**Controls/Numeric**
Diagram	*For Loop*	**Functions/Structures**
	Numeric Constant	**Functions/Numeric**
	Random Number (0–1)	**Functions/Numeric**
	Increment (+ 1)	**Functions/Numeric**

This VI sequentially generates three random numbers from zero to "1.0." After the number is generated, a value of one ("+1") is added, and the sum is displayed in the cell in a front panel *Indicator Array.*

The ***single-step*** method permits a ***step-by-step*** procedure for identifying and rectifying logic errors. On the task bar at the top of the screen, click on the **Highlight Execution** icon (lightbulb), the fifth icon from the **Run** arrow. Note that the icon changes to a yellow color. To the right of this icon is the **Start Single Stepping** button. With **Highlight Execution** turned on, run the VI, and note that the entire VI will ***blink,*** signaling that debugging mode is turned on. Now click on the **Start Single Stepping** button. The first element of the VI (*Random Number (0-1)* generator (i.e., a pair of dice) is highlighted and begins to blink. Note also that a red or orange ball appears. Each time the **Start Single Stepping** button is clicked, the ball progresses to the ***next*** VI element, demonstrating the ***logical flow*** of information to and from program elements. Also note that functions that generate ***numerical*** or **string** data display that data in a ***box*** overlying the function. In this case, the first number displayed is a random number ("0–1.0"). Progressing to the next step, the +**1** function is highlighted and a number is displayed (i.e., the initial random number plus "1"). Click the **Start Single Stepping** button again until each function has been highlighted and each iteration of the VI has been completed. In this VI, three random numbers are generated and displayed in the front panel array; therefore the VI executes three times. After the last iteration, the entire block diagram is highlighted, indicating the VI has run completely, signaling that the VI can be stopped.

To animate the debugging process and watch the ***step-by-step*** execution of functions work ***sequentially*** until the VI has completed running, click on the ***second***

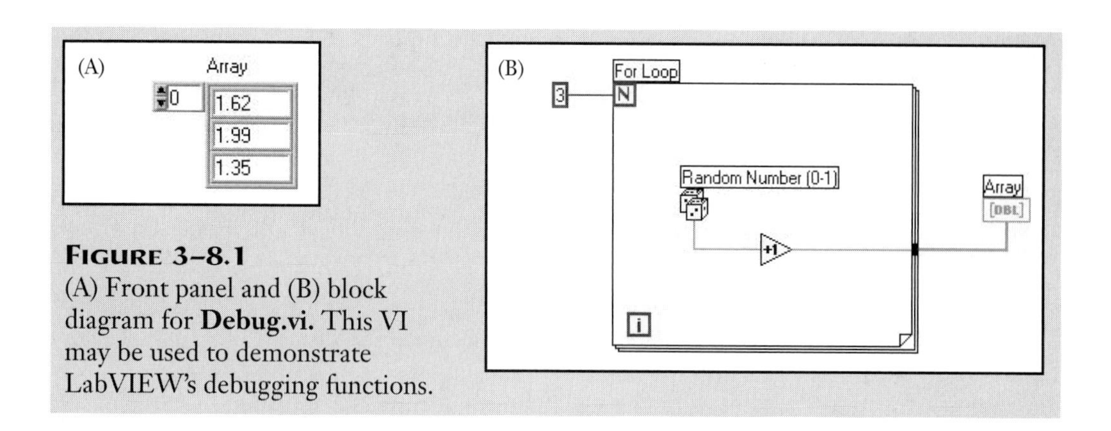

FIGURE 3–8.1
(A) Front panel and (B) block diagram for **Debug.vi.** This VI may be used to demonstrate LabVIEW's debugging functions.

Start Single Stepping button to the right of the **Highlight Execution** icon. This demonstrates the ***step-by-step*** progression of the VI in continuous ***slow motion.***

To indicate the value of control or indicator variables, arrays, etc., a *Probe* variable displaying a numeric value or string may be popped up on a wire leading to/from a variable. Place the *Arrow Tool* on a wire, and right-click. A menu will appear. Choose the *Probe* menu item and note that a probe indicator will be displayed and its corresponding number inserted into the wire leading to/from a function. *Probes* display data in engineering notation by default. Selecting the *Custom Probe* menu item permits the selection of other types of tools such as a *Numeric Indicator* from the **Controls/Numeric** palette that displays data as numbers (decimal precision definable) or integers. Run the VI with the **Highlight Execution** icon turned ***on*** in either step-by-step or continuous mode, and observe that *Probe* values change with each new iteration of the VI (Figure 3–8.2).

Finally, ***break*** one or several of the wires using the *Arrow Tool*, and run the VI. When the **Error List** message appears, highlight an error message, and click on the **Find** button.

SUMMARY

LabVIEW has a built-in ***error-handling*** capability that is automatically activated when a broken **Run** arrow is returned. The VI will not run, and an **Error List** will pop up immediately, identifying the source(s) of the problem. Highlighting an error message and clicking on the **Find** button will bring the user into the block diagram where the potential problem is highlighted.

Several debugging techniques are available to the programmer. Clicking on **Highlight Execution** and one of several ***stepping action*** buttons on the task bar will activate the debugging process.

Diagnostic *Probes* may be inserted into wires permitting the programmer to measure data while the VI runs to verify a logical flow of information or diagnose potential logic errors.

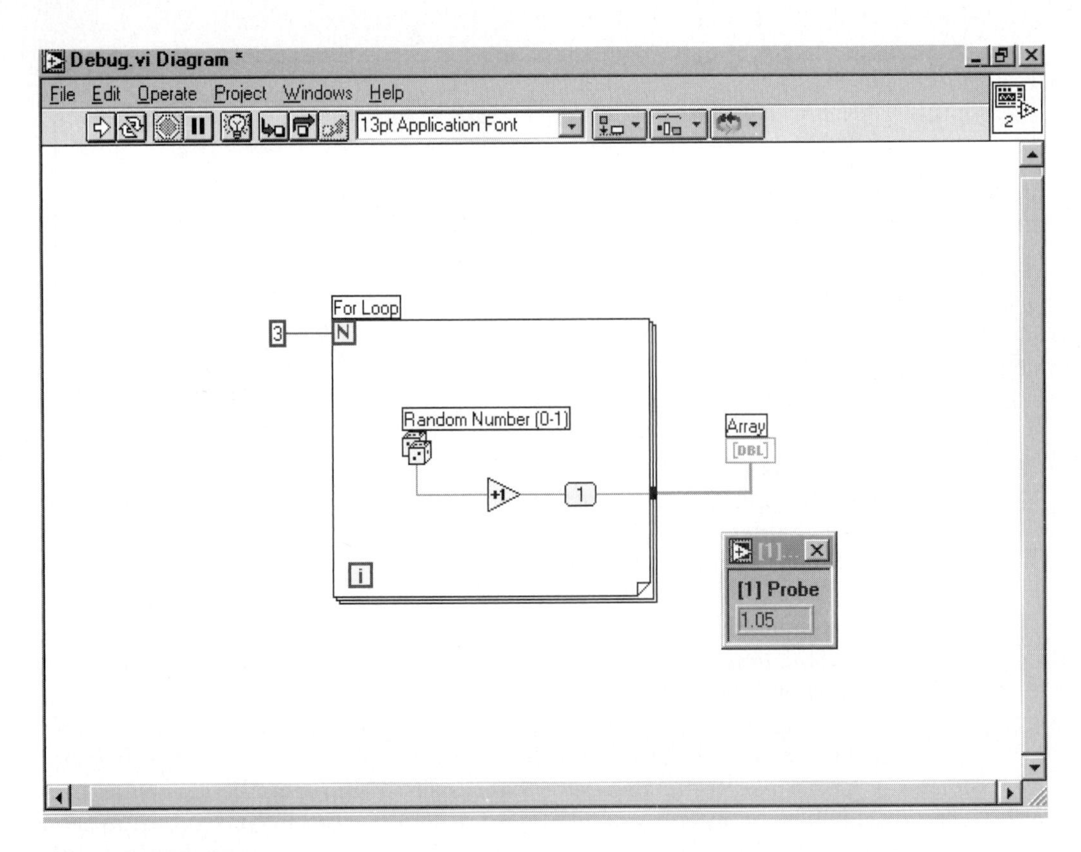

FIGURE 3–8.2
Block diagram demonstrating the use of *Probes* for analyzing VI logic and debugging.

PRACTICE EXERCISE

Bring up the file called **Broke.vi** from the **CD ROM disk directory.** The purpose of this VI is to generate two sets of random numbers and display each set in an *Indicator Array* and on a *Waveform Graph* in the front panel. One set of numbers ranges from "0 to 1" and the second ranges from "1 to 10". Note that the **Run** arrow is ***broken,*** indicating that a number of programming errors are in the VI. Using the techniques and methods described previously, evaluate and repair the VI so that it will run properly. The VI called **Fixed.vi,** in the **CD ROM disk directory,** is the same VI in proper running order. If problems are experienced diagnosing an error, it may be helpful to call up and/or print out this VI to compare with the one currently being evaluated.

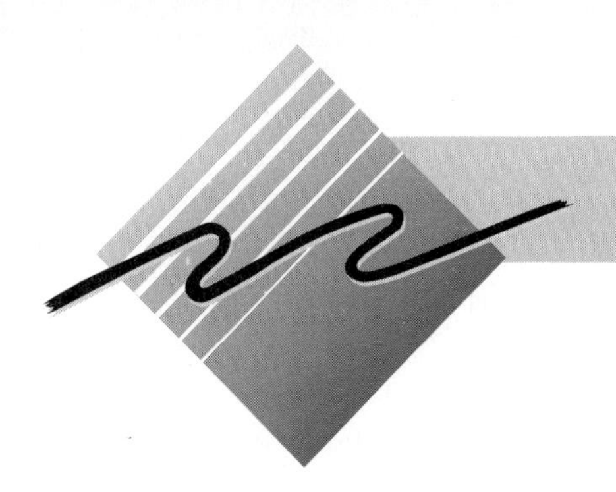

STRINGS

OBJECTIVES

- Construct several VIs using string control and indicator variables.
- Save string data to a tab-delimited spreadsheet file.

STRING CONTROL AND INDICATOR VARIABLES

The preceding discussion of *Control* and *Indicator* variables has involved ***numbers.*** Data may also be handled as **strings.** Strings are groups of ASCII (American Standard Code for Information Exchange) characters and may be ***text, numbers,*** or ***both.*** All ***text data*** are inherently treated as strings. ***Numerical*** data may also be converted to a string, and ***mixed*** data, including both ***text*** and ***numbers,*** are treated as a string. From a programming standpoint, string variables act in much the same way as numeric variables, requiring their own unique control and indicator functions. String functions are found in both the front panel (**Controls/String & Table** palette) and block diagram (**Functions/String** palette) and are wired and otherwise handled like numeric functions.

CONCATENATING STRINGS

Figure 3–9.1 demonstrates the use of the *Concatenate Strings* function found in the block diagram in the **Functions/String** palette. ***Concatenating*** string ***data groups inputs string data*** (i.e., from *String Controls*) and ports this information to a *String Indicator. Concatenate Strings* is initially configured with two input (i.e., left side of icon) terminals. Additional terminals are added by clicking and dragging either lower corner of the icon downward. Note that an *End of Line* function

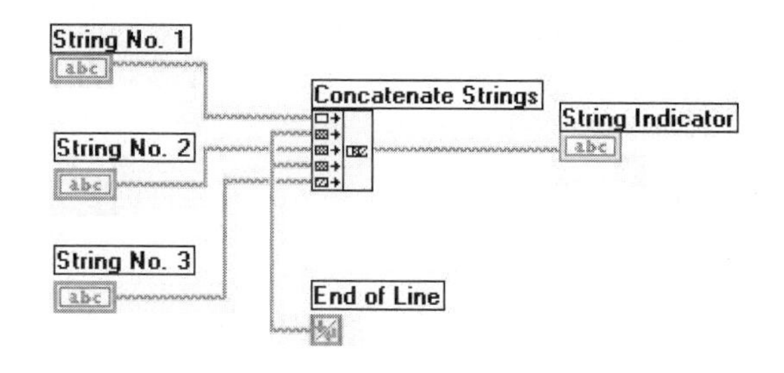

FIGURE 3–9.1
The *Concatenate Strings* function merges string variable contents into a single string indicator. The *End of Line* function acts like a carriage return and separates the contents of each string variable into three separate lines of information in the *String Indicator.*

OBJECT/FUNCTION OR SUBVI LOCATOR
STRINGS1.VI

Panel	Object/Function or SubVI	Palette/Menu or Directory
Front	*String Control* × 3	**Controls/String &Table**
	Numeric Indicator × 3	**Controls/Numeric**
	String Indicator × 3	**Controls/String &Table**
Diagram	*Concatenate Strings*	**Functions/String**
	String Length × 3	**Functions/String**
	End of Line	**Functions/String**

(**Functions/String** palette) has been wired ***between*** each *String Control* variable terminal. This has the same effect as pushing the Enter key of the keyboard and inserting a ***carriage return*** between each line of data. If the *End of Line* is not used, each string will be connected together in a single line. Substituting a *Tab* for an *End of Line* function creates a space between each string or locates the next string data in a series to the next column in a spreadsheet saved in a ***tab-delimited (text)*** format (see example following).

SAMPLE VIS

Strings1.vi (Figure 3–9.2) demonstrates ***basic string operations.*** Write or call up this VI from the **CD ROM disk directory.** On the front panel and to the left are three *String Controls* that are used to input three lines of ***string data.*** Next to the controls are three *Digital Indicators* that ***count*** the number of string characters (including spaces) in each string. After the VI is run, the string data are displayed in a *String Indicator* to the left. Note that each string resides on a separate line as if the line had been typed on a word processor and a carriage return had been inserted after each line. The *String Length* function, in the block diagram, is wired to each *String Control* variable and ports its result to a *Numeric Indicator* configured as

FIGURE 3–9.2
(A) Front panel and (B) block diagram of **Strings1.vi.** This VI takes the contents of three separate *String Controls* and merges the information into a single *String Indicator* using the *Concatenate Strings* function.

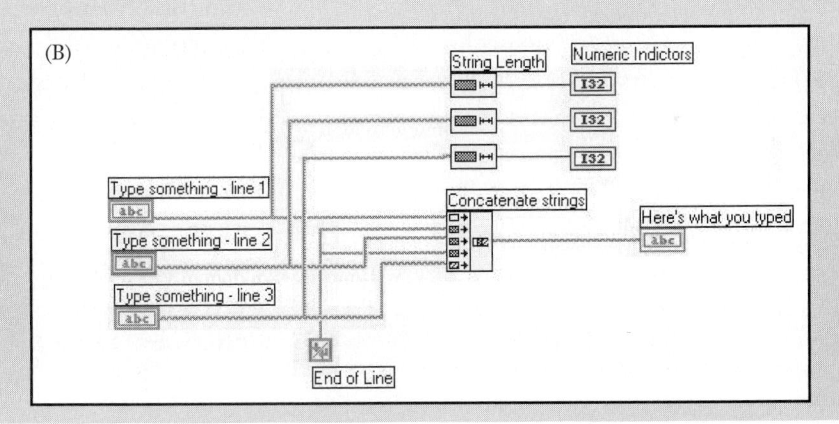

an integer (I32). When the VI is run, the number of characters in each *String Control*, including spaces, is displayed. To see how the VI works, type in information (use letters and numbers) in each control ("Type something . . .") and **Run** the VI several times. If you constructed this VI, save it using a unique identifying name into a convenient directory.

String functions are used to continuously update the collection of simulated temperature data in **Strings2.vi** (Figure 3–9.3). Each time a temperature is registered and plotted on the *Waveform Chart*, the ***day, date, and time*** are posted in a *String Indicator* above the graph. Write or bring up this VI from the **CD ROM disk directory.**

In the block diagram, the *Concatenate Strings* function is used in a similar way as with the previous example. In this case, the simulated temperature data are generated as a ***number*** from the central output terminal of **Promon1.vi.** Since the ***number*** will be displayed as a ***string*** in the front panel, it must be ***converted to string format*** using the *To Fractional* function. Note that the ***decimal precision*** has been set (default = 2) by wiring a *Numeric Indicator* to a terminal in the lower left

OBJECT/FUNCTION OR SUBVI LOCATOR
STRINGS2.VI

Panel	Object/Function or SubVI	Palette/Menu or Directory
Front	*String Indicator*	**Controls/String &Table**
	Round Stop Button	**Controls/Boolean**
	Vertical Toggle Switch	**Controls/Boolean**
	Dial	**Controls/Numeric**
	Digital Control × 2	**Controls/Numeric**
	Waveform Graph	**Controls/Graph**
Diagram	*While Loop*	**Functions/Structure**
	Promon1.vi	**Functions/Select a VI . . .**
	To Fractionate	**Functions/String**
	Get Date/Time String	**Functions/Time & Dialog**
	Concatenate Strings	**Functions/String**
	Tab	**Functions/String**
	End of Line	**Functions/String**
	Wait Until Next ms Multiple	**Functions/Time & Dialog**

corner of the icon. The converted number is then wired to the first input terminal in *Concatenate Strings.* The ***date*** and ***time*** when each temperature point is registered are generated by the *Get Date/Time String* function. This function provides the option of showing the ***second*** at which the data point is generated. In this case, a *Boolean Toggle Switch* (defaulting to the ***false/no*** condition) on the front panel has been wired to this terminal. Note that a space between each descriptor in the *String Indicator* (i.e., temperature, day, date, and time) is created by wiring a *Tab* function between each string terminal.

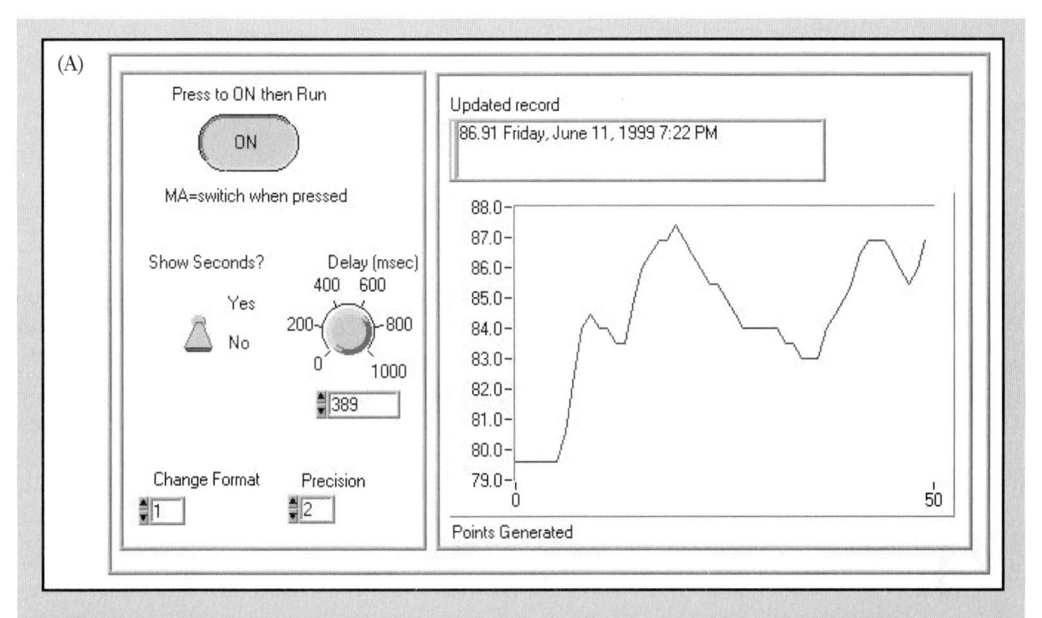

FIGURE 3–9.3
(A) Front panel and (B) block diagram of **Strings2.vi.** Note that the *String Indicator* above the *Waveform Chart* in the front panel documents the data point being generated with the day, date, and time. Simulated temperatures (numeric data) must be converted into a string format by the *To Fractional* function in the block diagram.

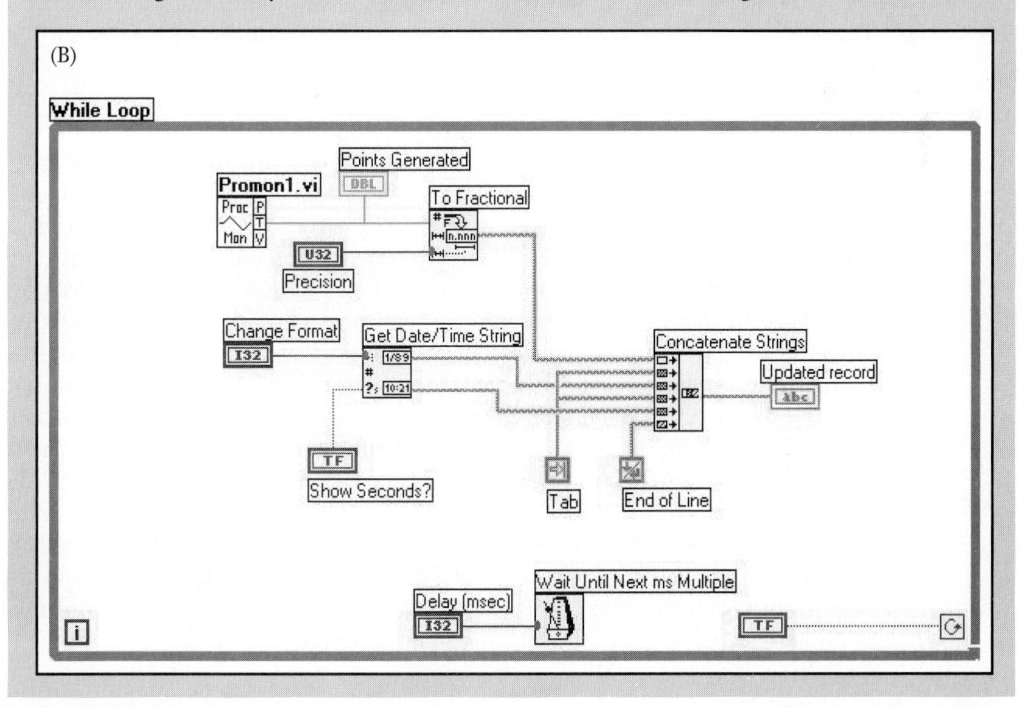

The ***rate*** at which each temperature point is generated is controlled by enclosing the VI in a *While Loop* toggled with a *Boolean Labeled Oblong* button using the *Wait Until Next ms Multiple* function. **Run** the VI several times, changing the default values on the front panel to understand how this VI works. If you constructed this VI, save it using a unique identifying name into a convenient directory.

SUMMARY

Strings are groups of text and/or numeric data (ASCII characters) that are handled and manipulated in much the same way as numeric data using *String Controls* and *Indicators*. ***Numbers*** that are to be treated as ***Strings*** must be converted to ***string format*** using the *To Fractional* function. ***String data*** are grouped using the *Concatenate Strings* function. ***Spacing*** and ***location*** of ***string data*** on ***another line*** are handled by using the *Tab* and *End of Line* functions, respectively.

PRACTICE EXERCISES

Call up **Strings2.vi** from the **CD ROM disk directory.** In the block diagram, ***remove*** some or all of the *Tab* and/or *End of Line* functions wired to *Concatenate Strings*. Note that when wires are removed from terminals, a broken **Run** arrow appears, indicating a problem with the VI. Unwired terminals will cause this error. The problem may be corrected by right-clicking the *Arrow Tool* on the terminal to be removed and choosing the *Remove Input* option from the menu. ***Remove all unwired terminals***, and note that the **Run** arrow appears whole again, signifying that the VI is ready to operate. **Run** the VI, and see the result of these changes on the way the **string data** are displayed in the *String Indicator*.

Call up **Strings3.vi** from the **CD ROM disk directory,** and examine the front panel and block diagram. Note that this VI has many of the same features described in **Strings2.vi** plus some added capabilities for analyzing and saving data. **Strings3.vi** will generate a predetermined number (default = "100") of simulated temperatures using the **Promon1.vi** subVI. When the VI is **Run,** note that a ***prompt window*** appears asking the operator to create a ***filename*** and to identify a ***directory*** in which the data file should be saved. The recommended ***file extension*** is ***.dat*** (for ***data*** file); however, any extension will be accepted. Once the filename is created and the **Save** button is pressed, the VI generates and plots data points while updating the data record of the temperature, and the day, date, and time it was collected in the *String Indicator* above the graph. Note also that this VI has a ***comparison*** function that compares the current temperature to a ***threshold value*** that's set on the front panel using a *Dial* ("High Limit"). If the threshold is exceeded, an *LED* lights, and a ***beep*** signal is heard. A message in the *String Indicator* reports that the temperature is "Over" the threshold. If the temperature is less than threshold, an "Under" message is returned. Move to the block diagram, review the upper right corner of the *For Loop*, and note that the *Greater?* function and two *Boolean Case Structures* provide the comparison function.

Data files are saved by wiring together three **File I/O** (Input/Out) icons. The subVI called *Open/Create/Replace File.vi* provides the option of opening or replacing a file. Note the *Numeric Constant* 2 (open or replace) is wired to the *function* terminal on the left side of the icon. When the filename is determined, *Write File* saves the data in a ***tab-delimited*** (text file) format. *Close File* closes the file after the data are saved.

Run the VI using the front panel default values, and save the file with a convenient filename and directory. Next, using ***spreadsheet software*** (e.g., Excel™, Quattro Pro™, etc.), open the previously saved data file. Most current spreadsheet programs automatically detect the file as a ***tab-delimited*** (text) file and guide the user through an opening procedure. If this feature is not available, choose the **Open as a Text File** option, and the file should open. Note on the spreadsheet that ***four columns*** of data are present. The ***first*** column includes the ***simulated temperature*** readings. Confirm that the predetermined number of data points have been collected by scrolling down to the last cell. The cell number should be the same as the number of data points identified on the front panel ("No. of Points?") *Digital Control* (assuming the first cell is numbered "1"). The ***second*** column returns the day and date, and the ***third*** column returns the time the temperature was recorded. The ***last*** column indicates whether the temperature was "Under" or "Over" the predetermined threshold. Note that when the spreadsheet is first opened, some of the columnar data may be ***compressed.*** Using the cursor, expand the columns to the appropriate width to view all the data. Rerun the VI with several combinations of front panel control options, and observe changes in the *String Indicator*, graph, and spreadsheet files.

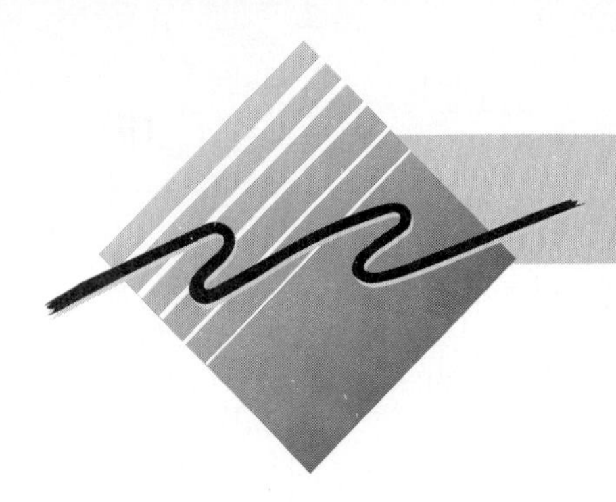

INDEXING

OBJECTIVES

- ❖ Call up, configure, and wire the *Index Array* function in a simple VI.
- ❖ Manipulate arrays of data using indexing.

MANIPULATING ARRAYS OF DATA AND FUNCTIONS WITH INDEXING

Indexing is an important function that allows the user to choose single cells or groups of cells from an array of data. Manipulating data arrays in this fashion is often handled in the front panel. In the block diagram, indexing is also used to select for a specific operation using the *Index Array* function located in the **Functions/Array** palette.

SAMPLE VI

Index.vi demonstrates the use of indexing functions in both the front panel and block diagram (Figure 3–10.1). This VI may also be found in the **CD ROM disk directory.** This VI reads a previously saved data file consisting of 2 columns and 20 rows (Figure 3–10.2). These data are also available in the **CD ROM disk directory.** The filename is **Index.dat.**

The main component of this VI is the *Index Array* function placed in a *Case Structure* in the block diagram. When *Index Array* is first called up and placed in the block diagram, a single ***indexing terminal*** (small black rectangle in the lower left corner) is present. Using the *Arrow Tool,* an ***additional*** terminal may be selected by clicking and dragging down on either lower corner of the icon. In its two-terminal configuration, *Index Array* permits the indexing (i.e., selection) of either a ***row*** (top terminal) or ***column*** (bottom terminal) of spreadsheet data. Note that both terminals cannot be ***enabled*** at the same time. That is, if one is selected, the other must be ***disabled*** by right-clicking on the terminal and using the *Disable Indexing* menu option. *Index Array* is configured to index rows or columns by wiring a *Digital Control* in the front panel to this terminal. Remember that a "zero" value by default means that the ***first*** row or column will be accessed. Selecting a value of "1" in the digital control accesses the ***second*** row or column, etc. In the *Case Structure*, the ***true*** condition (toggle either arrow at the top using the *Arrow Tool*) configures *Index Array* to read ***row*** data, while the ***false*** condition permits ***column*** data to be read. Toggling between the two conditions is achieved using a *Boolean Vertical Switch* in the front panel. When the switch is in the ***down*** (default) position, "Column(s)" are read. In the ***up*** position, "Row(s)" are read. Note that the VI must be ***rerun*** each time the switch is ***reset.*** Column or row data are displayed in the front panel using a *1D Array*. Note that the *1D Array* has its own ***indexing control*** (to the left of the top cell with an up and down arrow). This control allows the user to select a specific cell for inspection and is most useful when the *Array* is closed up as a single cell when front panel space is at a premium.

To demonstrate the use of indexing, write this VI or call it up from the **CD ROM disk directory. Run** the VI with the front panel switch in its default (down) position to index on column data and with the *Digital Control* in its default ("0") position to access the first column. At the prompt, select the data file called **Index.dat** from the **CD ROM disk directory,** and click on the **Open** button. Compare what is seen on the monitor in the *1D Array* with the data in Figure 3–10.1. Note that the first cell has a value of "12.00," the second "15.00," and the last "21.00." Now, using the *Hand Tool*, change the value of the *Digital Control* to "1," and rerun the VI. Now the values of the first, second, and last cells in the second column are "123.00" (first), "543.00" (second), and "459.00" (last), respectively. Finally, set the switch to the ***up*** position, reset the *Digital Control* with a value of "0," and rerun the VI. This time, only two cell values appear in the *1D Array*. The first cell number is "12.00," and the second is "123.00." The remaining cells in the array are empty and not highlighted. In this case, the ***first row*** of data has been accessed (i.e., as if reading ***across*** a spreadsheet).

To see how the ***indexing control*** on the *1D Array* is used, close up the array to a single-cell configuration by left-clicking on either lower corner of the array with the *Arrow Tool* and dragging the last cell toward the first. Reset the switch to the ***down*** position to access "Column" data again, and rerun the VI. With the indexing control of the array set at "0" (default), the value of the cell to the right is "12.00." Now click on the indexing control, set the value to "5," and note that the cell value is "45.00."

SUMMARY

Indexing allows the user to access ***row*** or ***column*** data in a tabular (spreadsheet) format. On the front panel, a particular cell is accessed in a data array by clicking on the indexing control of an *Array* using the *Hand Tool*. *Index Array* is used in the block diagram to access a ***row*** (upper terminal) or ***column*** (lower terminal) either by wiring a *Constant* (block diagram) or variable *Control* device (front panel) to the terminals of *Index Array*.

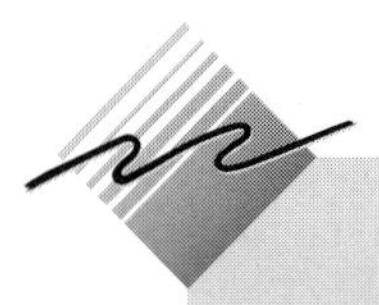

OBJECT/FUNCTION OR SUBVI LOCATOR
INDEX.VI

Panel	Object/Function or SubVI	Palette/Menu or Directory
Front	*Vertical Switch*	**Controls/Boolean**
	Array	**Controls/Array & Cluster**
	Digital Control	**Controls/Numeric**
Diagram	*Case Structure*	**Functions/Structures**
	Read From Spreadsheet File.vi	**Functions/File I/O**
	Index Array × 2	**Functions/Array**

FIGURE 3–10.2
A previously saved spreadsheet with three columns of data (**Index.dat**) used to demonstrate indexing functions in **Index.vi** (see Figure 3–10.1).

Row	Column 1	Column 2
1	22	43
2	23	44
3	24	45
4	25	46
5	26	47
6	27	48
7	28	49
8	29	50
9	30	51
10	31	52
11	32	53
12	33	54
13	34	55
14	35	56
15	36	57
16	37	58
17	38	59
18	39	60
19	40	61
20	41	62
21	42	63

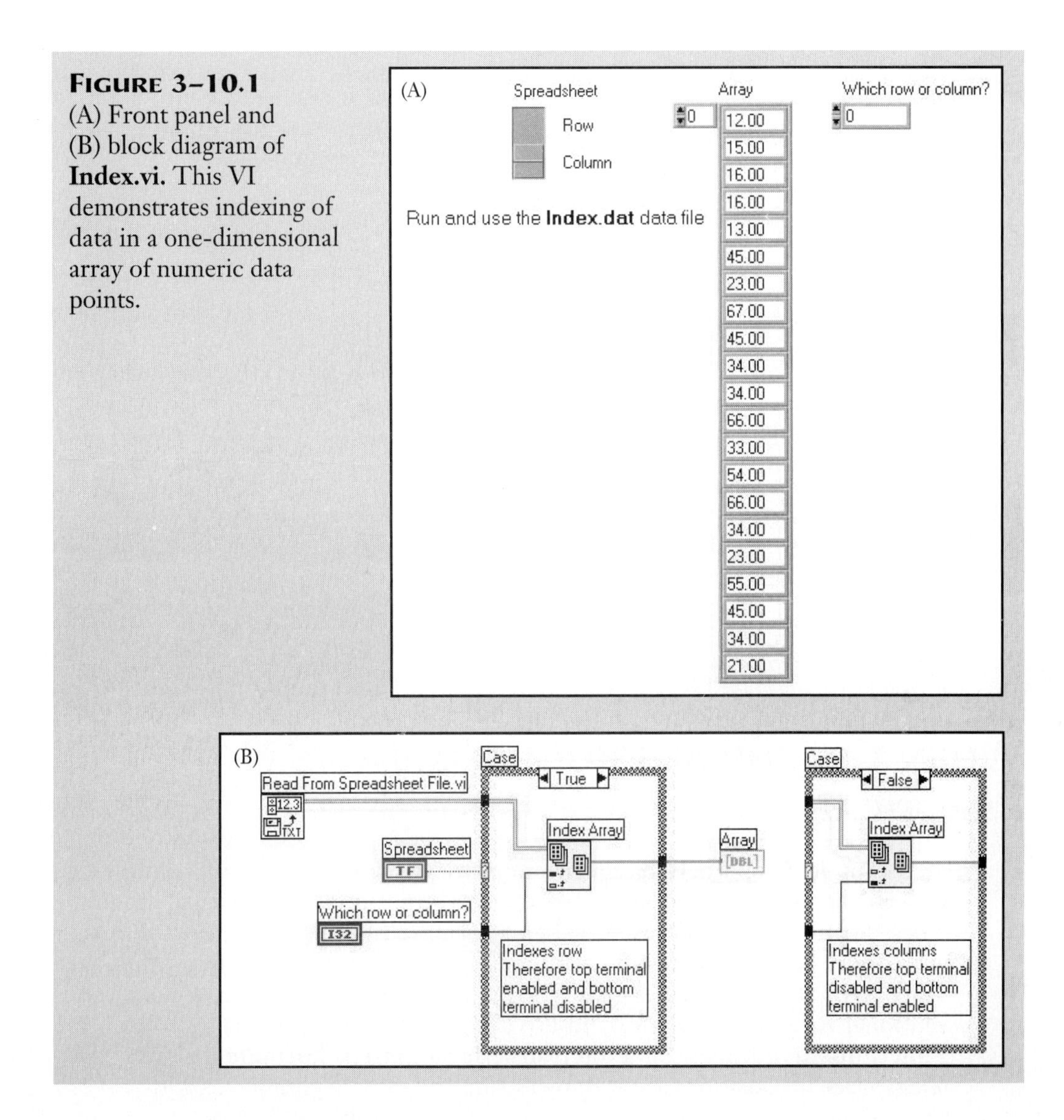

FIGURE 3–10.1 (A) Front panel and (B) block diagram of **Index.vi.** This VI demonstrates indexing of data in a one-dimensional array of numeric data points.

PRACTICE EXERCISE

Using a spreadsheet program (Excel™, Quattro Pro™, etc.), call up the data file named **Index.dat** from the **CD ROM disk directory.** Note that data have been (and should always be) saved in a ***tab-delimited*** (text file) format. Add several additional columns of data, and resave the file using a filename such as **Index2.dat.** It is important ***not*** to add column ***headers*** to the raw spreadsheet data. Be sure that when saving the new spreadsheet, the ***tab-delimited*** (text file) format option is used. Now **Run Index.vi,** and practice accessing additional columns and rows of data.

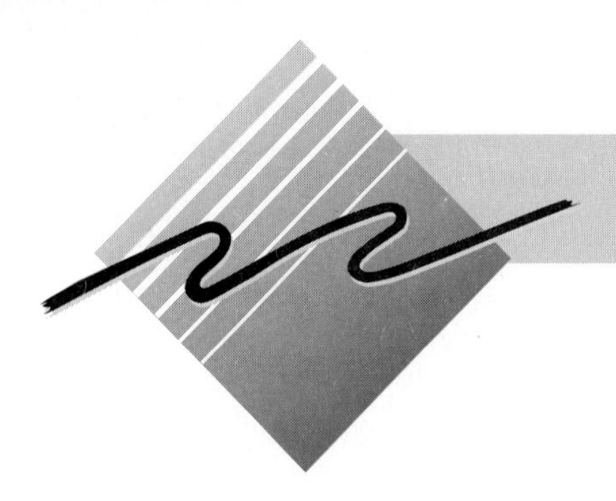

SECTION 3–11

FORMULA NODES

OBJECTIVES

- Construct and use *Formula Nodes*.
- Compare the use of *Formula Nodes* vs. LabVIEW's conventional methods for handling mathematical formulas.

WHEN GRAPHICAL PROGRAMMING IS NOT PRACTICAL

To this point, when there has been a need to write mathematical formulas (e.g., basic arithmetic statements), icons from the **Functions/Numeric** palette in the block diagram have been used. When a formula is ***long*** or ***complicated***, it may make more sense to write the formula in the conventional manner rather than using LabVIEW icons. *Formula Nodes* permit the programmer to insert conventional formulas into a VI and are accessed in the block diagram from the **Functions/Structures** or **Functions/Mathematics/Formula** palettes. *Formula Nodes* are positioned and drawn using the same technique as with a *While* or *For Loop*.

A *Formula Node* (Figure 3–11.1—block diagram) is essentially a box in which a formula is written using standard operator values from the keyboard (e.g., + = plus; − = minus; * = multiply; / = divide, etc.). *Inputs* and *Outputs* to the *Formula Node* are created by placing the *Arrow Tool* on the left or right border and right-clicking to pop-up a menu. Select "Add Input" or "Add Output" from the menu. Note that an empty terminal (box) appears. Using the *Lettering Tool*, insert a variable in each terminal consistent with the intent of the formula. In this example, a *Digital Control* has been wired to the "X" *Input* terminal. This will be the variable on which several operations are performed. For example, in Case 1 the value for

"X" is divided by "2" and then "1" is added to the quotient. The result (Y) is then ported to a *Digital Indicator* via the "Y" *Output* terminal. The formula must ***end*** with a ***semicolon*** (;). If ***multiple formulas*** are included, a semicolon must separate each formula.

SAMPLE VI

Write or call up **Formula.vi** from the **CD ROM disk directory** (see Figure 3–11.1). Three *Formula Nodes* have been inserted into a numerically controlled *Case Structure*. A *Dial* is used to choose between one of three cases. Three cases are used for writing formulas. *Case 0* uses a formula written with LabVIEW icons. *Case 1* uses the same formula written in ***conventional format*** using a *Formula Node*. Obviously, the result will be the same for both methods. *Case 1* includes an audible signal (*Beep.vi*) that helps to differentiate this method from *Case 0*. *Case 2* also uses a *Formula Node* that performs a different operation on input variable "X." The result is displayed on both a *Digital Indicator* and a *Meter* on the front panel.

To observe how this VI works, insert the number "134.6" into the *Digital Control* labeled "Choose a number (x)." Alternately, select "Method 0" and "Method 1" using the *Dial* on the front panel, and **Run** the VI. Note that a result of "68.3" is returned when either method is selected. When "Method 2" is selected, a result of "284.6" is returned.

SUMMARY

Formula Nodes are used to insert mathematical formulas that may be too complicated or cumbersome to program using LabVIEW icons. Input and output of variables to and from the *Formula Node* are handled by wiring control and indicator functions that are configured on the border of the node.

PRACTICE EXERCISES

Modify **Formula.vi** by adding another *Formula Node* that will ***square the input*** variable, and then subtract "360" from it. Hint: To ***square a number***, use the ∧ symbol. This modification will require that a fourth *Case* be added to the *Case Structure*. Reconfigure the *Dial* on the front panel to handle a fourth operation. To verify that your VI is working properly, confirm that inputting "12.3" returns a value of "-208.7." Depending on the magnitude (and sign) of the result, the *Meter* may have to be numerically ***rescaled***. Call up and/or print out the VI named **Square.vi** from the **CD ROM disk directory** to compare it with the reconfigured VI.

Bring up the VI called **Formnode.vi** from the **CD ROM disk directory.** This is the same VI described in Figure 3–11.1. Move to the block diagram, study the formulas in the *Formula Nodes* in Cases "0" and "1," and confirm that they represent the ***same*** operation. From the front panel, start the VI in continuous **Run** mode, insert several input variables in the *Digital Control*, and note that the ***same value*** appears in both *Digital Indicators*. For example, if the number "2.00" is input, the result is 3.91; if "26.78" is input, the result is "376.65," etc.

OBJECT/FUNCTION OR SUBVI LOCATOR
FORMULA.VI

Panel	Object/Function or SubVI	Palette/Menu or Directory
Front	*Digital Control*	**Controls/Numeric**
	Digital Indicator	**Controls/Numeric**
	Dial	**Controls/Numeric**
	Meter	**Controls/Numeric**
Diagram	*Case Structure*	**Functions/Structures**
	Formula Node × 3	**Functions/Structures**
	Divide	**Functions/Numeric**
	Increment (+1)	**Functions/Numeric**
	Numeric Constant	**Functions/Numeric**
	Beep.vi	**Functions/Graphics & Sound/Sound**

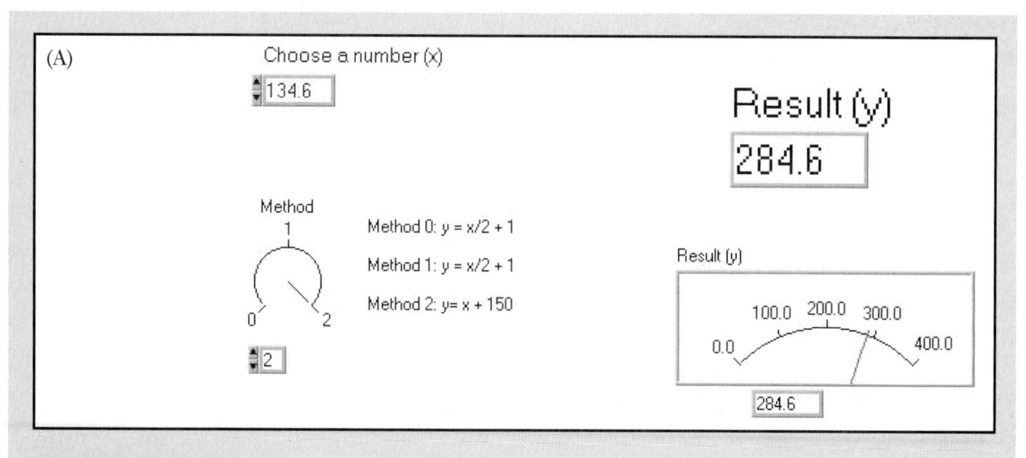

FIGURE 3–11.1
(A) Front panel and (B) block diagram of **Formula.vi.** *Formula Nodes* are used to write conventional mathematical formulae when LabVIEW icons are impractical to use.

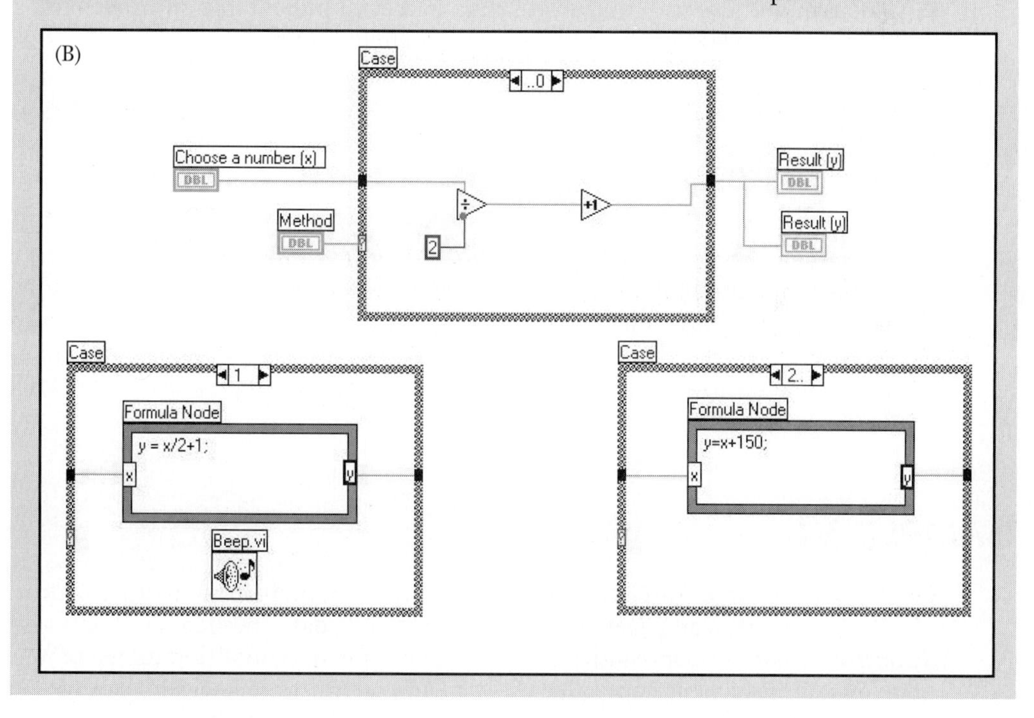

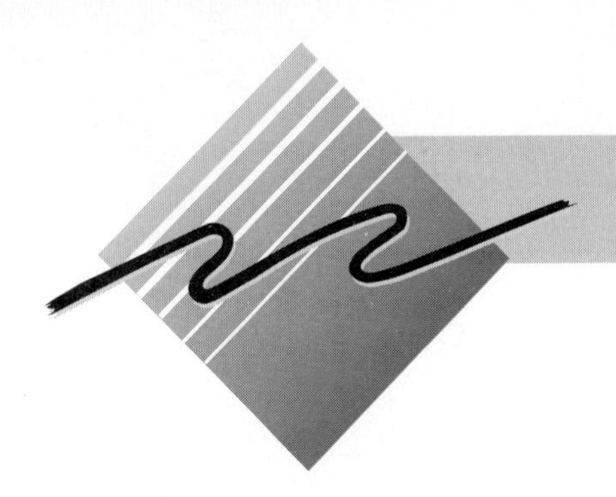

SECTION 3–12

TABLES

OBJECTIVES

- ❖ Construct and use a VI that stores data in a front panel table and saves the same data to a spreadsheet file in a tab-delimited format.

INTRODUCTION

A LabVIEW *Table* is essentially a ***spreadsheet*** inserted into the front panel. The *Table* may be configured to display multiple columns and rows (Figure 3–12.1). When the number of columns or rows physically exceeds the bounds of the table, *Scroll Bars* appear, allowing access to the out-of-view data. *Tables* are configured using *Attribute Nodes*, wired in the block diagram, to apply physical and functional characteristics to the *Table* (number of rows or columns; use of headers; captions, etc.).

SAMPLE VI

Gen3col.vi generates three columns of scaled random numbers and displays them in a *Waveform Graph* and *Table* in the front panel. The data are then saved, in a ***tab-delimited*** format, to a spreadsheet. The number of generations (iterations) of random numbers is variably controlled using a *Dial* on the front panel and displayed in *a Digital Indicator*. The user is given the option of including *Column Headers* in the saved spreadsheet using a *Boolean Labeled Oblong Button* that toggles a *Case Structure*. Pressing the control button to "YES" (i.e., the **true** condition) causes three ***headers*** to be inserted at the top of the three columns in the saved spreadsheet.

Tables are created from the front panel and block diagram. Working first in the front panel, select *Table* from the **Controls/String & Table** palette. Locate and resize the table so that ***three columns*** and ***ten rows*** are visible. Column width may be adjusted by left-clicking and dragging the column border left (narrower) or right (wider) as would be done in most spreadsheet software (Excel™, Quattro Pro™, etc.). Note that no *Scroll Bars* are visible at this time. Place the cursor anywhere on the *Table;* pop-up a menu by right-clicking the mouse, and select *Create/Attribute Node* from the menu choices. Move to the block diagram, and note that an icon (the *Attribute Node*) labeled "Visible" lies next to the *Table* icon. Right-click the lower corner of the *Attribute Node*, and ***expand it down one cell.*** The lower cell just created will be labeled "Disabled." Place the cursor on "Disabled," and right-click. From the menu, choose *Select Item*, and then select *Column Header [ ].* Right-click on the upper cell, and from *Select Item*, choose *Col Headers Vis.* Again, right-click on the upper cell, and select *Create Constant.* Note that a *Boolean Constant* pops up to the left. Using the *Hand Tool*, select the true (T) condition. Create three *String Constants* (these will serve as the column headers for the *Table*) from the **Functions/String** palette, and type in "Random no. 1,2,3," respectively. Wire the three *String Constants* into a *Build Array* function (expand it three levels), and wire its output terminal to the lower cell of the *Attribute Node* (*Column Headers []*).

The ***three sets of random numbers*** will be generated by the **Rxscale.vi** subVI from Section 3–5 and scaled to "5, 15, and 15," respectively, using *Numeric Constants* wired to the terminal on the left side of the icon. In addition to displaying the data on a front panel *Table*, the three sets of random numbers will be saved to a ***tab-delimited spreadsheet*** using the same programming techniques used to construct **Strings3.vi** in Section 3–9, "Strings." Note that the VI gives the user the option of inserting headers into the spreadsheet with the same labels that appear in the *Table.* This option is provided by including a *Sequence Structure* ***inside*** of *a Case Structure* toggled by a front panel *Boolean* button. When the button is pressed to the "YES" (true condition) position before the VI is run, ***headers*** will be saved into a spreadsheet file by the *Write File* function (Figure 3–12.1—block diagram). The ***tabular data*** will then be saved to the spreadsheet file by another *Write File* function and then closed.

Build and save the remainder of the VI into a convenient directory using the filename **Gen3col.vi.** To test the VI, press the "Use Headers in Spreadsheet" button to the "YES" position, set the number of "Iterations" of random numbers to be generated using the *Dial*, and **Run** the VI in the usual manner. At the prompt, select a ***directory,*** and ***name*** the data file **Col3.dat.** When the VI stops running, note that the numbers have been inserted into the front panel *Table* (see Figure 3–12.1). Use the *Scroll Bar* in the *Table* to view data that appear after row 10. Next, using a spreadsheet program, open the saved **(Col3.dat)** data file (Figure 3–12.2) and note that the same columns of random numbers inserted into the front panel *Table* appear in the spreadsheet. Column width may have to be expanded using the click-and-drag method.

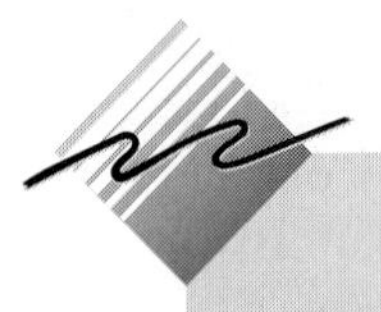

OBJECT/FUNCTION OR SUBVI LOCATOR
GEN3COL.VI

Panel	Object/Function or SubVI	Palette/Menu or Directory
Front	*Waveform Graph*	**Controls/Graph**
	Table	**Controls/String & Table**
	Labeled Oblong Button	**Controls/Boolean**
	Dial	**Controls/Numeric**
	Digital Indicator	**Controls/Numeric**
Diagram	*Case Structure*	**Functions/Structures**
	Sequence Structure	**Functions/Structures**
	Concatenate Strings × 2	**Functions/String**
	String Constant × 6	**Functions/String**
	Tab × 2	**Functions/String**
	End of Line × 2	**Functions/String**
	Open/Create/Replace File.vi	**Functions/File I/O**
	Write File × 2	**Functions/File I/O**
	Close File	**Functions/File I/O**
	Simple Error Handler.vi	**Functions/Time & Dialog**
	Increment (+1)	**Functions/Numeric**
	For Loop	**Functions/Structures**
	Rxscale.vi × 3	**SubVI Library** or **CD ROM disk directory**
	Numeric Constant × 4	**Functions/Numeric**
	To Fractional × 4	**Functions/String/ Additional String to Number Functions**
	Bundle × 2	**Functions/Cluster**
	Build Array × 2	**Functions/Array**
	Boolean Constant	**Functions/Boolean**

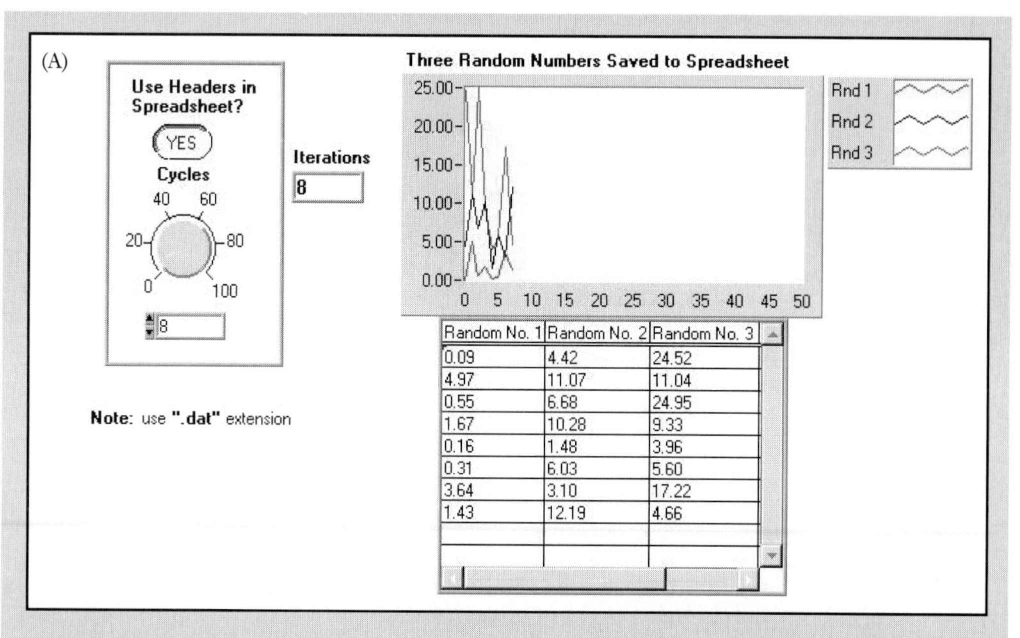

Random No. 1	Random No. 2	Random No. 3
0.09	4.42	24.52
4.97	11.07	11.04
0.55	6.68	24.95
1.67	10.28	9.33
0.16	1.48	3.96
0.31	6.03	5.60
3.64	3.10	17.22
1.43	12.19	4.66

FIGURE 3–12.1
(A) Front panel and (B) block diagram of **Gen3col.vi.** This VI generates three sets of scaled random numbers using the **Rxscale.vi** subVI and plots them in real time on a *Waveform Chart* and three-column *Table* in the front panel.

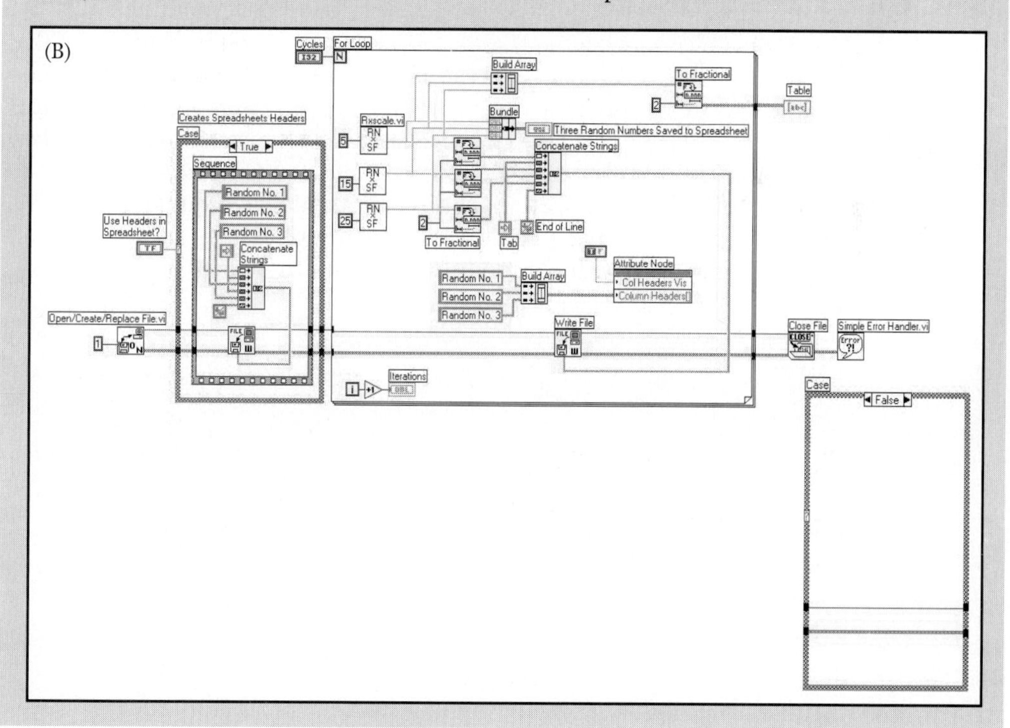

FIGURE 3–12.2
Three columns of data saved by **Gen3col.vi** in spreadsheet format. Note that the data are the same as in the *Table* in Figure 3–11.2.

Random No. 1	Random No. 2	Random No. 3
0.09	4.42	24.52
4.97	11.07	11.04
0.55	6.68	24.95
1.67	10.28	9.33
0.16	1.48	3.96
0.31	6.03	5.6
3.64	3.1	17.22
1.43	12.19	4.66

SUMMARY

Spreadsheets may be inserted into the front panel of VIs as *Tables. Tables* are configured using *Attribute Nodes* that convey physical and functional characteristics. Column and row data that exceed the physical bounds of the *Table* are accessed using *Scroll Bars.*

PRACTICE EXERCISE

Modify **Gen3col.vi** by removing the *Waveform Graph* and expanding the *Table* so that at ***least 20 rows*** are visible. ***Add two more columns of data,*** and ***label*** them "***Random No. 4 and 5,***" respectively. ***Scale*** the random numbers in ***columns 4*** and ***5*** by factors of "1" and "100," respectively. Add the ***same capabilities*** to the saved ***spreadsheet data file.*** Finally, change the ***precision*** of the numbers to ***one decimal place.***

Save the modified VI to a convenient directory, and give it a unique filename. In the **CD ROM directory file** is a VI named **Gen5col.vi.** Call up and/or print out this VI, and compare it with the modified version just created.

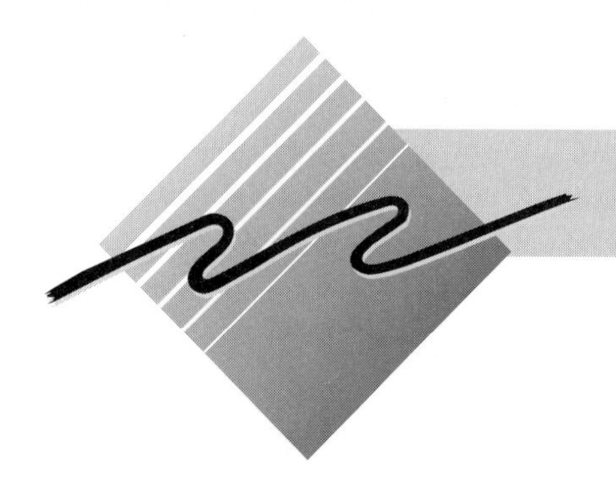

SECTION 3–13

DATA ACQUISITION

OBJECTIVES

- ❖ Understand how physiological signals are represented as electrical output voltages.
- ❖ Understand how output voltages are acquired and converted to digital signals and read by LabVIEW VIs.
- ❖ Understand several hardware options for acquiring data using LabVIEW.
- ❖ Learn how to build a simple interface device for acquiring signals from an isokinetic dynamometer.

INTRODUCTION AND THEORY OF OPERATION

As has been suggested, in some ways LabVIEW may be thought of as a very sensitive and sophisticated ***voltmeter***. ***Analog*** signals from biomechanical or kinesiological measurement devices are first collected by ***sensors,*** then ***amplified*** and ***conditioned,*** and then passed on to a computer for ***digital conversion*** and ultimate use by LabVIEW. The entire process is referred to as ***analog-to-digital*** (i.e., A-to-D) conversion.

Sensors include electrodes, force transducers, probes, strain gauges, and dynamometer input arms. The output voltages of these devices are often very small. For example, electromyographic electrodes measure voltage outputs from muscle as either microvolts or millivolts. As such, these small potentials need to be ***amplified*** and ***conditioned*** (e.g., filtered) before digital conversion. In the case of electromyography, signals are usually amplified by a ***preamplifier*** and again by a ***driver amplifier*** to provide sufficient ***signal gain.*** Signals from other types of sensors such as a force transducer or dynamometer may require only one-stage amplification. ***Signal conditioning*** may be achieved using hardware or software or a combination

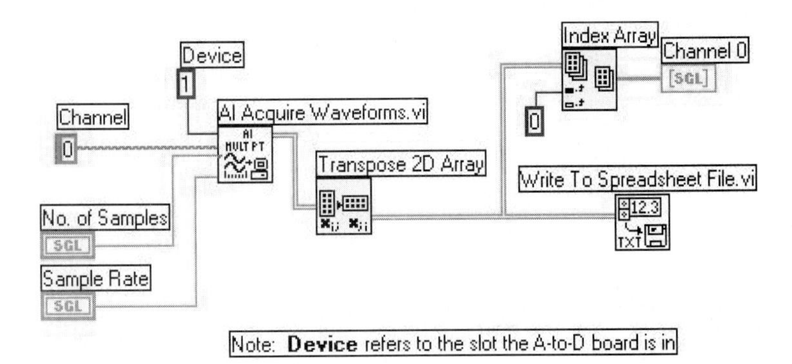

FIGURE 3–13.1
The *AI Acquire Waveforms.vi* subVI is used to acquire multiple channels of data from the computer's A-to-D board. A single channel version of this subVI is also available.

of both. If conditioning is not a hardware option, then LabVIEW may be used for this purpose. For example, in Section 3–6, "More SubVIs," digital filtering using a *Butterworth filter* was discussed, and a software filter was constructed as a subVI to offer lowpass, bandpass, and bandstop filtering options. Many of the VIs described in the sections that follow will include a signal filter.

After signals are amplified, hardware ***interface devices*** are used to acquire these signals and pass them on to a computer for digital conversion by an A-to-D board. Several options for this process will be discussed in the next section. After the signals have been digitized, they are ready to be accessed by LabVIEW functions. Figure 3–13.1 is the block diagram of a simple VI that will acquire multiple channels of data from the computer's A-to-D board. The heart of this VI is the *AI Acquire Waveform.vi* found in the **Data Acquisition/Analog Input** menu from the **Functions** palette. This VI communicates with the computer's A-to-D board and acquires data from a measurement tool (e.g., the torque channel of a dynamometer). A single channel version of this VI is also available. Note that there are terminals that may be wired to block diagram digital and string constants (e.g., "Device"—slot number in the computer—and "Channel") or front panel digital controls (e.g., "No. of Samples" and "Sample Rate"). The acquired signal is then output to a *Waveform Graph* and stored in spreadsheet format using the *Write to Spreadsheet File.vi.* This code will be used to construct a two-channel version of this VI called **Write2ch.vi** in Section 3–14, "Writing and Reading Data."

HARDWARE OPTIONS AND SETUP

The hardware setup used to collect data by VIs written for this book is one of several common configurations used in research laboratories. This discussion is not intended to be a comprehensive review of all data acquisition hardware options but rather to provide a practical guide to hardware selection that will permit the first-time user of LabVIEW to begin collecting and analyzing data. Hardware choice is

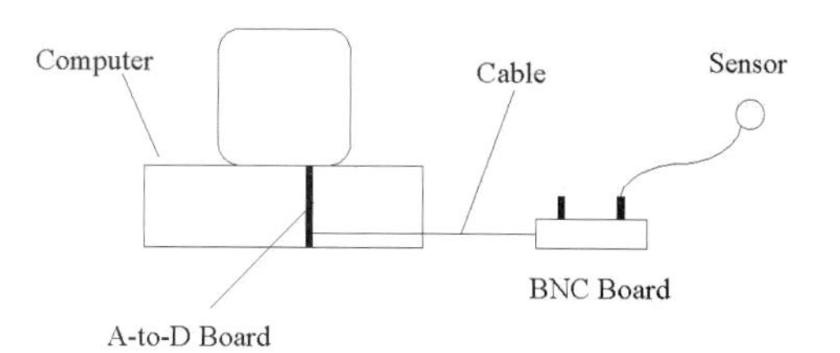

FIGURE 3–13.2 Hardware connections between the computer's A-to-D board, a BNC interface board, and a sensor.

a matter of matching specific devices to experimental needs, which are obviously varied and numerous. I recommend that the reader consult with technical support and sales representatives for the specific hardware being used to ensure compatibility. An enormous number of sensors and signal conditioning options are provided by many companies that produce electronic instrumentation. Thus, the user is not limited to equipment produced by a single proprietary provider. Using hardware from the National Instruments Corporation does offer the advantage of ensuring software and hardware compatibility. On the other hand, many other sensors and signal conditioning systems made by other suppliers may be considered for data collection, many of which are supported (i.e., instrument drivers are provided) by National Instruments.

National Instruments Corporation offers a wide variety of plug-in **data acquisition** (DAQ) boards (i.e., A-to-D boards) for a number of platforms including Windows, Macintosh, and Sun workstations. Boards manufactured by other companies may also be suitable. For this book, the "AT-MIO-16E-10 multifunction I/O" board for Windows NT/95/3.1 was used (Figure 3–13.2). This board offers 16 channels using 12-bit resolution with trigger capability and a total sampling rate of 110,000 Hz. All instruments and sensors used to make measurements output their amplified/conditioned signals via standard BNC connectors and coaxial cables. Data input to the DAQ board was via a "BNC-2080" adapter interface board and was connected with a 68-pin cable. "NI-DAQ™ v6.5.1" software was used to configure the DAQ board. This board has Windows "plug and play" capability, making board configuration relatively easy. The DAQ board is automatically detected by the computer, and a Windows setup Wizard guides the user through several setup procedures assigning device numbers and channel interrupts (IRQs). Manual setup is also available for experienced users with unique hardware configurations.

While the hardware described here is commonly used for data collection, National Instruments Corporation offers alternate hardware configurations including "Signal Conditioning for eXtensions for Instrumentation" (SCXI™) systems. In this system, sensor-specific ***terminal blocks*** attach to ***signal conditioning modules*** which in turn slide into a multislotted "chassis" (Figure 3–13.3). SCXI™ systems offer a number of input options to the computer including A-to-D boards (see preceding description) and serial and parallel port connections. Connections to laptop computers are also possible via a credit-card–sized "Personal Computer

FIGURE 3–13.3
An alternate hardware setup for data acquisition using an SCXI chassis and signal-conditioning modules.

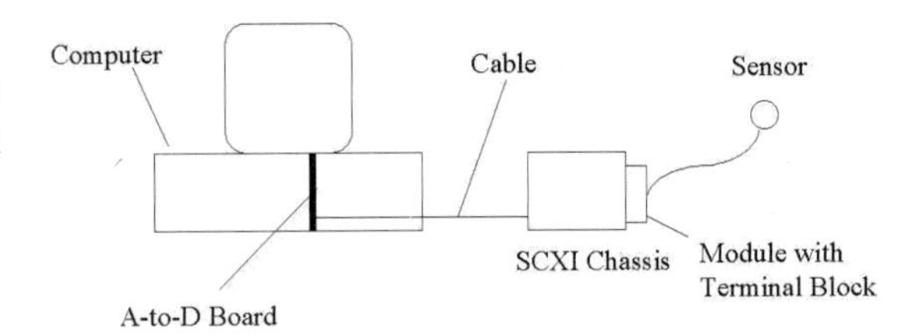

Memory Card International Association" (PCMCIA) expansion card permitting a greater degree of portability than with conventional desktop computers.

A DO-IT-YOURSELF DATA ACQUISITION INTERFACE DEVICE

Measurement devices often use proprietary technology to acquire and process data and may not provide a means of exporting the signal or data to LabVIEW. In such cases, it may be necessary to construct a custom ***interface device.*** What follows is a description of a device used to acquire torque and angle data from an isokinetic dynamometer. The interface was constructed of commonly found components that are readily available from electronics parts suppliers. Obviously, the design and construction of the device will vary depending on the specific dynamometer being used.

In this case, the dynamometer had a ***diagnostic multipinned signal output port*** (37-pin D-sub connector) included in the back panel of the device-controller unit. The port is used by service technicians to test hardware and software functions. The technician's diagnostic computer is plugged into this port. If an output port is not included, the device-controller's case will need to be opened and the appropriate terminal connectors identified. This obviously requires some experience with electronics components and should only be attempted by those individuals who have a working knowledge of electronics/computer circuitry.

Of the 37 pins provided on the terminal connector, 3 are of particular importance and include the pins for the ***torque*** and ***angle channels*** and a ***ground.*** In many cases, the ***pin-outs*** will be described in technical manuals provided with the device. If this information is not available, technical support departments may be willing to provide this information. If this is not the case, pin-outs may be determined using a voltmeter. While an assistant manually operates the input arm of the dynamometer, touch the voltmeter's positive terminal to each terminal pin. A positive voltage indicates that the pins being tested are used for the torque and angle channels. It may not be immediately obvious which of the pins provides the torque signal and which provides the angle signal. After data are collected using LabVIEW VIs (see Section 3–14, "Writing and Reading Data"), it will become obvi-

On the front panel, the user may control the ***sampling rate*** (default = "1000 Hz") and the ***number of samples*** collected. In the example in Figure 3–14.1, ***6000 samples*** will be acquired at a ***sampling rate of 1000 Hz.*** Thus, 6 seconds of data will be collected and saved.

When the VI is **Run,** a dialog window prompts the user for a ***filename*** and ***directory.*** It's a good idea to append a **.dat** (for ***data file***) extension to the filename.

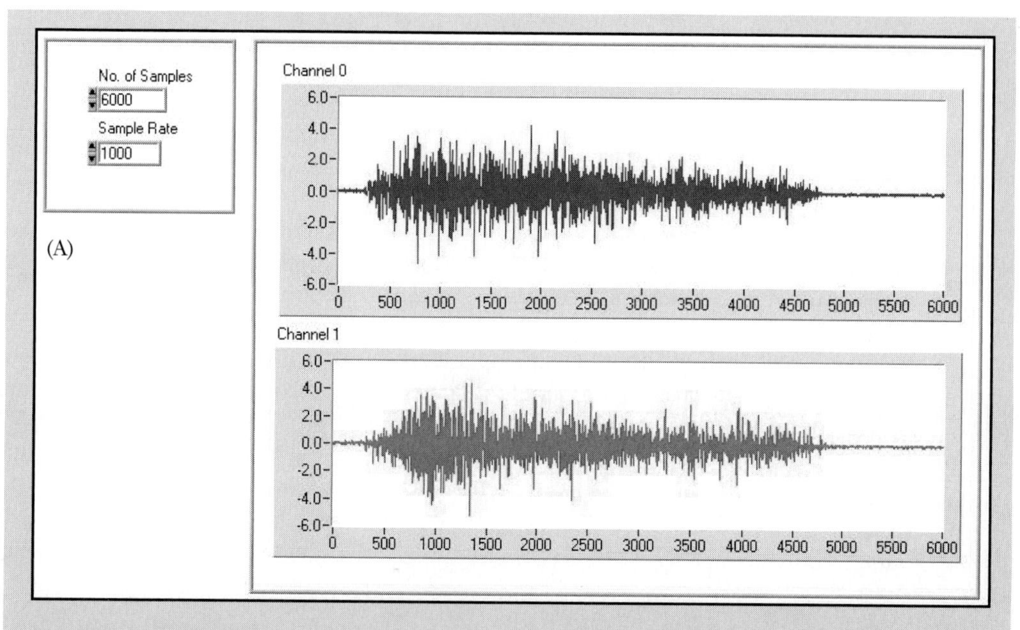

FIGURE 3–14.1
(A) Front panel and (B) block diagram of **Write2ch.vi** used to acquire two channels of data from the computer's A-to-D board using the *AI Acquire Waveforms.vi* subVI. In this case, two channels of EMG data are acquired and displayed on a front panel *Waveform Graph* and saved in spreadsheet format.

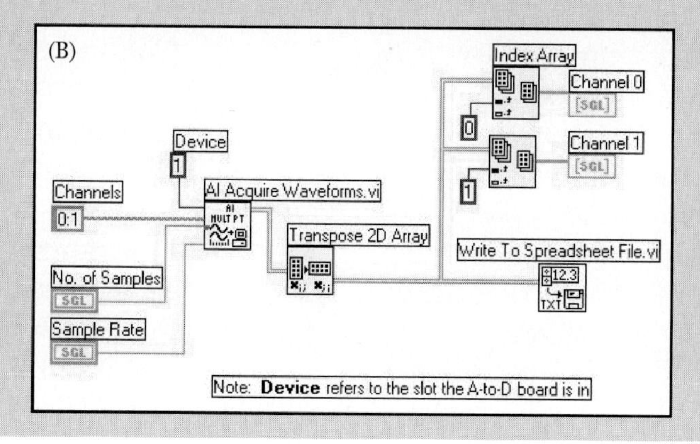

This will help to differentiate data from executable files (i.e., with **.com** or **.exe** extensions), especially if both types of files are saved and mixed in the same directory.

READING DATA IN SPREADSHEET FORMAT

The data that were saved to disk using **Write2ch.vi** may be displayed using the VI called **Read2ch.vi** (Figure 3–14.2). Write or call up this VI from the **CD ROM disk directory.** In addition to displaying the saved data on two *Waveform Graphs*, the user has the option of filtering the signals using the **Filter.vi** subVI that was constructed in Section 3–6, "More SubVIs." Recall that **Filter.vi** permits the on/off toggling of a *Butterworth filter* that can be set as a ***lowpass, bandpass,*** or ***bandstop*** filter. Filter selection is achieved using a *Dial* on the front panel.

In the block diagram, note that a file is selected for display and filtering using the *Read From Spreadsheet File.vi* function. The thick (orange) multiple-array wire leading from *Read From Spreadsheet File.vi* contains ***both*** channels of saved data. Two *Index Array* functions divide off each channel of data, sending the respective signals to the **Filters.vi** subVI. The data are, in turn, ported to *Waveform Graphs* for display on the front panel. **Save** this VI to a convenient directory using the **Write2ch.vi** filename.

OBJECT/FUNCTION OR SUBVI LOCATOR
READ2CH.VI

Panel	Object/Function or SubVI	Palette/Menu or Directory
Front	*Digital Control* × 2	**Controls/Numeric**
	Dial	**Controls/Numeric**
	Boolean Vertical Toggle Switch	**Controls/Boolean**
	Waveform Graph × 2	**Controls/Graph**
	Recessed Frame × 2	**Controls/Decorations**
Diagram	*Read From Spreadsheet File.vi*	**Functions/File I/O**
	Index Array × 2	**Functions/Array**
	Numeric Constant × 2	**Functions/Numeric**
	Filters.vi	**SubVI Library or CD ROM disk directory**

If the computer being used for this exercise is configured with an A-to-D board, practice collecting and saving two channels of data using **Write2ch.vi.** Remember to save the file using a **.dat** extension. Next, call up and display the data using **Read2ch.vi.** Rerun the VI several times using various filtering options. If your

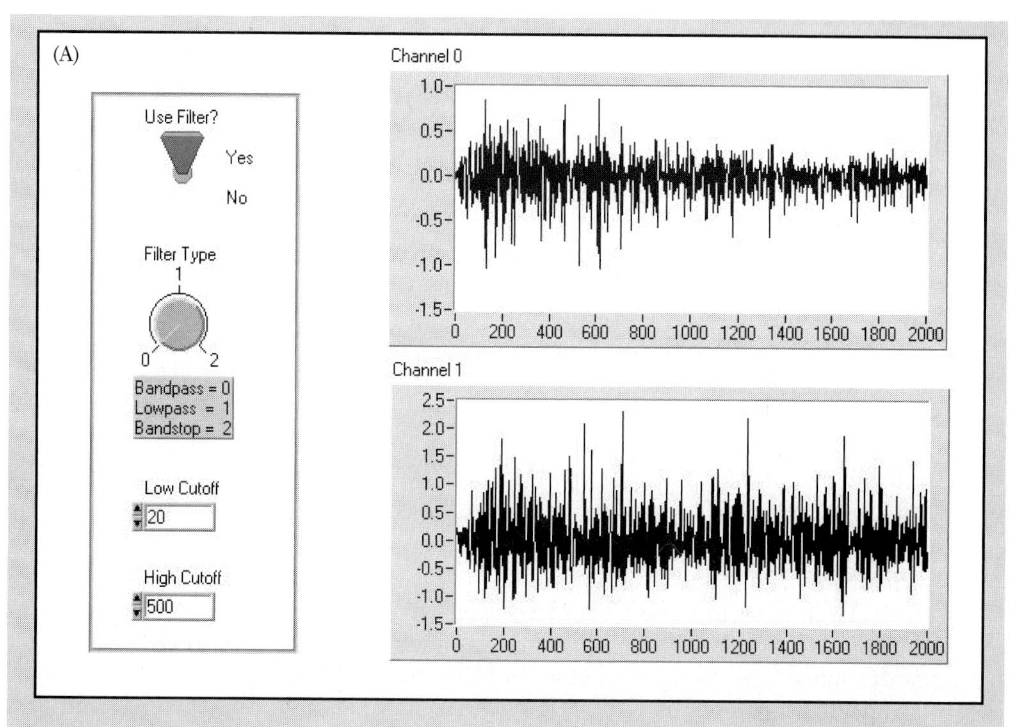

FIGURE 3–14.2
(A) Front panel and (B) block diagram of **Read2.ch.vi.** This VI reads two channels of previously saved data in spreadsheet format using the *Read From Spreadsheet File.vi* subVI in the block diagram and displays it in two front panel *Waveform Graphs.*

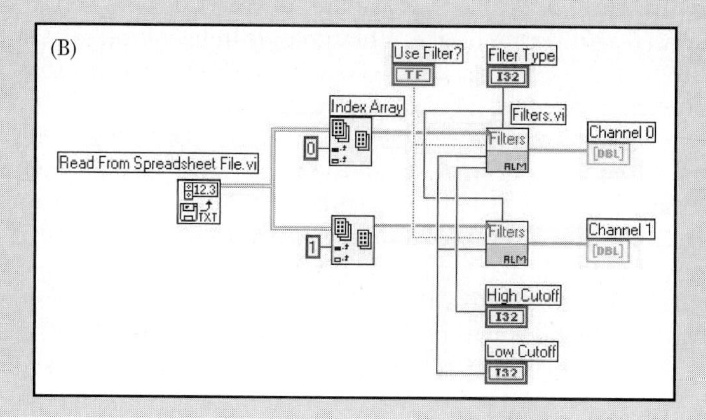

computer does not have an A-to-D board, confirm that the **Read2ch.vi** operates properly using one of the two channel sample data files (e.g., **EMGx22s.dat**).

SUMMARY

Data collected from sensors are acquired and digitized by the computer's A-to-D board and may be saved, conditioned, and displayed by LabVIEW using either a ***tab-delimited spreadsheet*** or ***binary*** file format. VIs that save data as a ***tab-delimited*** spreadsheet file are generally less complicated to program and offer the added advantage of porting data to most spreadsheet packages. Saving and processing data using ***binary*** format is inherently more efficient, and while more complicated in terms of programming structure, uses less hard drive storage space. Saving data in ***binary*** format should be considered when data will be collected for relatively long periods of time. Two VIs used to write (save) and read data in ***tab-delimited*** spreadsheet format were discussed.

PRACTICE EXERCISES

Using **Read2ch.vi** as a template, add a third channel to this VI to give it the capability of reading and displaying three data sets at one time. Note that in **Read2ch.vi** data were displayed as ***volts.*** Using the **Disvolts.vi** subVI described in Section 3–6, "More SubVIs," add the ability to display data as ***volts, millivolts,*** or ***microvolts.*** If this subVI is not built, it is available in the **CD ROM disk directory.** To confirm that the VI is wired properly and will run, use the data file called **3Chan.dat.** ***Channel 0*** is an ***isometric torque curve,*** and ***channels 1*** and ***2*** are ***EMG*** signals. All were saved at a ***sampling rate*** of "1000 Hz" for 8 seconds. Call up and/or print out **Read3ch.vi** from the **CD ROM disk directory,** and compare it with the VI just revised.

As an introduction to VIs that read data in ***binary*** format, open the VI called **Hread.vi** from the **CD ROM disk directory.** This VI displays and measures ***M-wave*** and ***H-reflex*** amplitudes. ***H-reflexes*** are elicited by stimulating nerves, leading from muscle spindles and proceeding toward the spinal cord, with a galvanic stimulator. ***H-reflexes*** are used as a physiologic index of the excitability of neurons (i.e., motoneurons) exiting the spinal cord. Two EMG waveforms are elicited during this testing procedure: (1) An ***M-wave,*** the result of direct muscle stimulation, is always elicited ***first,*** followed by (2) an ***H-reflex*** (Figure 3–14.3). The time between the two waveforms varies with the nerve/muscle being studied.

Hread.vi (Figure 3–14.3) was constructed using a National Instruments VI as a template in the **Examples Library.** Open this file from the **CD ROM disk directory,** and switch to the block diagram. The code in the upper right corner of the *While Loop* was added to the original VI. Several modifications to the front panel were also made including a *Digital Indicator* to display the "Maximal Amplitude" of the waveforms being studied and a "Scale Factor" to ***reverse polarity*** of

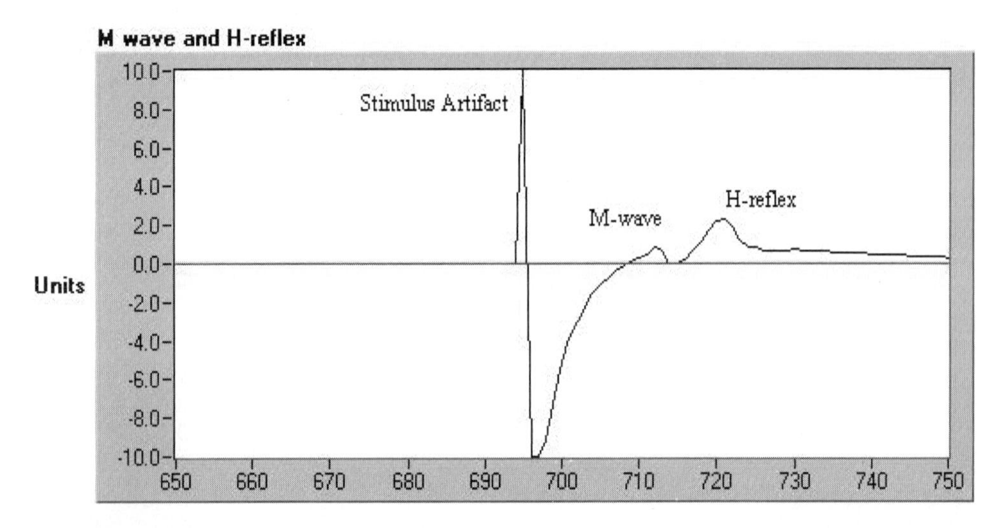

FIGURE 3–14.3
Waveform Graph used to display an M-wave and H-reflex. The first spike is a stimulus artifact documenting when an electrical stimulus is applied to a nerve.

the signal. By default, the VI will read 1000 data points (i.e., "scans") at a time. Each block of 1000 data points is advanced using the "SHOW NEXT" button. ***String data*** such as ***data filename***, the ***sampling rate***, and ***stimulator parameters*** are displayed in a *String Indicator* called "User Header" in the lower left corner.

Review the front panel and block diagram as an introduction to ***binary*** format programming. To use the VI, left-click the **Run** arrow, and a dialog window will prompt you for a data file. In the **CD ROM disk directory** is a file called **Hreflex.bin.** Highlight this file, and press the **Open** button. Note that the first visible set of waveforms will start approximately ***6000*** data points (msec) from the beginning of the file. Advance the signal by pressing the "SHOW NEXT" button under the graph with the *Hand Tool* **6** times until a complex waveform appears.

Note that the waveforms appear ***compressed.*** To ***elongate*** the waveform, swipe the *Lettering Tool* over the ***zero*** point on the ***x-axis*** of the graph, and type "600." Swipe over point "999" (last on right), type in "750," and press the Enter key. This has the effect of ***zooming-in*** on the signal and separating the waveforms for visual inspection (see Figure 3–14.3). The ***first*** sharp upward deflection is the ***stimulus artifact*** (i.e., the point when the muscle is activated with a galvanic stimulator.) The ***second*** upward deflection is the ***M-wave,*** and the ***third*** is the ***H-reflex.*** Continue to cycle through the remainder of the signal by left-clicking on the "SHOW NEXT" button until an "End of File" message appears in the lower right corner of the screen just above the "# of Scans Read from File" *Digital Indicator.* Note that "106000" scans will have been read.

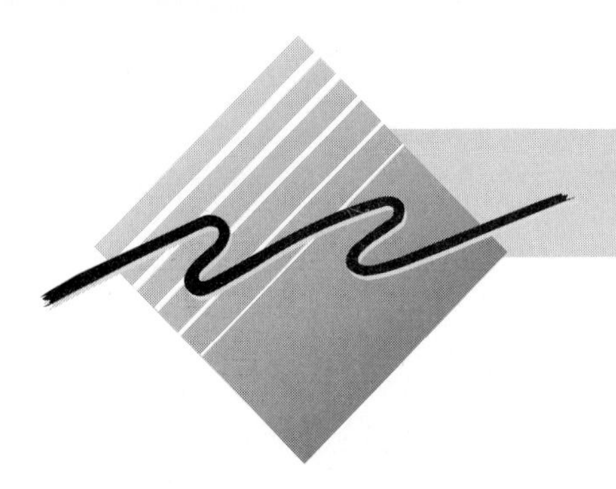

SECTION 3–15

ELECTROMYOGRAPHY

OBJECTIVES

- ❖ Write a VI that collects four channels of EMG data.
- ❖ Write a VI that filters EMG data and computes the maximal integral of a variably selected segment of the signal.
- ❖ Write a two-channel VI that computes the maximal integral of EMG signals.
- ❖ Write a VI that normalizes two channels of EMG data against a predetermined maximal contraction.
- ❖ Write a VI that rectifies and bandpass filters an EMG signal and calculates the median and mean power frequencies.
- ❖ Write a two-channel VI that calculates the median and mean power frequencies.

INTRODUCTION

Electromyographic (EMG) analysis has been a mainstay of kinesiological study for the past 50 years. Originally, EMG was used to document the ***on/off*** phenomenon during normal and abnormal movement patterns. For example, one would expect a burst of electrical activity in the quadriceps femoris during normal walking at a self-selected pace in the interim between heel-strike and foot-flat. The quadriceps eccentrically guides the knee into 20° of flexion, to absorb the impact of the forward and downward momentum of the body. A second burst is seen during push-off to prevent the knee from collapsing into flexion as the path of the ground reaction force moves behind the knee, creating a flexion moment.

Electromyography has also been used to ***quantify*** muscle activity. For example, there is an approximate linear relationship between muscle force output and EMG activity during ***isometric*** contractions. Quantification of the EMG signal involves ***full-wave rectification*** (i.e., adding the negative deflection of the signal to the positive signal and displaying it on one side of the baseline) and ***integrating*** the signal by quantifying the ***area under the curve.*** This makes successive contractions comparable to one another. More recently, EMG has been used to study ***fatigue characteristics*** of muscle fiber types (e.g., Type I, tonic/slow twitch or Type II, phasic/fast twitch). The method commonly employed is a ***power spectral analysis*** of muscle fibers' frequency of firing. For example, during a sustained fatiguing contraction, Type II fibers' (less endurant relying on anaerobic metabolic pathways) firing frequency would be expected to decrease before the more endurant Type I fibers, causing a ***spectral shift to the left.*** The ***mean*** or ***median power frequency*** would be expected to decrease concurrently.

Following are a number of VIs built to measure EMG activity that employ the measurement characteristics just described. All VIs and subVIs may be found in the **CD ROM disk directory.**

4CHANEMG.VI

4Chanemg.vi is fundamentally a four-channel version of **Write2ch.vi** described in Section 3–14 "Writing and Reading Data." Write or call up this VI from the **CD ROM disk directory.** Use **Write2ch.vi** as a template, and ***add*** two channels. **4Chanemg.vi** (Figure 3–15.1) collects four channels of EMG data from the computer's analog-to-digital (A-to-D) board for a ***specified time period*** at a ***predetermined sampling rate.*** Once the data are collected, the raw signals are displayed on four *Waveform Graphs*, and the data are saved in a ***spreadsheet format*** using a filename and directory of the user's choosing.

Before running the VI, the user specifies the ***sampling rate*** and ***number of samples*** to be collected in two *Digital Controls.* The ***default*** settings are a sample rate of "1000" for "2000" samples. In other words, 2 seconds of data will be collected. Values in both controls may be changed using the *Hand Tool* by clicking on the up (increase) or down (decrease) controller arrows. Or, using the *Lettering Tool,* left-click on the control, and edit the values.

At the top of the front panel are *String* and *Numeric* controls labeled "Channels" and "Device Number," respectively. The "Channels" control defaults to "0:3," meaning that data from channels 0 through 3 will be collected. The "Device" control defaults to "1" in this case. The "Device" number refers to the slot number inside the computer that the A-to-D converter occupies. Channel and device control may also be handled in the block diagram by wiring *String* and *Numeric Constants* to their respective terminals on the *AI Acquire Waveforms.vi* subVI that acquires the signal from the A-to-D board. If only a single LabVIEW device is installed, the "Device number" will never change, and so it may be more logical to handle this in the block diagram with *Constants,* especially if front panel space is limited. The same is true of the "Channel" *String Control.*

In this VI, all three *Numeric Controls* deal with parameters that are logically recognized as ***integers.*** That is, it is inappropriate to describe these values (e.g., number of sample, sample rate, and device number) as less than whole numbers. To change the numeric content of each control to integers, right-click the cursor on the control, and choose the *Representation/I32* menu option. When the cursor is released, values will change to integers. Also note, on the block diagram, the icon representing a *Numeric Control* has changed to a ***blue*** color and has the label "I32" inside of it.

The heart of this VI in the block diagram is the *AI Acquire Waveform.vi* subVI that is the communications link between the A-to-D board in the computer and the data collection VI. Note that input terminals on the ***left*** of the subVI are provided for the "device (number)," "channels," "number of samples," and "scan (sampling) rate" controls. A single *2D* (multiple channel) *Array* wire connects to a terminal on the ***right*** (output) side. An *Index Array* function selects each data channel from the array and displays it on *Waveform Graphs* on the front panel. Simultaneously, the data will be saved in ***spreadsheet format*** by the **Write File.vi** subVI.

FILT&INT.VI

Raw physiological signals often need to be quantified so that direct comparisons may be made either between successive trials of an activity or between subjects. ***Integration*** permits a segment of a signal to be quantified and involves ***measurement***

OBJECT/FUNCTION OR SUBVI LOCATOR
4CHANEMG.VI

Panel	Object/Function or SubVI	Palette/Menu or Directory
Front	*Digital Control ×4*	**Controls/Numeric**
	String Control	**Controls/String & Table**
	Waveform Graph × 4	**Controls/Graph**
Diagram	*AI Acquire Waveforms.vi*	**Functions/Data Acquisition/Analog Input**
	Index Array × 4	**Functions/Array**
	Numeric Constant × 4	**Functions/Numeric**
	Transpose 2D Array	**Functions/Array**
	Open/Create/Replace File.vi	**Functions/File I/O**
	Write File	**Functions/File I/O**
	Close File	**Functions/File I/O**
	Simple Error Handler.vi	**Functions/Time & Dialog**
	String Constant	**Functions/String**

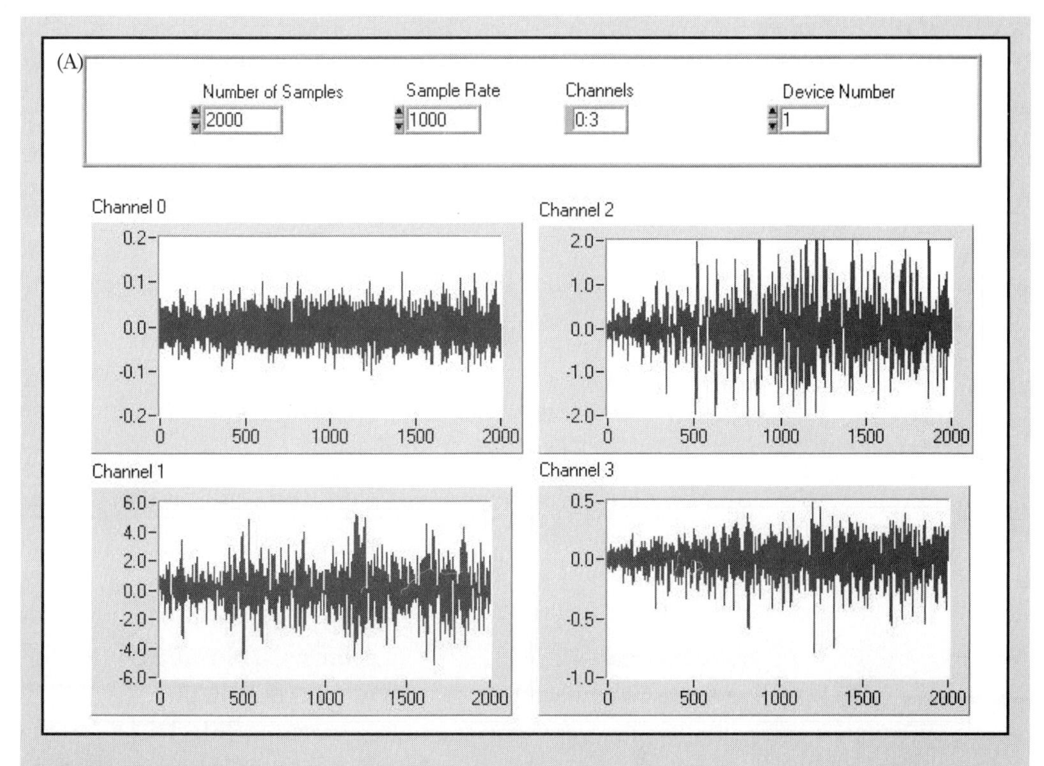

FIGURE 3–15.1
(A) Front panel and (B) block diagram of **4Chanemg.vi.** This VI acquires four channels of EMG data from the computer's A-to-D board and saves the data to disk using the *Write File* and related functions in the block diagram. Note that this is essentially a four-channel version of **Write2ch.vi** (see Figure 3–14.1).

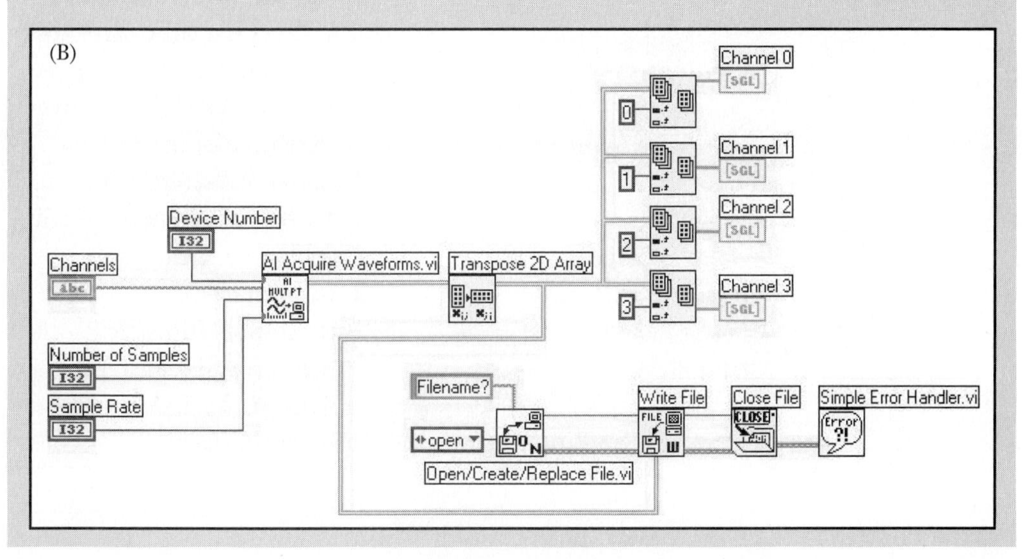

of the area under a curve. Once the segment has been assigned a numerical value, the data may be compared with other similarly treated data, or it may be submitted to some type of statistical manipulation. EMG signals are often quantified using various ***integration algorithms.*** Typically, the signal is first ***rectified*** and ***filtered,*** and then the segment of the signal of interest is ***integrated.*** **Filt&int.vi** is a VI that performs these operations on a single channel of data and then ***computes*** and ***graphs*** the ***integral*** on the front panel (Figure 3–15.2).

OBJECT/FUNCTION OR SUBVI LOCATOR
FILT&INT.VI

Panel	Object/Function or SubVI	Palette/Menu or Directory
Front	*Labeled Oblong Button*	**Controls/Boolean**
	Digital Control × 3	**Controls/Numeric**
	Digital Indicator × 2	**Controls/Numeric**
	Vertical Pointer Slide	**Controls/Numeric**
	Waveform Graph × 4	**Controls/Graph**
Diagram	*Read From Spreadsheet.vi*	**Functions/File I/O**
	Positive Infinity	**Functions/Numeric/ Additional Numeric Constants**
	Index Array	**Functions/Array**
	Disvolts.vi	**Functions/Select a VI . . . / CD ROM disk directory**
	Segment.vi	**Functions/Select a VI . . . / CD ROM disk directory**
	Boolean Constant	**Functions/Boolean**
	Filters.vi	**Functions/Select a VI . . . / CD ROM disk directory**
	Numeric Constant × 9	**Functions/Numeric**
	Array Size	**Functions/Array**
	Absolute Value	**Functions/Numeric**
	Integrl2.vi	**Functions/Select a VI . . . / CD ROM disk directory**
	Array Max & Min	**Functions/Array**

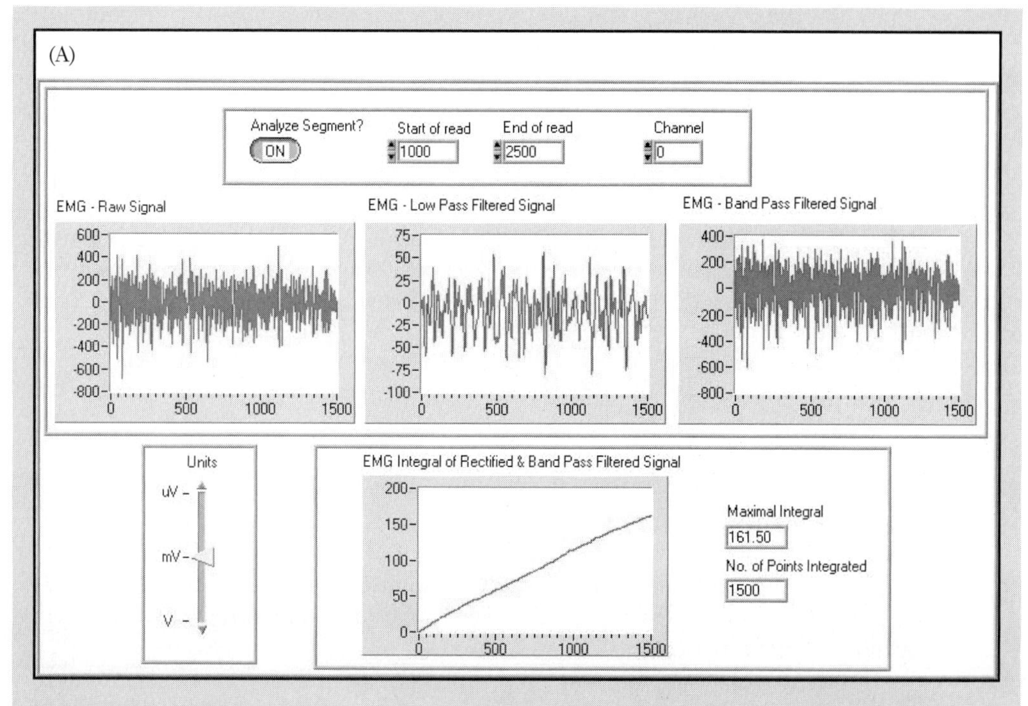

FIGURE 3–15.2
(A) Front panel and (B) block diagram of **Filt&int.vi.** This VI reads a previously saved EMG file and filters and integrates it. The raw and filtered signals and its integral are plotted on four *Waveform Graphs* in the front panel.

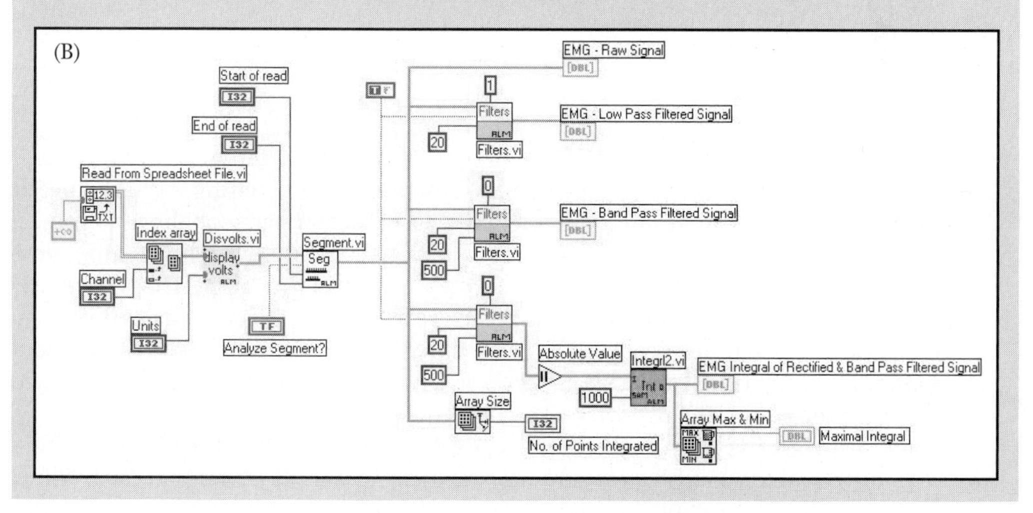

When the VI is **Run,** the *Read From Spreadsheet File.vi* subVI prompts for a data filename. The user has the option of displaying the signal as ***millivolts*** (default), ***microvolts,*** or ***volts*** using the **Disvolts.vi** subVI in the block diagram. The **Segment.vi** subVI provides the option of displaying a portion of the complete signal by inputting the "Start" and "End" values of the segment in two front panel *Digital Controls.* The **Filters.vi** subVI is used to create lowpass (20-Hz cutoff) and highpass filters (20-Hz low cutoff and 500-Hz high cutoffs). Raw and filtered signals are displayed on three front panel *Waveform Graphs.* The ***maximal integral*** is calculated using a ***bandpass filtered*** and ***rectified*** signal and displayed in a front panel *Digital Indicator.* The ***maximal integral*** is also graphed on a fourth *Waveform Graph.*

IEMGX2.VI

Iemgx2.vi (Figure 3–15.3) is essentially a two-channel version of **Filt&int.vi.** On the front panel, two *Waveform Graphs* are used to display each EMG channel. The upper graph displays the complete ***raw*** signal, and the lower graph uses a ***bandpass-filtered*** and ***-rectified*** signal to compute the ***maximal integral,*** which is displayed in a *Digital Indicator.*

On the block diagram, note that, since the *Read From Spreadsheet.vi* subVI reads an array of data with two channels, two *Index Array* functions—configured to read channels "0" and "1," respectively—with *Numeric Constants,* are used to partition each signal from the array.

NORMALX2.VI

During between-subjects comparisons, certain measurement parameters are context sensitive and only make sense when the parameter is referenced to a measurement that is common among all subjects. ***Normalization,*** stating one measure as a function of another, permits valid between subjects comparisons. For example, if the height of a step is measured as a foot is lifted (e.g., while ascending a step), ***normalization*** might be used to standardize step height so that all persons of varying height, leg length, or some other measure related to a person's physical stature, could be compared. Typically, the ***measurement parameter is divided by the normalizing measure.*** The resultant ***ratio*** is then used as a dependent measure to compare the status or function of one person against others in the same study.

Normalx2.vi (Figure 3–15.4) is a VI used to ***normalize*** EMG signals from two muscles during ***submaximal isometric*** contractions. The value against which these signals are normalized is a ***maximal isometric*** contraction.

In the front panel, each EMG channel displays the raw signal in the ***top*** *Waveform Graph* and the ***rectified*** and ***bandpass filtered*** signal in the ***lower*** graph. In the lower left corner are two *Digital Indicators* displaying the "Max(imal)" and "Normalized Integral," respectively. Before running the VI, the user inputs "Max(imal)" voluntary contraction ("MVC") integrals into two *Digital Controls* in the lower left corner of the front panel. These values would already have been determined using another VI such as **Iemgx2.vi** (see preceding discussion).

SPEC.VI

Spec.vi (Figure 3–15.5) uses a ***Fast Fourier Transform*** procedure to convert ***time domain*** EMG signals into ***frequency domain*** data using a previously saved data file. Four *Waveform Graphs* on the front panel display the ***raw*** and ***conditioned*** signal. The ***two top*** graphs show the ***raw*** and ***bandpass filtered*** and ***rectified*** signals, respectively. The ***largest*** graph displays the ***power spectrum*** of the signal, while the ***fourth*** graph shows the ***integrated spectrum*** of frequencies. A *Digital Indicator* to the left displays the "Max(imal) Integral." Four *Digital Indicators* report the "Median," "Mean Power Frequencies," "Est(imated) Peak Frequency," and "Est(imated) Peak Power," respectively.

The main component of this VI is the **Powspec.vi** subVI, which uses a number of National Instruments' spectral analysis subVIs to compute and display the power spectrum (see "Practice Exercises," later).

PSPECX2.VI

Pspecx2.vi (Figure 3–15.6) uses a two-frame *Sequence Structure*—again using the **Powspec.vi** subVI—to compute and plot the ***power spectrum*** of two data sets on two front panel *Waveform Graphs.* "Median" and "Mean Power" frequencies are also computed and displayed in *Digital Indicators.* The plots and data in Figure 3–15.6 are from the biceps brachii during a fatigue experiment involving the elbow flexors. The data in "Power Spectrum 0" represent the ***prefatigue*** condition. The subject was then given a fatiguing exercise using a weight and did elbow flexion exercises until exhaustion. Immediately afterward, an EMG from the biceps was recorded, and a second analysis ("Power Spectrum 1") was ***compared*** with the ***prefatigue*** condition.

Muscle fatigue manifests as a reduction in firing of fast-twitch (Type II—phasic), high-frequency motor units. Accordingly, after fatigue the ***mean*** or ***median power frequency*** should ***decrease,*** reflecting a shift in use to more endurant (Type I—tonic), lower frequency units. In Figure 3–15.6, note that ***mean*** and ***median***

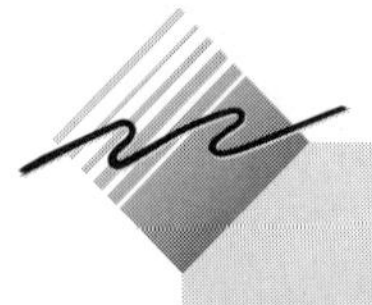

OBJECT/FUNCTION OR SUBVI LOCATOR
IEMGX2.VI

Panel	Object/Function or SubVI	Palette/Menu or Directory
Front	*Dial*	**Controls/Numeric**
	Digital Control	**Controls/Numeric**
	Digital Indicator × 2	**Controls/Numeric**
	Waveform Graph × 4	**Controls/Graph**
Diagram	*Read From Spreadsheet File.vi*	**Functions/File I/O**
	Positive Infinity	**Functions/Numeric/ Additional Numeric Constants**
	Index Array × 2	**Functions/Array**
	Numeric Constant × 2	**Functions/Numeric**
	Disvolts.vi × 2	**Functions/Select a VI . . . / CD ROM disk directory**
	Bpass.vi × 2	**Functions/Select a VI . . . / CD ROM disk directory**
	Absolute Value × 2	**Functions/Numeric**
	Integrl2.vi	**Functions/Select a VI . . . / CD ROM disk directory**
	Array Max & Min	**Functions/Array**

power frequencies decreased in the ***fatigued*** vs. ***prefatigue*** conditions. Note also a visual ***shift-to-the-left*** in ***the overall pattern*** in the lower (fatigue condition) graph, again reflecting a decrease in firing of higher frequency units.

SUMMARY

Several VIs were constructed that save multiple channels of EMG to disk in a ***spreadsheet format*** and process the saved signals. Two VIs demonstrated basic ***filtering*** and ***integration*** procedures, while a third ***normalized*** integrated EMG signals to a predetermined maximal value. The last VIs in this chapter demonstrated basic single and two-channel ***power spectral*** analysis procedures where the power spectra were displayed on graphs and the ***median*** and ***mean*** power frequencies were computed.

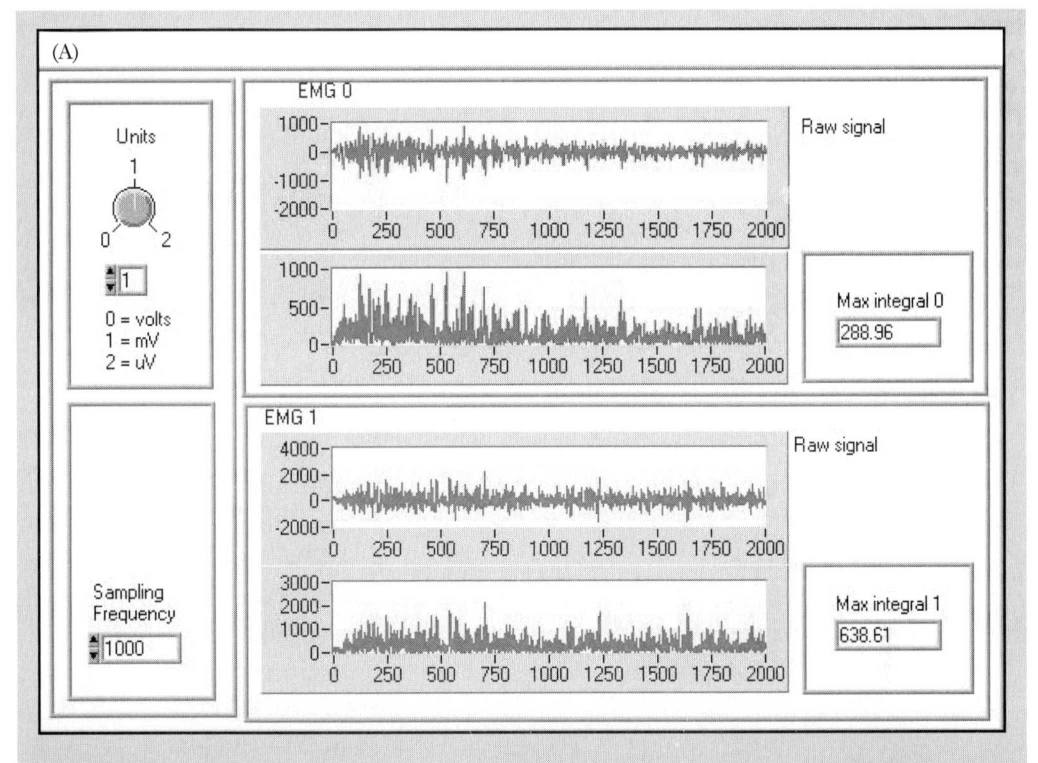

FIGURE 3–15.3
(A) Front panel and (B) block diagram of **Iemgx2.vi.** This VI reads a previously saved file with two EMG channels and integrates them after being bandpass filtered. The raw and rectified signals for each channel are plotted on front panel *Waveform Graphs*, and the maximal integrals for each channel are displayed in *Digital Indicators*.

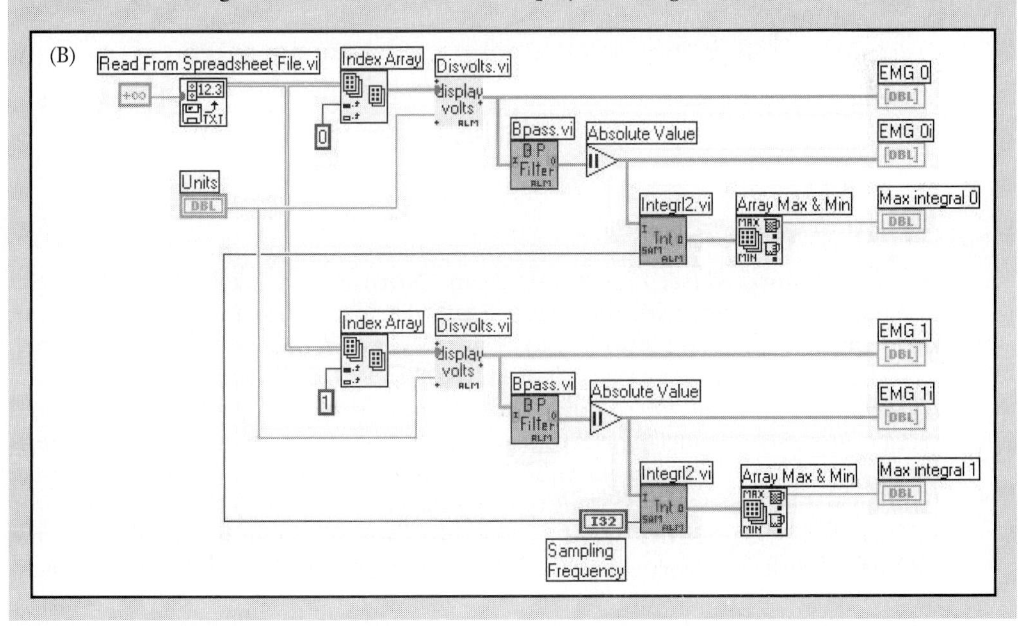

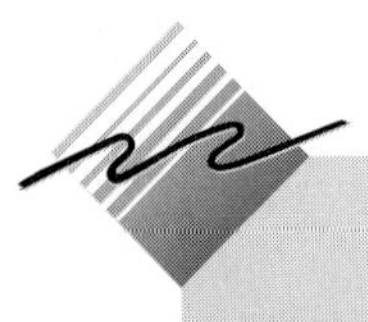

OBJECT/FUNCTION OR SUBVI LOCATOR
NORMALX2.VI

Panel	Object/Function or SubVI	Palette/Menu or Directory
Front	*Dial*	**Controls/Numeric**
	Digital Control × 4	**Controls/Numeric**
	Digital Indicator × 4	**Controls/Numeric**
	Waveform Graph × 4	**Controls/Graph**
Diagram	*Read From Spreadsheet File.vi*	**Functions/File I/O**
	Positive Infinity	**Functions/Numeric/ Additional Numeric Constants**
	Index Array	**Functions/Array**
	Disvolts.vi	**Functions/Select a VI . . . / CD ROM disk**
	Bpass.vi	**Functions/Select a VI . . . / CD ROM disk**
	Absolute Value	**Functions/Numeric**
	Integrl2.vi	**Functions/Select a VI . . . / CD ROM disk**
	Numeric Constant × 2	**Functions/Numeric**
	Array & Index	**Functions/Array**
	Divide × 2	**Functions/Numeric**

PRACTICE EXERCISES

Note that **Iemgx2.vi** (see Figure 3–15.3) and **Normalx2.vi** (see Figure 3–15.4) can integrate and/or normalize the ***entire*** EMG data file being analyzed. That is, in their current form, there is no way to analyze a ***segment*** or ***segments*** of each signal.

Build or call up these two VIs from the **CD ROM disk directory,** and add a ***segment analysis capability*** to each VI for the ***lower graph*** (i.e., bandpass filtered and rectified) for each channel. This is probably most easily achieved by wiring in the **Segment.vi** subVI that was created in Section 3–6, "More SubVIs," in the appropriate location in the block diagram. Some type of ***front panel control(s)*** will also be required to operate the **Segment.vi** subVI. If this subVI was not built, it is available in the **CD ROM disk directory.** After the VIs are modified, save them into a convenient

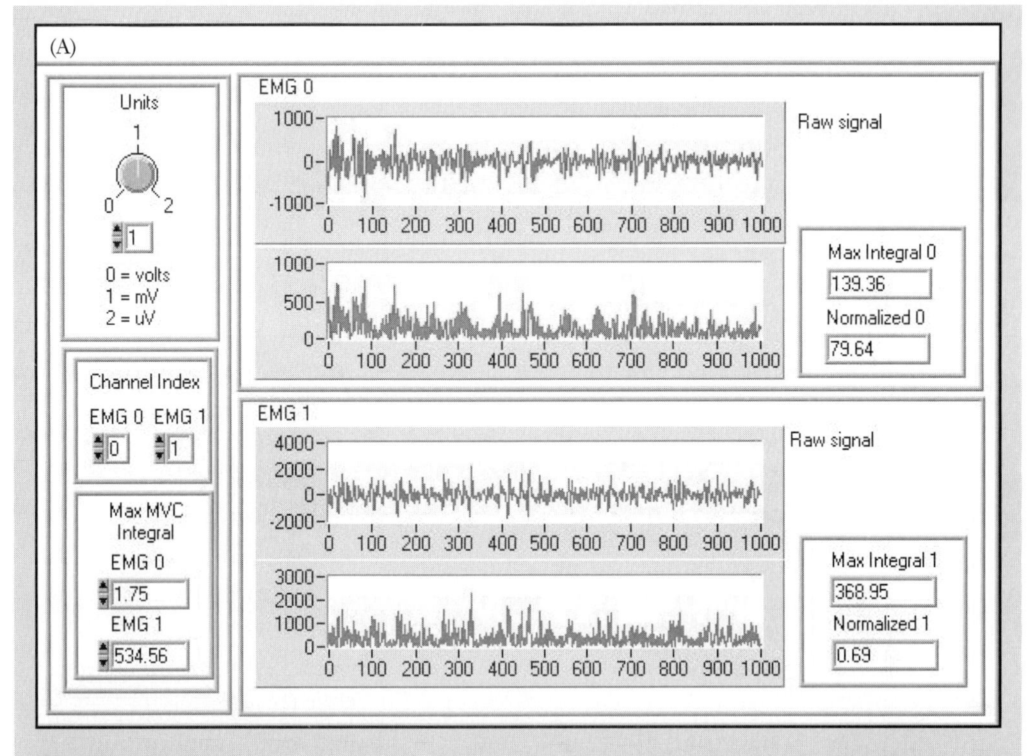

FIGURE 3–15.4
(A) Front panel and (B) block diagram of **Normalx2.vi** used to normalize two channels of isometric EMG data against the maximal integrals during a maximal voluntary contraction of the same muscle.

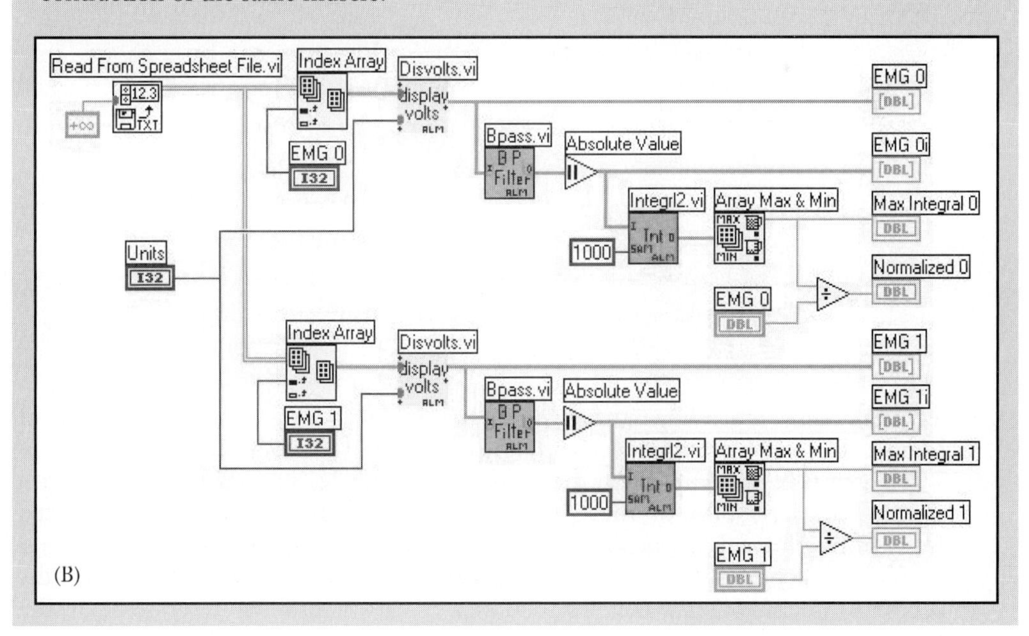

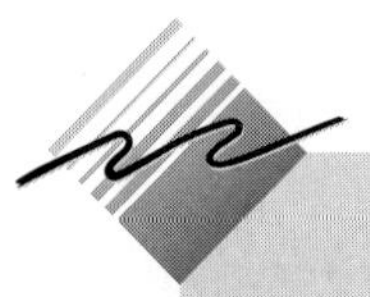

OBJECT/FUNCTION OR SUBVI LOCATOR
SPEC.VI

Panel	Object/Function or SubVI	Palette/Menu or Directory
Front	*Digital Control* × 3	**Controls/Numeric**
	Digital Indicator × 5	**Controls/Numeric**
	String Indicator	**Controls/String & Table**
	Waveform Graph × 4	**Controls/Graph**
Diagram	*Read From Spreadsheet File.vi*	**Functions/File I/O**
	Positive Infinity	**Functions/Numeric/ Additional Numeric Constants**
	Index Array	**Functions/Array**
	Bpass.vi	**Functions/Select a VI . . . / CD ROM disk**
	Disvolts.vi	**Functions/Select a VI . . . / CD ROM disk**
	Powspec.vi	**Functions/Select a VI . . . / CD ROM disk**
	Absolute Value	**Functions/Numeric**
	Unbundle	**Functions/Cluster**
	Bundle	**Functions/Cluster**
	Integral x(t).vi	**Functions/Signal Processing/Time Domain**
	Reciprocal	**Functions/Numeric**
	Numeric Constant	**Functions/Numeric**
	Array Max & Min	**Functions/Array**

directory using the following filenames: **Iemgmod.vi** (i.e., a modified version of **Iemgx2.vi**) and **Normod.vi** (i.e., a modified version of **Normalx2.vi**).

Print out, or compare on the monitor screen, the versions just created with the ***modified versions*** of these VIs in the **CD ROM disk directory** called **Iemg_mod.vi** and **Nor_mod.vi.** To confirm that the ***segment analysis*** function works, run each modified VI using the ***sample data file*** in the **CD ROM disk directory** called **EMGx21.dat.** See Section 3–6, "More SubVIs," to review how the **Segment.vi** subVI works. For the modified version of **Normalx2.vi,** remember to

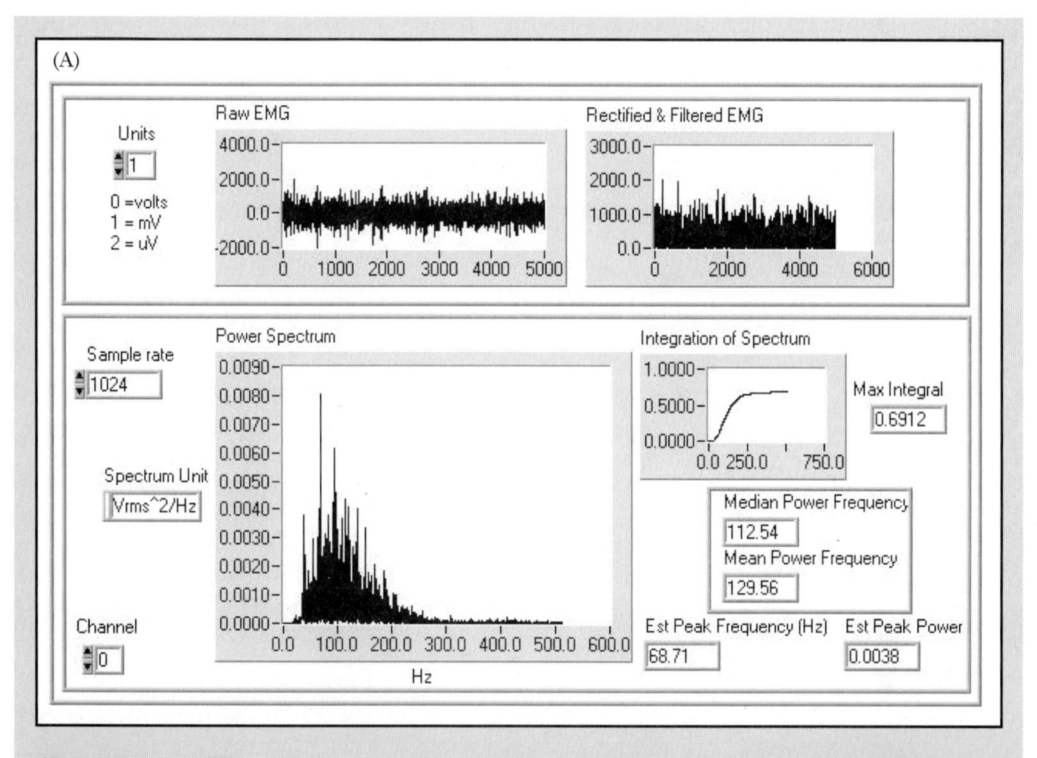

FIGURE 3–15.5
(A) Front panel and (B) block diagram of **Spec.vi.** This VI computes the power spectrum of a signal from a previously saved data file in spreadsheet format using a fast Fourier transform procedure to convert time to the frequency domain. Raw, rectified, and bandpass-filtered signals, the power spectrum, and integration of the spectrum are displayed in *Waveform Graphs* in the front panel. The median and mean power frequencies are also calculated and displayed in front panel *Digital Indicators.*

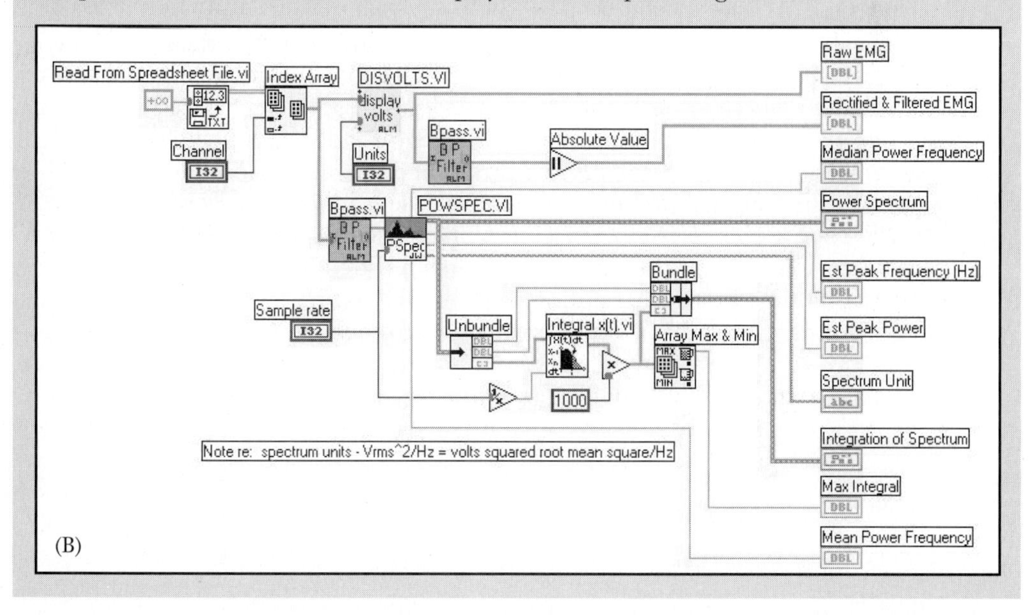

OBJECT/FUNCTION OR SUBVI LOCATOR
PSPECX2.VI

Panel	Object/Function or SubVI	Palette/Menu or Directory
Front	*Digital Indicator* × *4*	**Controls/Numeric**
	Waveform Graph × *2*	**Controls/Graph**
	File Path Indicator	**Controls/Path & Refnum**
Diagram	*Sequence Structure*	**Functions/Structures**
	Read From Spreadsheet File.vi × *2*	**Functions/File I/O**
	Index Array × *2*	**Functions/Array**
	Numeric Constant × *4*	**Functions/Numeric**
	Bpass.vi × 2	**Functions/Select a VI . . . / CD ROM disk directory**
	Pspec.vi	**Functions/Select a VI . . . / CD ROM disk directory**

input values for "Max MVC Integrals" in the front panel *Digital Controls* in the ***lower left corner*** before running the VI (use arbitrary values for testing purposes).

As noted, **Spec.vi** and **Pspecx2.vi** were constructed using the **Powspec.vi** subVI, which was, in turn, constructed using a number of National Instruments' subVIs. Call up the **Spec.vi** subVI from the **CD ROM disk directory,** and switch to the block diagram. Locate the **Powspec.vi** subVI, and left-double click on it using the *Arrow Tool,* which is on the front panel of the subVI. Switch to the block diagram, and explore the subVIs and other functions required to operate it. Note especially the National Instruments' subVIs called: *Scaled Time Domain Window.vi, Auto Power Spectrum.vi, Spectrum Unit Conversion.vi,* and *Power & Frequency Estimate.vi* subVIs and how they are wired. When finished, **Close** out the **Powspec.vi** subVI using the **File** task bar option. If prompted to save any inadvertent changes that might have been made while exploring, left-click on the "No" button.

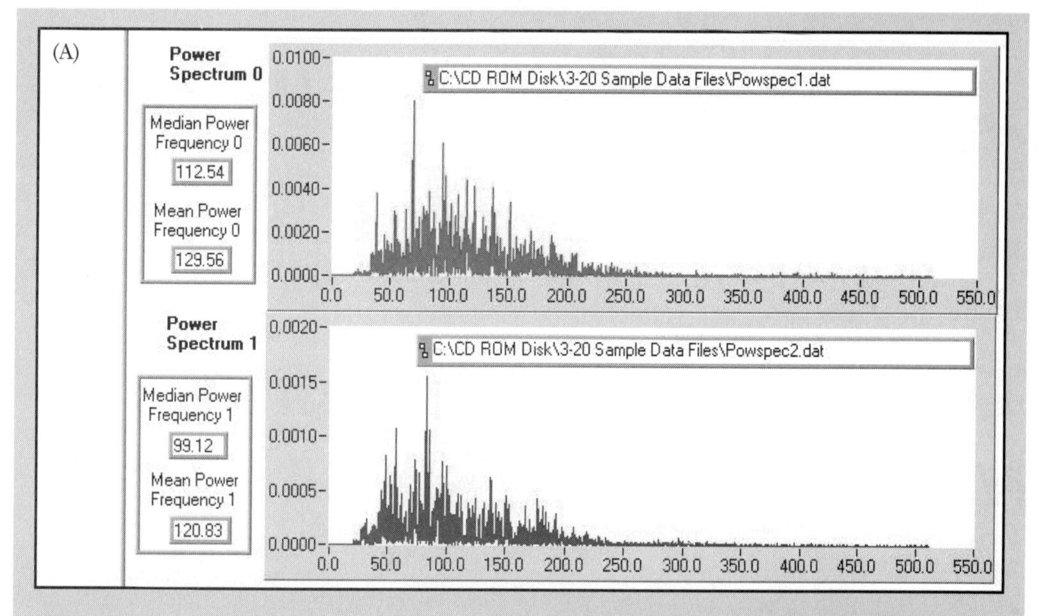

FIGURE 3–15.6
(A) Front panel and (B) block diagram of **Pspecx2.vi.** This VI computes the power spectrum of two signals from a previously saved data file in spreadsheet format and displays the power spectrum in two *Waveform Graphs* in the front panel. Note that a *Sequence Structure* with two frames is used in the block diagram to read and process the signals.

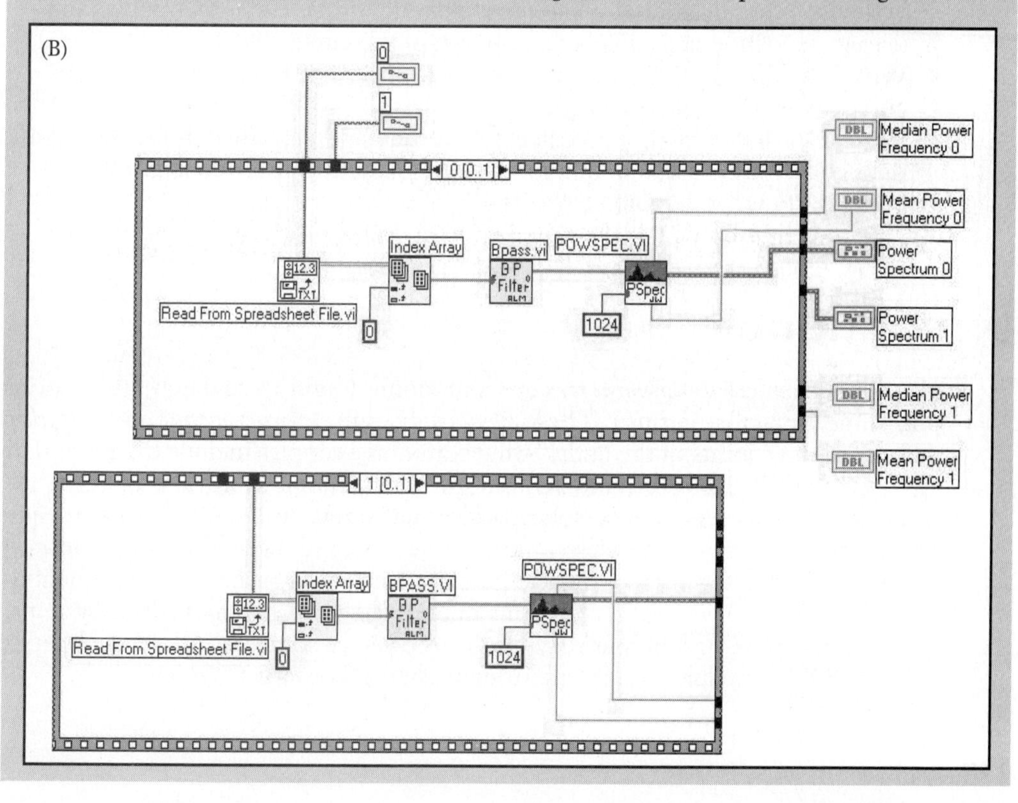

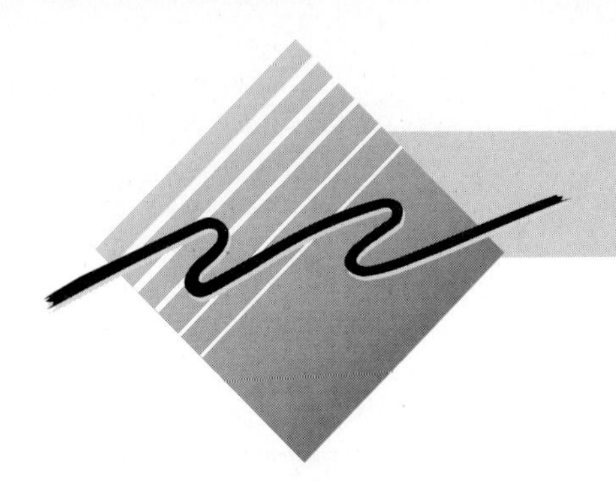

SECTION 3–16

Torque and Velocity Measurements

Objectives

- ❖ Write a VI that displays a torque curve and measures isometric torque parameters using a previously saved data file.
- ❖ Write a VI that displays a complete isokinetic torque curve that allows the user to simultaneously display a segment of the curve.
- ❖ Write a VI that displays a complete torque curve and a segment of torque curve and calculates mean torque.
- ❖ Write a VI that displays and calculates torque and velocity parameters from data collected on a dynamometer during isokinetic muscle contractions.
- ❖ Write a VI that simultaneously plots three torque curves.

Introduction

Electromechanical ***dynamometers*** are commonly found in research laboratories and clinical practice settings. These devices measure ***torque output*** and ***angular velocity*** of most joints of the body. Some common examples include the BIODEX II™, CYBEX™, LIDO™, and KINCOM™ dynamometers. Most of these instruments take measurements isokinetically and isometrically. All measure torque and angular velocity as muscles contract concentrically (i.e., shortening contraction), and most also measure muscle performance eccentrically (i.e., lengthening reactions). Most of the newer versions operate electromechanical drive systems, make calculations, and output data using proprietary software to laser or laserjet printers. Older models output data to strip-chart recorders.

Typical types of data that are output include ***peak torque, time-to-peak torque,*** and ***angular velocity*** measures. While these data are useful to clinicians, researchers studying human performance often require more extensive data analysis such as calculating ***mean torque*** and ***velocity;*** the ability to study a ***segment*** of a data set; calculation of the ***area under a curve*** to quantify ***impulse, work,*** and ***power;*** and the ability to make calculations after a predetermined ***threshold torque*** or ***velocity*** has been achieved. Interfacing LabVIEW with conventional dynamometers gives the user more control and options for making these and other calculations.

Many computerized dynamometers today have serial, parallel, or other types of output ports connected to the device's central processing unit. Ports are often located on the back panel of the unit as either male or female multipin adapters. Using a voltmeter, the function of the torque and velocity data channels (and a common ground) are relatively easy to identify. In some cases, ***pin-outs*** are included in technical manuals. After the pin-outs have been identified, temporary or permanent ***interfaces*** can be constructed with common electrical components to port the dynamometer's torque and velocity signals to an analog-to-digital (A-to-D) converter and then on to LabVIEW VIs. Following is a series of VIs that measure torque and angular velocity in human joints.

TORQUE.VI

Torque.vi (Figure 3–16.1) is intended to analyze ***isometric*** torque curves. In this example, the right quadriceps femoris was tested during a ***maximal voluntary contraction*** while the knee was maintained in 20° of flexion for 8 seconds. The ***sampling rate*** was ***1000 Hz;*** thus, each tick on the x-axis is 1 msec.

The torque signal is displayed on the front panel on two *Waveform Graphs.* The larger of the two graphs includes a *Cursor Display* with two cursors that may be operated independently or together to analyze either ***amplitude*** (y-axis) or ***temporal*** aspects (x-axis) of the signal. The second *Waveform Graph* displays the ***slope*** of a preselected segment of the torque curve. "Slope Start" and "End" points are determined using two *Digital Controls* and default to "1000" and "2500," respectively. In this example, "Cursor 0" is set at the "1073"-msec point, slightly after the torque signal's rise point from the baseline and reads "13.73" Newton-meters. "Cursor 1" is at the "5643"-msec point and reads "271.42" Newton-meters. Slope parameters for "y1" and "y2" are "13.73" and "212.72," respectively. The "x1" and "x2" values are "1073" and "1550," respectively, yielding a "Slope" of "0.42" when the VI is run using the **Torq3.dat** data file in the **CD ROM disk directory.** Build this VI, or call it up from the **CD ROM disk directory.**

On the front panel, a number of ***torque*** and ***time-dependent*** parameters are calculated automatically and displayed in *Digital Indicators* including ***peak torque, mean torque,*** and ***standard deviation; peak torque index; time-to-peak torque;***

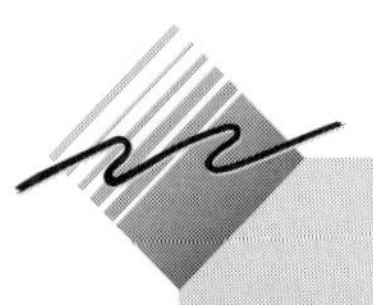

OBJECT/FUNCTION OR SUBVI LOCATOR
TORQUE.VI

Panel	Object/Function or SubVI	Palette/Menu or Directory
Front	*Labeled Oblong Button* × 2	**Controls/Boolean**
	Dial	**Controls/Numeric**
	Digital Control × 13	**Controls/Numeric**
	Vertical Toggle Switch	**Controls/Boolean**
	Digital Indicator × 11	**Controls/Numeric**
	File Path Indicator	**Controls/Path & Refnum**
	Waveform Graph × 2	**Controls/Graph**
Diagram	*Read From Spreadsheet.vi*	**Functions/File I/O**
	Positive Infinity	**Functions/Numeric/ Additional Numeric Constants**
	Index Array	**Functions/Array**
	Multiply	**Functions/Numeric**
	Filters.vi	**Functions/Select a VI . . . / CD ROM disk directory**
	Array Subset	**Functions/Array**
	Numeric Constant × 3	**Functions/Numeric**
	Array Max & Min × 3	**Functions/Array**
	Add	**Functions/Numeric**
	Threshold Peak Detector.vi	**Functions/Signal Processing Measurement**
	Subtract × 3	**Functions/Numeric**
	Absolute Value × 4	**Functions/Numeric**
	Case Structure	**Functions/Structures**
	Segment.vi × 2	**Functions/Select a VI . . . / CD ROM disk directory**
	Mean.vi	**Functions/Mathematics/ Probability**
	SDsam.vi	**Functions/Select a VI . . . / CD ROM disk directory**
	Array Size	**Functions/Array**
	Divide × 2	**Functions/Numeric**

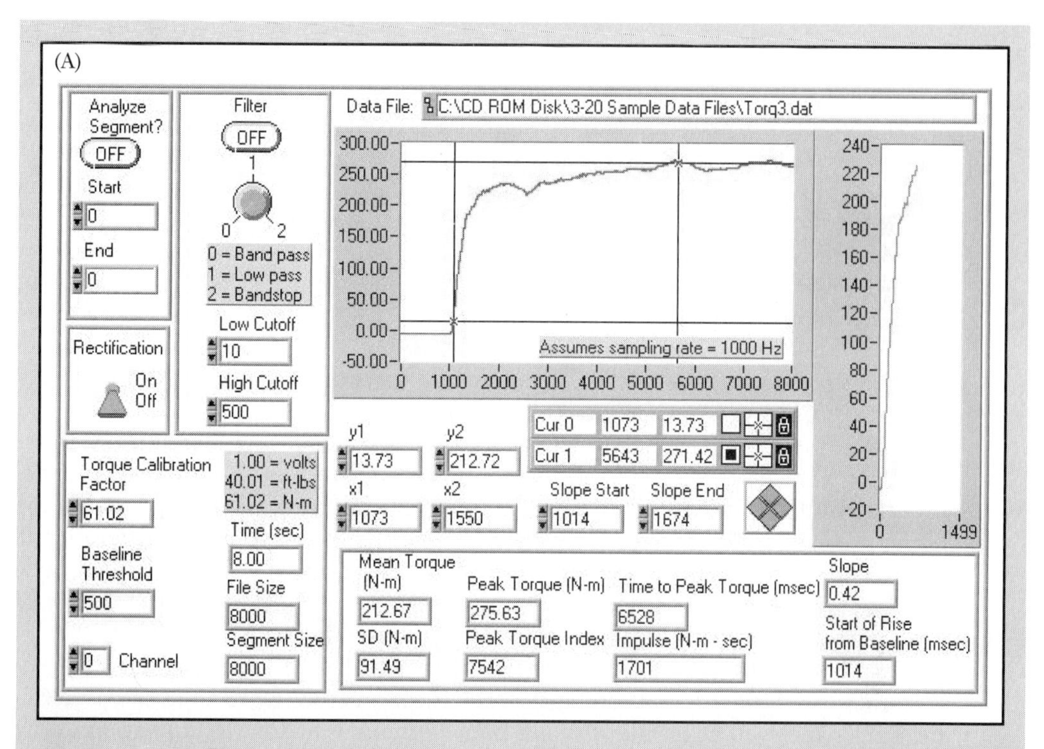

FIGURE 3–16.1
(A) Front panel and (B) block diagram of **Torque.vi** used to read a previously saved data file in spreadsheet format and to plot and calculate various torque parameters during an isometric muscular contraction performed on an isokinetic dynamometer.

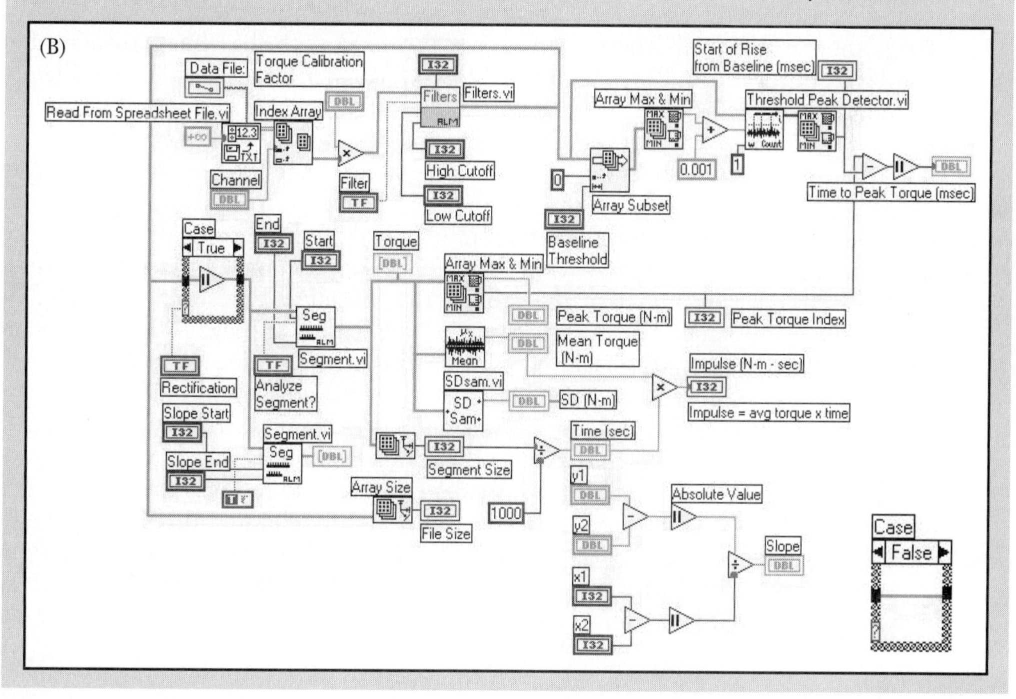

power; and the ***time index*** when the signal rises from the baseline. Amplitude may be read as ***volts, foot-pounds,*** or ***Newton-meters*** (default) by inputing a (predetermined) value in the "Torque Calibration Factor" *Digital Control.* For example, the calibration factor for the dynamometer used for this example for Newton-meters is 61.02 (i.e., 1 volt = 61.02 Newton-meters).

Data channels are selected using the "Channel" *Digital Control.* The ***segment analyzer*** and ***digital filter*** are used by pressing their respective "ON/OFF" buttons with the *Hand Tool.* The default setting for both is "OFF." These front panel controls are associated with the **Filters.vi** and **Segment.vi** subVIs created in Section 3–6, "More VIs," in the block diagram.

When the segment analyzer is used, the "Start" and "End" points are input into their respective *Digital Controls.* When the control button on the front panel is pressed "ON," the **Segment.vi** subVI is toggled on, permitting a ***segment*** of the entire data file to be analyzed. The size of the segment will be reported on the "Segment Size" *Digital Indicator* on the front panel. In Figure 3–16.1, the entire torque file is displayed and is "8000" msec long.

Signal "Rectification" (default = "Off") is provided by a *Boolean Vertical Toggle Switch,* which toggles a *Case Structure* in the block diagram between a "no rectification case" (***false*** condition) and a "rectification case" (***true*** condition). Rectification is achieved using the *Absolute Value* numeric function. Rectification of the signal may be useful when the polarity of the dynamometer input arm is reversed or when the opposite joint is tested when the subject moves to the opposite side (chair) of the dynamometer.

A fundamental concept in data analysis involves the ability of an instrument to differentiate between the ***system noise of a baseline*** and the ***true signal.*** In this VI, the point at which the isometric torque signal ***rises*** from the baseline is displayed in the "Start of Rise from Baseline (msec)" *Digital Indicator* on the front panel. Determining the ***rise point*** of the true signal is done using the *Threshold Peak Detector.vi* subVI in conjunction with the *Array Subset* function in the block diagram.

Before determining the rise point, a segment of the baseline ***before*** the rise point is analyzed to determine the maximal amplitude of the baseline signal. Note that the *Array Subset* function has an input terminal on the left side of the icon face wired with a *Numeric Constant* set at "zero." The portion of the baseline segment to be analyzed is determined by the value in the "Baseline Threshold" *Digital Control* on the front panel. The default value is "500," meaning that 500 msec of data beginning with point "zero" will be used for this analysis. The *Array Subset* function is wired to an *Array Max & Min* function. The maximal amplitude is read from the segment array, and a small amplitude voltage (in this case 0.001 volts) is added to the maximal value using an *Addition* function. This value is wired to an input terminal on the *Threshold Peak Detector.vi* subVI, which also receives the entire array of data points at another input terminal. The slightly elevated threshold voltage (i.e., a voltage slightly above baseline noise) is then compared by the *Threshold Peak Detector.vi* subVI, and that information is ported to another *Array Max & Min* function ***indexing*** the ***minimum voltage.*** The index value is displayed in a *Digital*

Indicator on the front panel as the "Start of Rise from Baseline (msec)." The next data point that follows will be in ***excess*** of the ***threshold voltage*** calculated and thus represents the ***beginning*** of the torque curve as it ascends from the baseline. Thus, the ***true*** torque signal has been differentiated from baseline ***noise.*** Save this VI using a convenient filename and directory. To confirm that the VI is operating properly, run the program using the **Torq3.dat** data file in the **CD ROM disk directory,** and compare the values in the VI just built with those in Figure 3–16.1.

TOR&SEG.VI

Tor&seg.vi (Figure 3–16.2) is intended to be used to analyze ***isokinetic*** (i.e., biphasic) torque production. The VI front panel has many of the same features and capabilities of **Torque.vi.** In this case, a second *Waveform Graph*, located under the first one, displays a ***rectified*** version of the data file rather than the slope. During isokinetic contractions, joint movement is permitted in ***both directions*** (e.g., flexion and extension). As such, the torque signal occurs above (e.g., positive/extension) and below (e.g., negative/flexion) the baseline. An unrectified signal displays the ***phasic*** activity of muscle contractions; to analyze a specific segment of the file, the user must ***rectify*** the signal. In Figure 3–16.2, ankle dorsiflexors and plantar flexors were studied for 12 seconds. In the upper graph, the ***first,*** positive deflection is for ankle dorsiflexors, and the ***second,*** negative deflection is for the ankle plantar flexors followed again by the dorsiflexors, etc. Since two ***movement phases*** are recorded, calculating torque and temporal parameters (e.g., peak torque, time-to-peak torque) is only valid when a ***segment*** of the entire file is analyzed. Cursors for the entire file are used to identify the "Start" and "End" points of the movement phase (e.g., plantar flexion). These values are input into the ***segment analyzer,*** and the file is **Run** again, this time, with the segment analyzer button toggled to the "ON" position. Now, only the ***segment*** of the file to be analyzed will be displayed in the ***lower*** graph. Calculated ***torque*** and ***temporal*** values are now valid for ***only*** the specified segment.

Note that controls, indicators, and calibration factors in the front panel and the block diagram are very similar to those used in **Torque.vi.** The second Practice Exercise (see later) involves building **Tor&seg.vi** using **Torque.vi** as a template.

MNTORQ.VI

Mntorq.vi (Figure 3–16.3) is a simpler version of **Torque.vi** that displays an ***isometric*** torque signal and a ***segment*** to be analyzed on two front panel *Waveform Graphs.* ***Mean torque*** and the ***standard deviation*** for the segment are calculated. Build this VI, or call it up from the **CD ROM disk directory.**

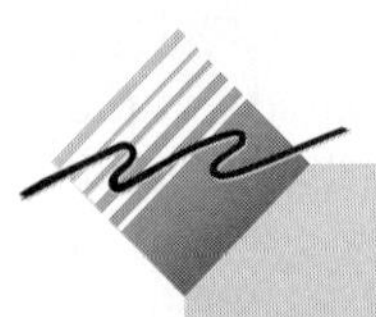

OBJECT/FUNCTION OR SUBVI LOCATOR
TOR&SEG.VI

Panel	Object/Function or SubVI	Palette/Menu or Directory
Front	*Labeled Oblong Button* × 2	**Controls/Boolean**
	Dial	**Controls/Numeric**
	Digital Control × 8	**Controls/Numeric**
	Digital Indicator × 10	**Controls/Numeric**
	Vertical Toggle Switch	**Controls/Boolean**
	File Path Indicator	**Controls/Path & Refnum**
	Waveform Graph × 2	**Controls/Graph**
Diagram	*Read From Spreadsheet File.vi*	**Functions/File I/O**
	Positive Infinity	**Functions/Numeric/ Additional Numeric Constants**
	Index Array	**Functions/Array**
	Multiply × 2	**Functions/Numeric**
	Filters.vi	**Functions/Select a VI . . . / CD ROM disk directory**
	Array Subset	**Functions/Array**
	Array Max & Min × 3	**Functions/Array**
	Add	**Functions/Numeric**
	Numeric Constant × 3	**Functions/Numeric**
	Threshold Peak Detector.vi	**Functions/Signal Processing Measurement**
	Subtract × 3	**Functions/Numeric**
	Absolute Value × 2	**Functions/Numeric**
	Case Structure	**Functions/Structures**
	Segment.vi	**Functions/Select a VI . . . / CD ROM disk directory**
	Mean.vi	**Functions/Mathematics/ Probability and Statistics**
	SDsam.vi	**Functions/Select a VI . . . / CD ROM disk directory**
	Array Size	**Functions/Array**
	Divide	**Functions/Numeric**

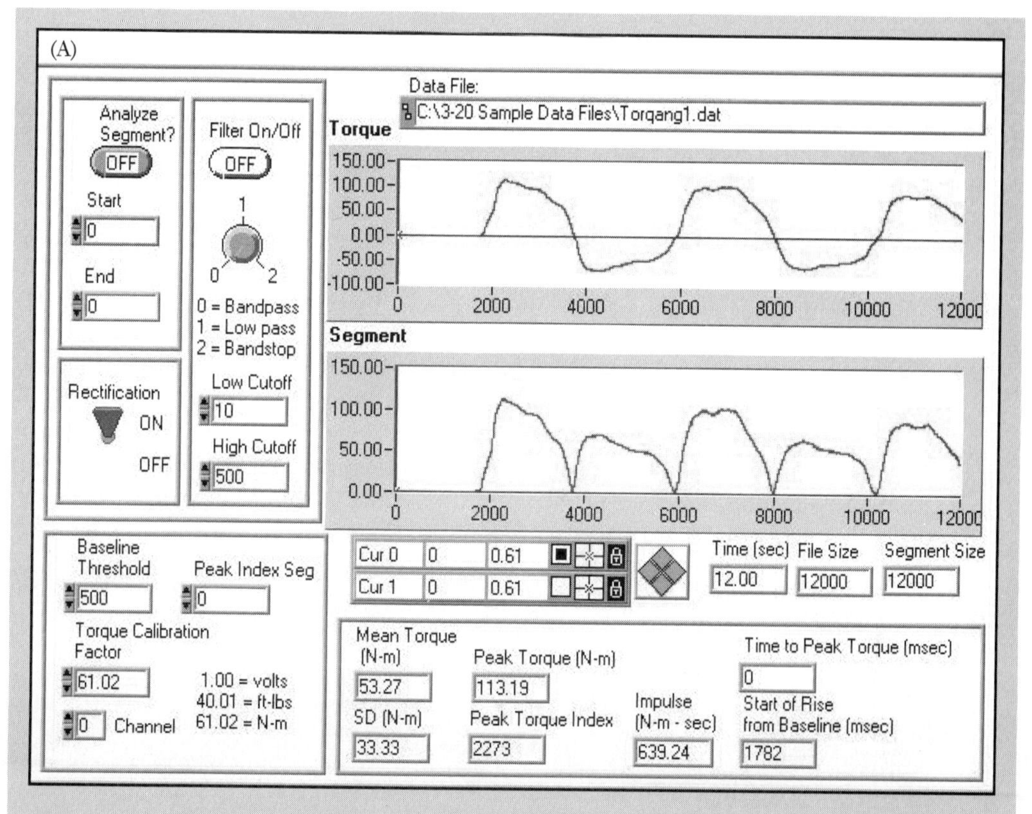

FIGURE 3–16.2
(A) Front panel and (B) block diagram of **Tor&seg.vi.** This VI reads a previously saved date file in spreadsheet format during an isokinetic muscular contraction performed on a dynamometer. The complete torque signal is displayed in a front panel *Waveform Graph*, while a segment of the complete file will be displayed in the graph underneath it.

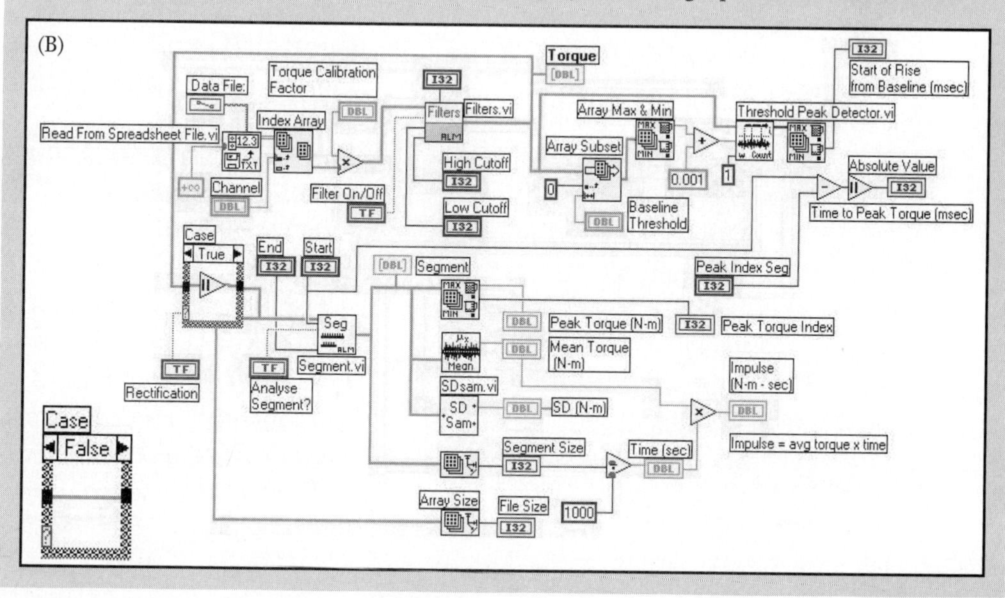

Two front panel *Vertical Pointer Slides* are used to index the data channel to be analyzed and to display signal units as ***Newton-meters*** (default), ***foot-pounds***, or ***volts.*** A *Cursor Display* associated with the *Waveform Graph* to the left is used to identify "Start" and "End" points for the ***segment*** to be analyzed. A *Boolean Labeled Oblong Button* activates the **Segment.vi** subVI created in Section 3–6, "More SubVIs," in the block diagram. Save the VI with a convenient filename and directory.

To confirm that the VI operates properly, **Run** it using the **Torq2.dat** data file set to "Channel 0" in the **CD ROM disk directory.** Before running it, input "855" in the "Start" and "3603" in the "End" *Digital Controls* using the *Lettering Tool*, and press the "ON/OFF" button of the ***segment analyzer*** to "ON" with the *Hand Tool.* "Mean Torque" should read "183.60" Newton-meters with a standard deviation of "67.92" in two *Digital Indicators* in the lower right corner of the front panel. Two *Digital Indicators* in the upper right corner should display a "File Size" of "8000" data points and a segment length of "2748" points.

OBJECT/FUNCTION OR SUBVI LOCATOR
MNSEG.VI

Panel	Object/Function or SubVI	Palette/Menu or Directory
Front	*Labeled Oblong Button*	**Controls/Boolean**
	Digital Control × 2	**Controls/Numeric**
	Digital Control × 4	**Controls/Numeric**
	File Path Indicator	**Controls/Path & Refnum**
	Vertical Pointer Slide × 2	**Controls/Numeric**
	Waveform Graph × 2	**Controls/Graph**
Diagram	*Read From Spreadsheet File.vi*	**Functions/File I/O**
	Index Array	**Functions/Index**
	Case Structure	**Functions/Structures**
	Multiply × 3	**Functions/Numeric**
	Numeric Constant × 3	**Functions/Numeric**
	Segment.vi	**Functions/Select a VI . . . / CD ROM disk directory**
	Array Size	**Functions/Array**
	Mean.vi	**Functions/Mathematics/ Probability and Statistics**
	SDsam.vi	**Functions/Select a VI . . . / CD ROM disk directory**

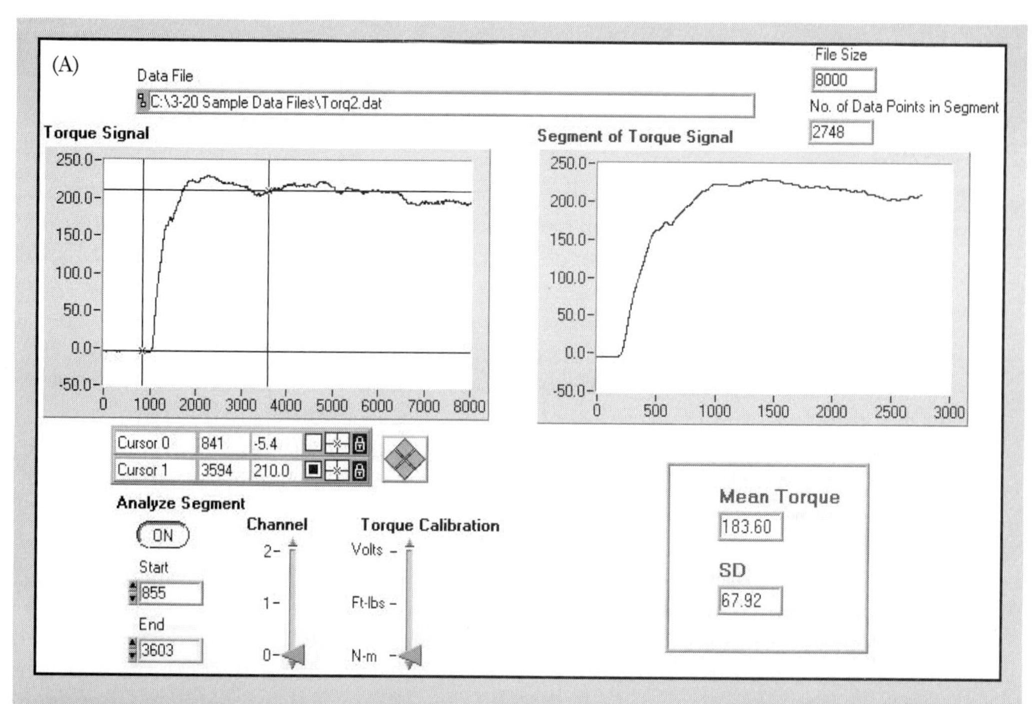

FIGURE 3–16.3
(A) Front panel and (B) block diagram of **Mntorq.vi.** This VI reads a previously saved data file in spreadsheet format during an isometric muscular contraction performed on a dynamometer and computes the mean torque amplitude from a preselected segment of the signal. The complete torque signal and the segment are plotted on two front panel *Waveform Graphs.* Note that a *Cursor Display* is used in the left graph to determine start and ending points for the segment of the signal to be analyzed.

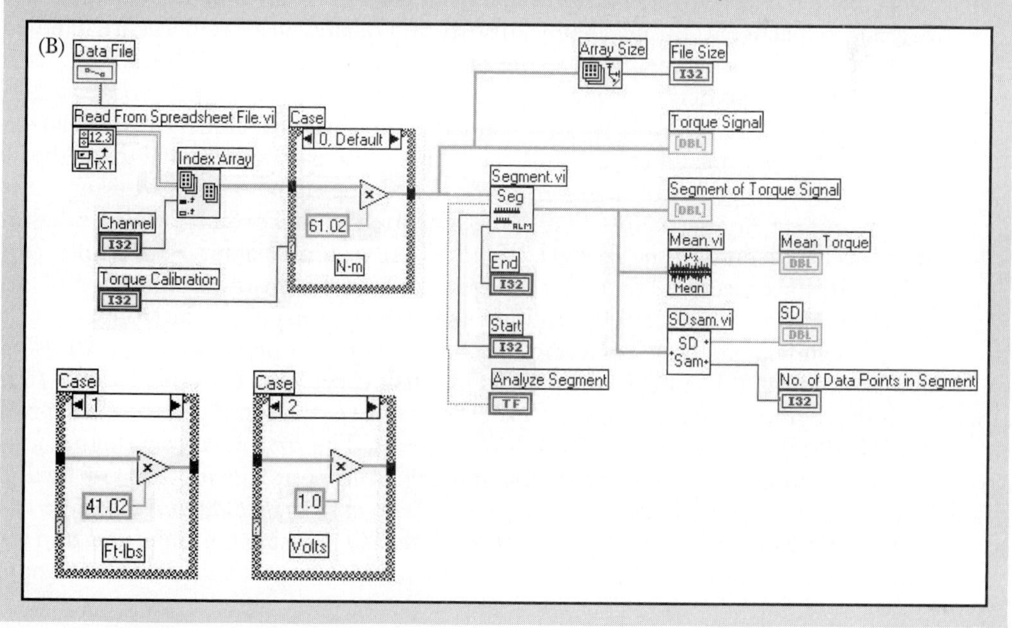

TOR&ANG2.VI

Tor&ang2.vi (Figure 3–16.4) permits the simultaneous display of the ***torque*** and ***angle*** channels of an isokinetic dynamometer and calculation of ***torque*** and ***angular displacement*** and ***velocity*** parameters. Build this VI, or call it up from the **CD ROM disk directory.** Use **Torque.vi** as a template to construct this VI. The ***top*** *Waveform Graph* displays the torque signal, and the ***lower*** one displays the angular displacement of the dynamometer's input axis. Each graph has a *Cursor Display.* Two *Boolean Vertical Toggle Switches* permit each signal to be ***rectified.*** Front panel elements dealing with torque measurements are essentially the same as described in the **Torque.vi** and **Tor&seg.vi** VIs described earlier, including a ***segment analyzer*** and ***digital filter.*** In this VI, the filter defaults to a ***bandstop filter*** with a ***low-frequency cutoff*** of "59 Hz" and a ***high cutoff*** of "61 Hz," making this a ***60-cycle*** filter. Lowpass and bandpass options are also available by inputting the appropriate number in a *Digital Control.* Channel ***selection*** for the "Torque" and "Angle" signals is likewise handled with *Digital Controls* that default to "0" and "1," respectively.

A predetermined "Angle Calibration Factor" of "0.053 volts/degree" is used to compute ***angular excursion*** and ***velocity*** measurements that are displayed in *Digital Indicators* on the front panel. Below and out-of-view of the main front panel elements on the monitor is a "Diagnostics Indicators" panel that displays voltage and time parameters in seven *Digital Indicators* and are rotated 90° and to the left (Figure 3–16.4—front panel). These should be located ***below*** the second *Cursor Display* when building this VI.

Switch to the block diagram, and note that torque and angle signals are first indexed from a data array and read by the *Read From Spreadsheet File.vi* function in the usual manner. Each channel is ***converted*** from ***volts*** to ***Newton-meters*** (default) and ***degrees,*** respectively. Torque channel display and related measurements are handled in the same way as in **Torque.vi.** Note that the **Segment.vi** and **Filters.vi** are used again. ***Rectification*** of the torque (and velocity) signal is achieved with a *Boolean*-toggled *Case Structure.* The "True" case computes the absolute value (i.e., rectifies) using the *Absolute Value* function, while the "False" case passes the signal through the *Case Structure* ***unprocessed. Integration*** of the torque signal is handled using a *For Loop* with *Shift Registers.* Note that in the **Torque.vi** and **Tor&seg.vi** VIs, integration was handled using the **Integrl2.vi** subVI created in Chapter 3–6, "More SubVIs." The lower section of the block diagram is concerned with computation of angular displacement and velocity parameters that are displayed on the front panel.

To understand how **Tor&ang2.vi** (Figure 3–16.4) operates, run the VI using the **Torang2.dat** data file in the **CD ROM disk directory. Run** the data file ***first*** with the ***segment analyzer*** turned "OFF," and note in the top *Waveform Graph* two sets of rectified knee extension and flexion curves. The ***first*** waveform (higher amplitude) demonstrates ***knee extension*** starting from approximately 90° of flexion and progresses to complete extension (zero degrees). To ***display one complete extension/flexion*** cycle, turn the ***segment analyzer*** "ON" using the *Hand Tool,* and input "Start" and "End" values of "1679" and "6204," respectively. Flip the "Angle

Rectification" toggle switch "ON," and **Run** the VI again with the ***same data file.*** This time, ***one extension/flexion cycle*** should be displayed in the upper *Waveform Graph.* ***Angular displacement*** will similarly be displayed in the ***lower*** graph and approximates a "V" shape. Confirm that the "Segment File Size" is "4525" points in the *Digital Indicator* in the upper right corner of the front panel. The complete "File Size" should read "12000" in another *Digital Indicator* to the left. Confirm also that the "Angular Excursion" for this cycle is "103°" and "Angular Velocity" is "43°/second." Also, confirm that voltage and time "Diagnostic Indicators" are the same in the framed panel. Finally, understand that the torque parameter measurements are calculated for both knee extension and flexion, and as such, these combined values are of little use. To ***compute torque*** parameters for ***either*** a ***knee extension*** or ***flexion phase,*** the segment analyzer has to be ***reset*** with "Start" and "End" points for the particular phase to be analyzed and the VI run again. The fifth Practice Exercise (see later) deals with this procedure and provides torque parameter measurements, using the same data file as just described, to compare with for the VI that was just constructed. **Save** this VI using a convenient filename and directory.

TORX3.VI

Torx3.VI (Figure 3–16.5) uses a ***three-frame*** *Sequence Structure* to retrieve and plot three arrays of torque data from three spreadsheet format data files and ***superimposes*** three ***torque curves*** on the same graph. A VI like this might be useful when the overall ***topology*** (form) of the curves needs to be analyzed. For example, if one of the three plots differs decidedly from the other two, a significant difference or trend may be suggested. Construct or call up this VI from the **CD ROM disk directory.**

In the front panel *Waveform Graph*, give each ***line plot*** a different ***color.*** After the graph is located and sized, right-click anywhere on the graph with the *Arrow Tool.* From the pop-up menu, select *Show/Legend.* Expand the *Legend* down two additional levels (total of three) by clicking and dragging the lower right corner downward. Reposition the legend as shown in Figure 3–16.5, and ***rename*** each plot "Trial 1," etc., using the *Lettering Tool.* With the *Paint Brush Tool*, right-click on each plot line, and select a distinguishing color for each.

In the block diagram, position and size a *Sequence Structure.* Add ***two additional frames*** by right-clicking anywhere on the frame with the *Arrow Tool*, and select *Add Frame After* from the pop-up menu. Add all elements for each frame as described in Figure 3–16.5.

Test the VI using ***three*** data files in the **CD ROM disk directory.** The files are **Torq1.dat, Torq2.dat,** and **Torq3.dat.** The point at which the torque curve ***rises from the baseline*** for each file will need to be determined. Determine this point by first running **Torque.vi** with each data file. The ***file length*** for each data file is "6000," and this value should be input into the "File Length" *Digital Control*

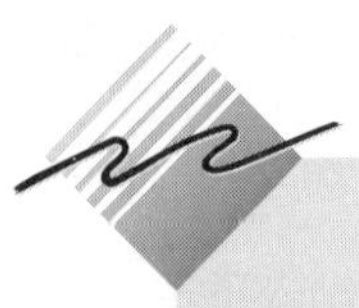

OBJECT/FUNCTION OR SUBVI LOCATOR
TOR&ANG2.VI

Panel	Object/Function or SubVI	Palette/Menu or Directory
Front	*Labeled Oblong Button* × 2	**Controls/Boolean**
	Digital Control × 10	**Controls/Numeric**
	Digital Indicator × 17	**Controls/Numeric**
	Vertical Toggle Switch × 2	**Controls/Boolean**
	File Path Indicator	**Controls/Path & Refnum**
	Waveform Graph × 2	**Controls/Graph**
Diagram	*Read From Spreadsheet File.vi*	**Functions/File I/O**
	Positive Infinity	**Functions/Numeric/ Additional Numeric Constants**
	Index Array × 2	**Functions/Array**
	Filters.vi × 2	**Functions/Select a VI . . . / CD ROM disk directory**
	Multiply	**Functions/Numeric**
	Case Structure × 2	**Functions/Structures**
	Absolute Value × 6	**Functions/Numeric**
	Segment.vi × 2	**Functions/Select a VI . . . / CD ROM disk directory**
	Array Size × 2	**Functions/Array**
	Array Max & Min × 2	**Functions/Array**
	For Loop	**Functions/Structures**
	Numeric Constant	**Functions/Numeric**
	Mean.vi	**Functions/Mathematics/ Probability and Statistics**
	SDsam.vi	**Functions/Select a VI . . . / CD ROM disk directory**
	Add	**Functions/Numeric**
	Subtract	**Functions/Numeric**
	Divide × 3	**Functions/Numeric**

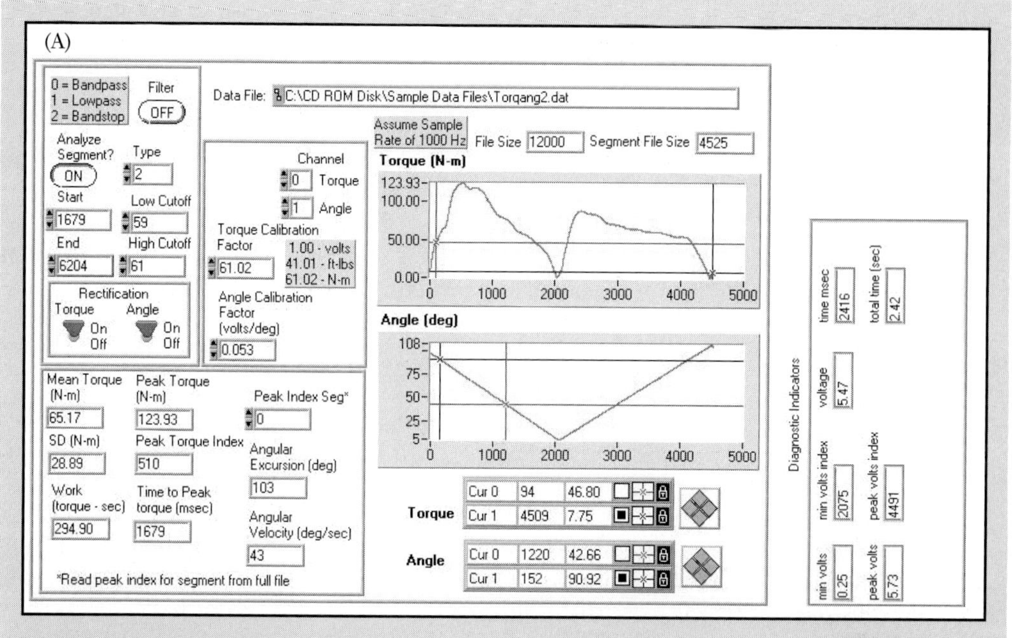

FIGURE 3–16.4

(A) Front panel and (B) block diagram of **Tor&ang2.vi.** Isokinetic torque and angle channels are read from a previously saved data file in spreadsheet format during an isokinetic muscular contraction and displayed on two *Waveform Graphs* in the front panel. Torque and joint angle parameters are calculated and displayed in *Digital Indicators* in the front panel.

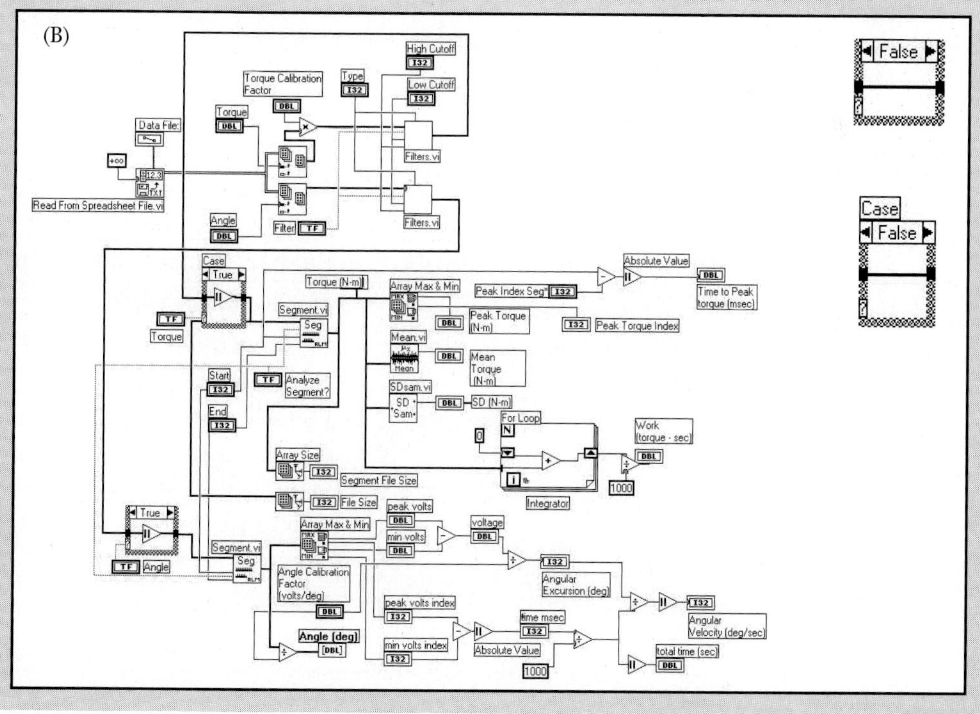

on the front panel. Insert the ***rise point*** value for each data file in the three *Digital Controls* labeled "Trial 1, 2 and 3." The values should be "1260," "1039," and "1014," respectively. When the VI runs, it will make three ***sequential*** prompts for the three data files before they are simultaneously plotted. Confirm that the three plots for the VI just constructed all start from the ***same*** "zero" point on the *Waveform Graph* and that the ***shape*** of each ***graph*** is the same as in Figure 3–16.5. **Save** the VI using a convenient filename and directory.

SUMMARY

LabVIEW VIs can be built to measure ***torque*** and ***velocity*** parameters from data collected on an isokinetic dynamometer. Both ***isometric*** and ***isokinetic*** (isotonic) contractions may be measured. In most instances, data files are run several times. During the first pass, the entire file is displayed to get the user oriented to the data. Next, ***cursors*** are used to identify the ***start*** and ***end*** point of a ***segment*** of the entire file for more detailed analysis. On subsequent passes, a ***segment analyzer*** is used to display and measure the segment of interest. Most of the VIs discussed can calculate a wide range of torque and velocity parameters such as peak and mean torque, time-to-peak torque, impulse, the point at which a torque signal rises from the baseline, angular displacement and velocity, and others. The last VI described permits the ***simultaneous*** display of up to three torque curves to analyze their overall ***topology***. Several practice exercises (next) review how the VIs are used, and various measurements are identified to confirm that the VIs have been written and are operating properly.

OBJECT/FUNCTION OR SUBVI LOCATOR
TORX3.VI

Panel	Object/Function or SubVI	Palette/Menu or Directory
Front	*Digital Control* × 5	**Controls/Numeric**
	Waveform Graph	**Controls/Graph**
Diagram	*Sequence Structure*	**Functions/Structures**
	Read From Spreadsheet File.vi × 3	**Functions/File I/O**
	Positive Infinity	**Functions/Numeric/ Additional Numeric Constants**
	Index Array × 3	**Functions/Array**
	Array Subset × 3	**Functions/Array**
	Build Array	**Functions/Array**

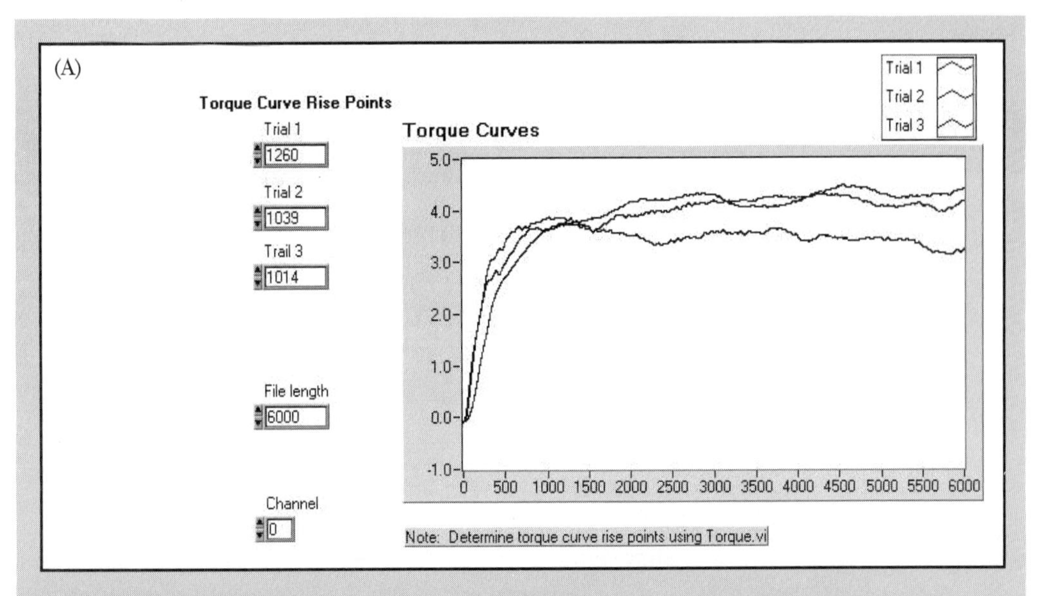

FIGURE 3–16.5
(A) Front panel and (B) block diagram for **Torx3.vi.** This VI superimposes three torque curves in a front panel *Waveform Graph* from a previously saved data file in spreadsheet format using a three-frame *Sequence Structure.*

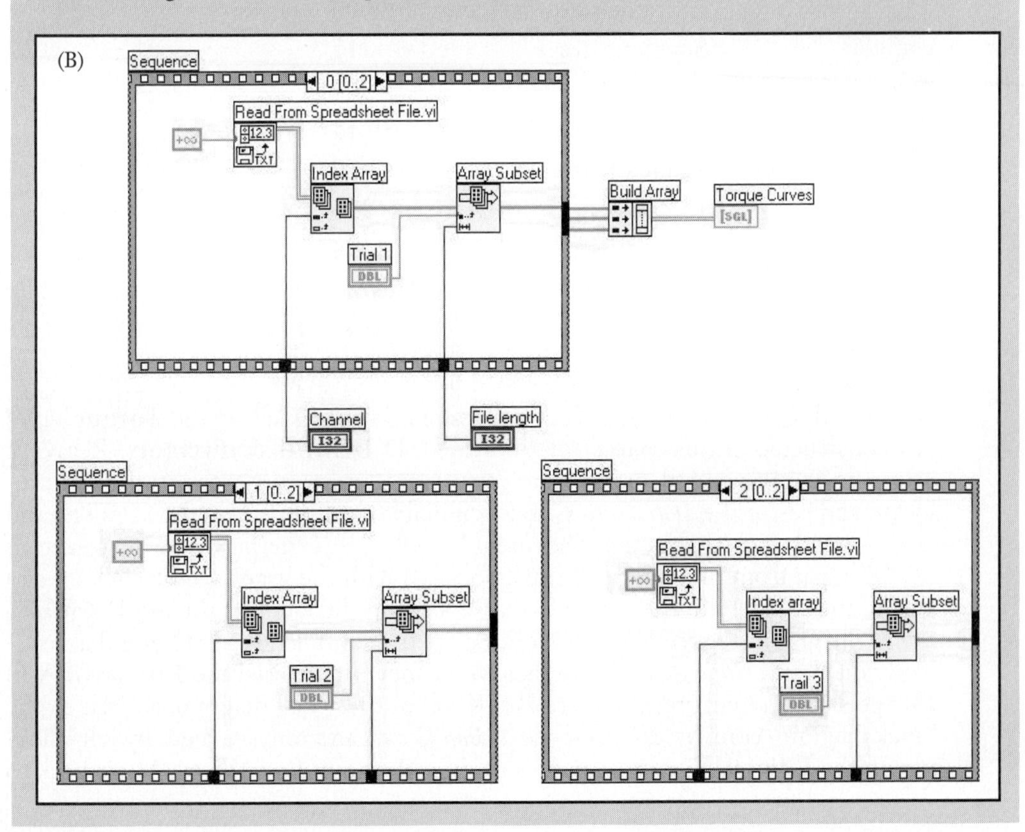

PRACTICE EXERCISES

Practice using **Torque.vi** with the **Torq1.dat** data file found in the **CD ROM disk directory.** Turn the segment analyzer "ON" using the *Hand Tool,* and input a "Start" and "End" values of "1426" and "1643," respectively. Input values for other controls on the front panel are as follows:

CONTROL	VALUE
y1	41.98
y2	144.19
x1	1426
x2	1643
Slope start	1426
Slope end	1643

Run the VI, and confirm the following ***torque*** and ***time*** measures:

INDICATOR	VALUE
Time (sec)	0.22
File size	8000
Segment size	217
Mean torque (N-m)	96.93
SD (N-m)	30.13
Peak torque (N-m)	143.89
Peak torque Index	216
Time to peak torque (msec)	1044
Impulse (N-m sec)	21
Slope	0.47
Start of rise from baseline	1260

Build **Tor&seg.vi** using **Torque.vi** as a template. Call up the **Torque.vi** VI just constructed in this chapter or from the **CD ROM disk directory.** Resave it using the **Tor&seg.vi** filename into a convenient directory. On the front panel, relocate and resize the *Waveform Graph* originally used to display the segment and the slope. Label the graph "Segment" with the *Lettering Tool* by selecting *Show/Legend* from the pop-up menu associated with the graph (right-click on any part of the graph with the *Arrow Tool*). Reposition the label on the ***upper left corner*** of the graph (Figure 3–16.3). Next, delete the seven *Digital Indicators* that originally displayed ***slope data.*** Note that when they are deleted the **Run** arrow will change shape, indicating there are *Bad Wires* in the block diagram. Switch to the block diagram, confirm the presence of *Bad Wires,* and remove them by left-clicking on the **Edit** task bar option and selecting **Remove Bad Wires.** Move back to the front panel, and relocate the *Cursor Display* to the left underneath the lower *Waveform Graph.* Also relocate the *Digital Indicators* for "Time (sec)," "File Size," and "Segment Size" underneath the lower *Waveform Graph* just to the right of the *Cursor Display.* Add a *Digital Control* labeled "Peak Index Seg" to the front panel, and locate it next to the "Baseline Threshold" *Digital Control.*

In the block diagram, disconnect the icon for the *Waveform Graph* labeled "Torque," and wire, in its place, the *Waveform Graph* labeled "Segment." Relocate the *Waveform Graph* labeled "Torque" toward the top of the block diagram, and wire it to the ***output side*** of the **Filters.vi** subVI. Delete the lower **Segment.vi** subVI previously associated with slope parameters and any *Bad Wires* that may occur. Check that the remaining icons are located approximately in the same positions as in Figure 3–16.3, and resave the VI.

To confirm that the VI is operating properly, run **Tor&seg.vi** using the **Torang1.dat** data file in the **CD ROM disk directory** with the segment analyzer turned "OFF" and the "Rectification" toggle switch turned "ON." Leave the filter "OFF." Compare the shape of the two graphs and values in the front panel *Digital Indicators* with those in Figure 3–16.3; they should be the same.

Add the capability in **Mntorq.vi,** built in this chapter, to measure ***peak torque*** and ***time-to-peak torque*** for an ***entire*** data file. This will require that the point at which the torque signal ***rises*** from the baseline be identified so that the ***time*** when ***peak torque*** occurs may be calculated. Add three front panel *Digital Indicators*, and label them "Peak Torque (N-m)," "Time to Peak Torque (msec)," and "Start of Rise from Baseline (msec)." Hint: Review the code in the upper right corner of the block diagram in Figure 3–16.1 (**Torque.vi**). Since this VI will read the ***entire*** data file, the ***segment analyzer*** should be ***removed.***

To confirm that the VI has been modified correctly, run it using the **Torq2.dat** data file in the **CD ROM disk directory.** "Peak Torque (N-m)" should read 230.29, "Time to Peak Torque (msec)" should read "1224," and the "Start of Rise from Baseline (msec)" should read "1039." "Mean Torque" and the standard deviation (SD) should be "176.37" and "75.34," respectively. **Save** the VI using the filename **Mtor_mod.vi** into a convenient directory. This VI may be compared with the VI called **Mtormod.vi** in the **CD ROM disk directory.**

Using **Tor&ang2.vi** built in this chapter, determine the ***mean torque*** (***and standard deviation***) and ***peak torque*** for the ***second knee extension phase*** using the data file named **Torqang1.dat** in the **CD ROM disk directory.** Use the following procedure. First, **Run** the VI with the ***segment analyzer*** and ***filter*** both turned "OFF." Identify the ***third*** waveform in the upper *Waveform Graph.* This is the ***second*** knee extension phase. Using the *Cursor Display* for the upper graph, confirm that the "Start" and "End" points of the ***third*** waveform are "5899" and "7971," respectively, and input these values into the ***segment analyzer*** *Digital Controls.* Using the *Hand Tool,* turn "ON" ***the segment analyzer,*** and run the data file again. Note that the upper *Waveform Graph* now displays only a single waveform specified in the segment analyzer. Confirm that “Mean Torque (N-m)” is “73.60” with a standard deviation (SD) of “30.95” and that “Peak Torque (N-m)” is “103.06.” Last, confirm that the “Segment File Size” is “2082” in the *Digital Indicator* in the upper right corner of the front panel.

Finally, modify **Torx3.vi** so that it can display ***four torque curves*** simultaneously. Use **Torq4.dat** in the **CD ROM disk directory** as the ***fourth data file*** to confirm that the VI is running properly. Save the modified VI using the filename **Torx_4.vi.** Compare this VI with the file named **Torx4.vi** in the **CD ROM disk directory.** Note that the ***rise point*** for the ***fourth*** channel (*Digital Control*) is the ***default value*** to help verify that it has been identified correctly.

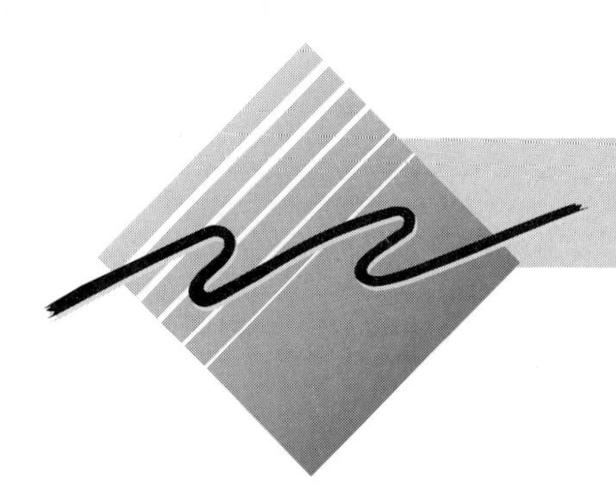

SECTION 3–17

Torque and EMG Measurements

Objectives

- Write a VI that collects one channel of torque and two channels of EMG data.
- Write a VI that reads a spreadsheet format data file and displays raw and bandpass filtered mean torque and two channels of integrated EMG at the point where peak torque is indexed.

Introduction

The simultaneous recording of torque output coupled with electromyography (EMG) has historically been a mainstay in kinesiological and biomechanical research and clinical practice. While a subject pushes against a dynamometer, muscles responsible for producing or restricting movement are studied. Torque may be measured ***isometrically***, ***isotonically***, or ***isokinetically***, depending on the experimental setup and measurement devices used. In the examples that follow, VIs permit ***isometric torque*** and ***two EMG*** signals to be collected and analyzed as a subject works against an isokinetic dynamometer. EMG signals are analyzed using the ***integration*** techniques described in Section 13–15 "Electromyography."

Tor&EMG2.vi

In Section 3–15, "Electromyography," **4Chanemg.vi** was constructed using the **Write2ch.vi.** In the case of **Tor&emg2.vi** (Figure 3–17.1), **Write2ch.vi** was used as a template to build a VI to record one channel of isometric ***torque*** and two channels of raw **EMG** data and save it to disk in a spreadsheet format. Call up the version of **Write2ch.vi** that was constructed in Chapter 3–15, "Electromyography," or call up the file from the **CD ROM disk directory,** and modify it to collect and save ***three channels*** of data. Note that the front panel layout is different compared with previous examples and that a ***different font size*** and ***style*** have been used to label controls and indicators. Font size, style, and color changes are handled by left-clicking on the **Text Settings** menu ring on the task bar. The ***default*** case uses a ***plain, 13-point, Times New Roman*** font. In this VI, a ***bold, 16-point Courier*** font was used. Note that when a font size for *Controls* or *Indicators* is larger than the default (13-point) setting, the size of the front panel elements ***automatically rescale*** themselves. In some cases, the *Control* or *Indicator* may have to be ***manually*** elongated by left-clicking and dragging either the upper or lower right corner and extending it to the right until the number or string is completely visible.

OBJECT/FUNCTION OR SUBVI LOCATOR
TOR&EMG2.VI

Panel	Object/Function or SubVI	Palette/Menu or Directory
Front	*Digital Control* × 2	**Controls/Numeric**
	String Control	**Controls/String & Table**
	Waveform Graph × 3	**Controls/Graph**
Diagram	*AI Acquire Waveforms.vi*	**Functions/Data Acquisition/Analog Input**
	Numeric Constant × 4	**Functions/Numeric**
	Transpose 2D Array	**Functions/Array**
	Index Array × 3	**Functions/Array**
	Write to Spreadsheet File.vi	**Functions/File I/O**

Three *Waveform Graphs* display the torque and EMG data after they have been recorded. As in previous examples, two *Digital Controls* were used to determine the "Sample Rate" (default = "1000") and "Number of Samples" (default = "2000") collected. A *String Control* specifies that the first three channels on the A-to-D board (i.e., 0 to 2) will be used to collect the data. "Device" number specification for the slot the A-to-D board resides in was handled using a *Digital Constant* in the block diagram. The device number could also be specified using a front panel *Digital Control* to provide the ability to select different A-to-D boards if more than one was installed or if other devices are periodically installed in that slot.

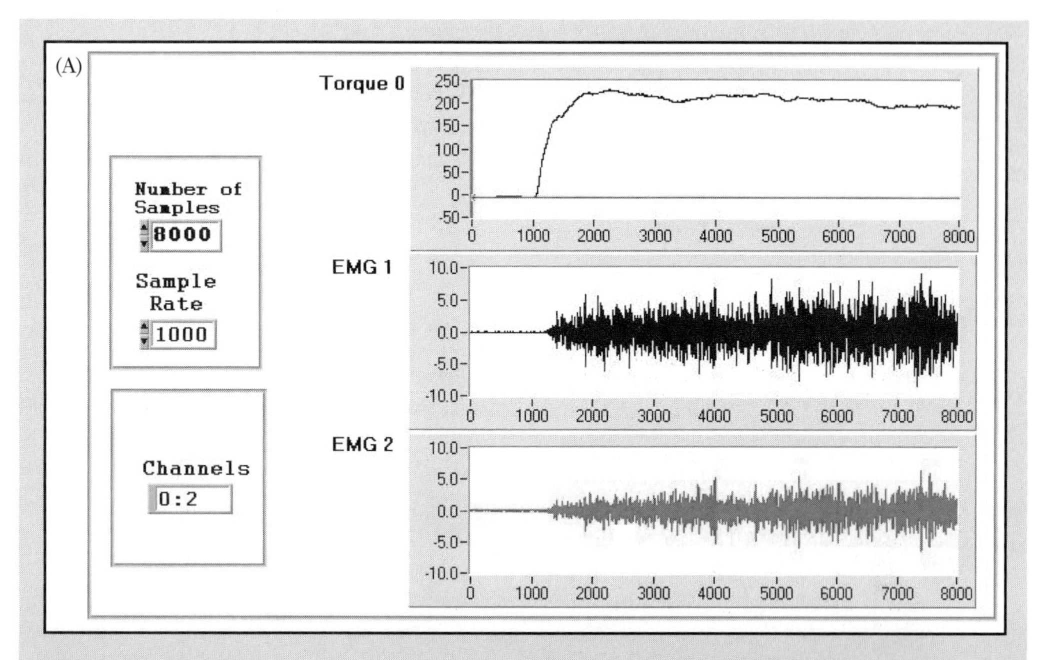

FIGURE 3–17.1
(A) Front panel and (B) block diagram of **Tor&emg2.vi.** A single-torque channel and two channels of EMG from the muscle working on a dynamometer are acquired from a computer's A-to-D board and displayed on three front panel *Waveform Graphs.*

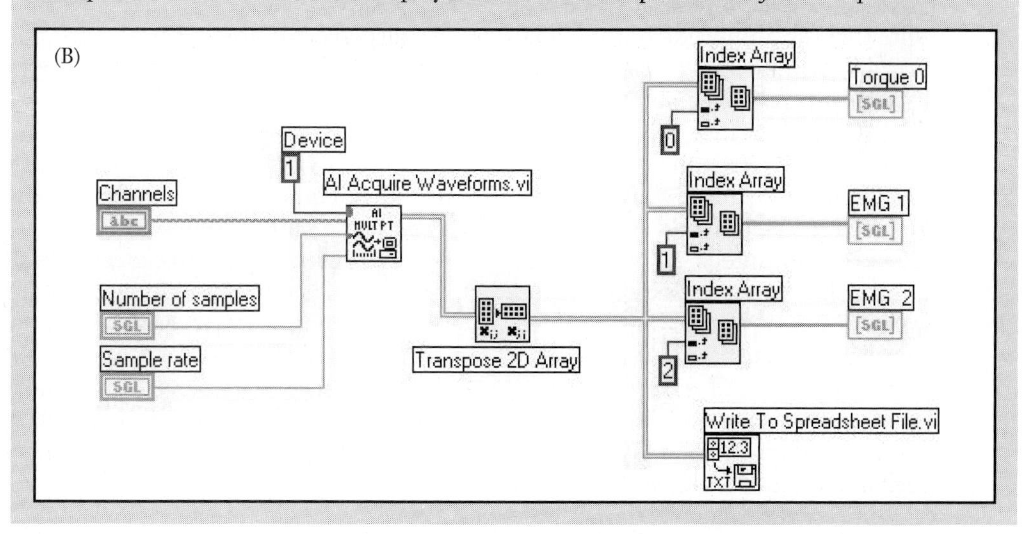

The block diagram for this VI is similar to that of **4Chanemg.vi** in Section 3–15, "Electromyography," with the exception that only three *Index Array* functions, with their corresponding *Numeric Constants,* were used to partition off the three channels of data collected by the *AI Acquire Waveforms.vi* function. Data are saved to disk using the *Write To Spreadsheet File.vi function.* **Save** the VI using a convenient filename and directory.

TOR&IEMG.VI

Tor&iemg.vi (Figure 3–17.2) analyzes files saved with **Tor&emg2.vi.** Build or call up this VI from the **CD ROM disk directory.** In the front panel, the upper *two Waveform Graphs* display "Raw" and "Mean Maximal" torque for 500 msec (default) from the point where ***peak torque*** is ***indexed*** in the ***segment*** specified by the "Start" and "End" values in two *Digital Controls.* The period when ***mean maximal torque*** is calculated and displayed may be adjusted by inputting a different value in the front panel *Digital Control* labeled "Time to Calculate Mean Value." In Figure 3–17.2, a ***maximal voluntary isometric contraction*** of the ***quadriceps femoris*** was performed for 8 seconds. Another *Digital Control* was used to input a torque ***calibration factor*** (1 volt = 61.02 Newton-meters). The ***torque signal*** may also be displayed as ***volts*** or ***foot-pounds.***

The lower two *Waveform Graphs* display the ***rectified*** and ***bandpass filtered*** EMG signals from two of the four quadriceps muscles (vastus medialis and vastus lateralis). A *Digital Indicator* below each graph displays the "Max(imal) Integral." Note that the amplitude of the signals may be displayed on the y-axis as volts, microvolts, or millivolts (default) using a *Vertical Pointer Slide* configured as a ***three-position integer*** (I32).

In the block diagram, the ***top*** section deals with torque channel manipulation, while the ***lower*** section processes and integrates the two channels of EMG. After a spreadsheet data file is read, the torque channel (channel 0) is selected using the *Index Array* function and converted to torque units (default = Newton-meters) using a predetermined conversion factor. A *For Loop* is used to calculate mean torque at the point where peak torque is indexed. *Subset Array* and *Mean.vi* functions are embedded in the *For Loop.* The *Array Subset* is indexed (lower left terminal) by the point in time when peak torque occurs. The "N" terminal of the *For Loop* is wired to an *Array Size* and *Subtract* function so that the *For Loop* will operate for the next "500" data points. An array of data is then output by the *For Loop* to an *Array Max & Min* function that displays the "Mean Maximal Torque Values" in a front panel *Digital Indicator.* "Start" and "End" indicies are also determined to index EMG integration in the lower section of the block diagram.

The "Max(imal) Integral" for each of the two EMG channels (i.e., channels 1 and 2) is calculated using essentially the same code and procedure described in **Iemgx2.vi** (see Figure 3–15.3). Two *Subset Array* functions, indexed by the value displayed in the "Start of Max Segment" *Digital Control* (see preceding discussion), determine the point at which the signals are integrated and the "Max(imal) Integral(s)" are displayed in the front panel for each muscle.

Save the VI using a convenient filename and directory. To confirm that the VI is operating properly, run the VI, and when prompted, use the ***data file*** named **TorqEMG3.dat.** Compare the values in the front panel *Digital Indicator(s)* and the graphs with those in Figure 3–17.2.

SUMMARY

Two VIs were constructed to collect, save, and analyze three channels of data. While torque is generated using a dynamometer, two channels of EMG are simultaneously recorded. **Tor&emg2.vi** is used to collect and save the data in a spreadsheet format and is essentially a three-channel version of a VI developed in a previous chapter. **Tor&iemg.vi** reads the data file saved using **Tor&emg2.vi** and calculates and displays raw and mean torque signals for 500 data points from the point where peak torque is determined. Simultaneously, two channels of EMG are integrated, starting at the peak torque index, and the maximal integrals are displayed on the front panel. *Waveform Graphs* display the raw and mean maximal torque signals and the filtered and rectified EMG signals.

PRACTICE EXERCISE

Modify **Tor&iemg.vi** by adding an additional channel of EMG to be integrated. In addition to displaying the filtered and rectified EMG signal in the front panel, add three more *Waveform Graphs* to display the raw (i.e., unrectified, unfiltered) EMG signals. Finally, add a front panel indicator that will display the directory and filename of the data file being processed. Save the VI into a convenient directory using the filename **T&i_mod.vi.** Compare the modified version just constructed with the VI called **Tor&iemg_mod.vi** in the **CD ROM disk directory.** To confirm that the VI is operating properly, run the VI, and when prompted, use the data file named **TorqEMG4.dat.** The following torque and integral values should be calculated and displayed:

PARAMETER	VALUE
Peak torque	74.51
Max mean torque	73.66
Start of max segment	1546
End of maximal segment	2046
Muscle No. 1 max integral	2071.43
Muscle No. 2 max integral	3352.03
Muscle No. 3 max integral	1746.20

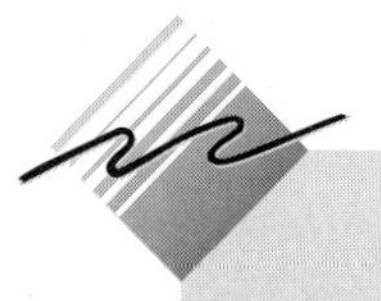

OBJECT/FUNCTION OR SUBVI LOCATOR
TOR&IEMG.VI

Panel	Object/Function or SubVI	Palette/Menu or Directory
Front	*Digital Control* × 2	**Controls/Numeric**
	Digital Indicator × 6	**Controls/Numeric**
	Vertical Pointer Slide	**Controls/Numeric**
	Waveform Graph × 4	**Controls/Graph**
Diagram	*Read From Spreadsheet File.vi*	**Functions/File I/O**
	Positive Infinity	**Functions/Numeric/ Additional Numeric Constants**
	Index Array × 3	**Functions/Array**
	Numeric Constants × 7	**Functions/Numeric**
	Multiply	**Functions/Numeric**
	Array Size	**Functions/Array**
	Subtract	**Functions/Numeric**
	Array Max & Min × 4	**Functions/Array**
	For Loop	**Functions/Structures**
	Add × 2	**Functions/Numeric**
	Array Subset × 3	**Functions/Array**
	Mean.vi	**Functions/Mathematics/ Probability and Statistics**
	Disvolts.vi × 2	**Functions/Select a VI . . . / CD ROM disk directory**
	Butterworth Filter.vi × 2	**Functions/Signal Processing/Filters**
	String Control	**Functions/String**
	Absolute Value × 2	**Functions/Numeric**
	Integrl2.vi	**Functions/Select a VI . . . / CD ROM disk directory**

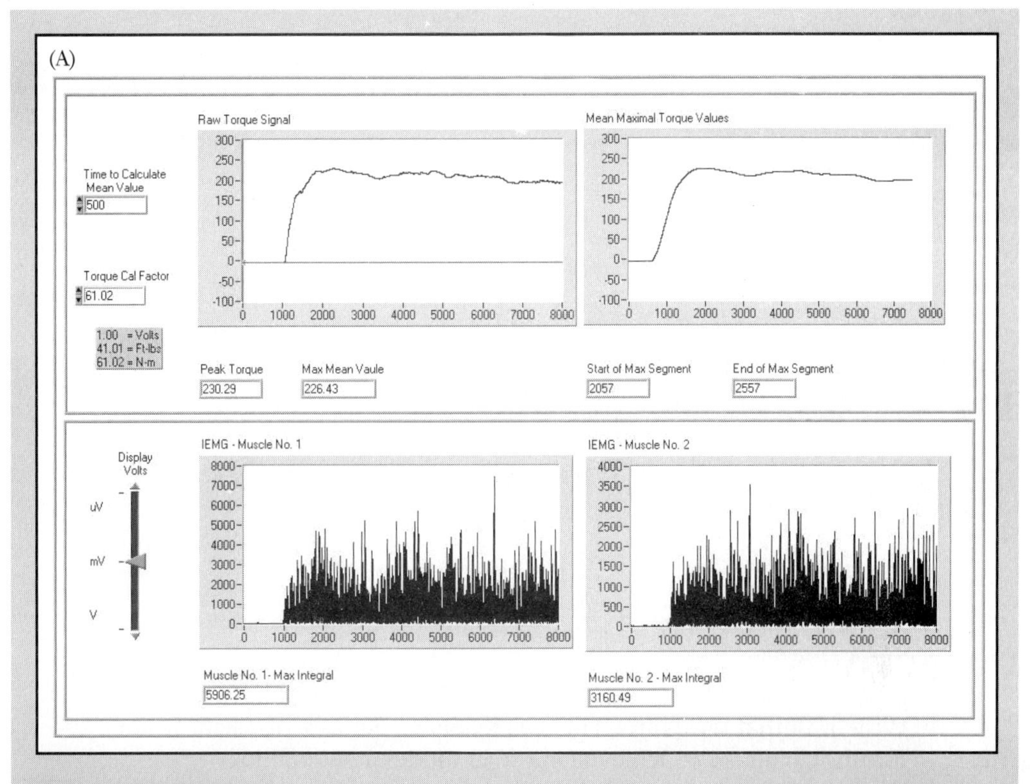

Figure 3–17.2
(A) Front panel and (B) block diagram of **Tor&iemg.vi.** This VI reads a previously saved file in spreadsheet format using the *Read From Spreadsheet File.vi* subVI in the block diagram. An isometric torque curve and two channels of simultaneous rectified filtered EMG are displayed on *Waveform Graphs*. The maximal integral is computed for each EMG channel. A second torque graph plots mean maximal torque for a preselected segment of the signal.

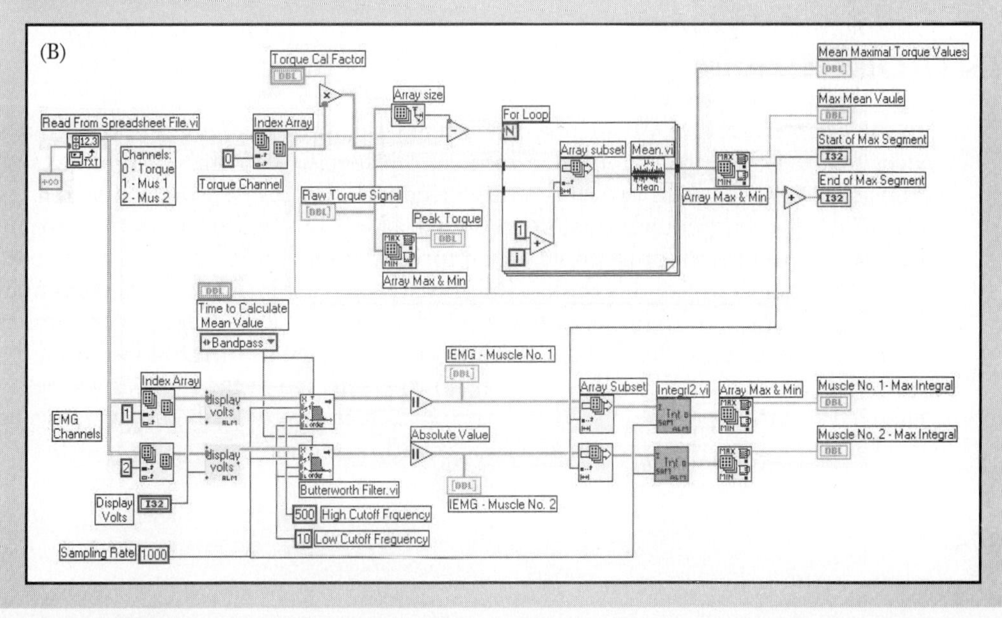

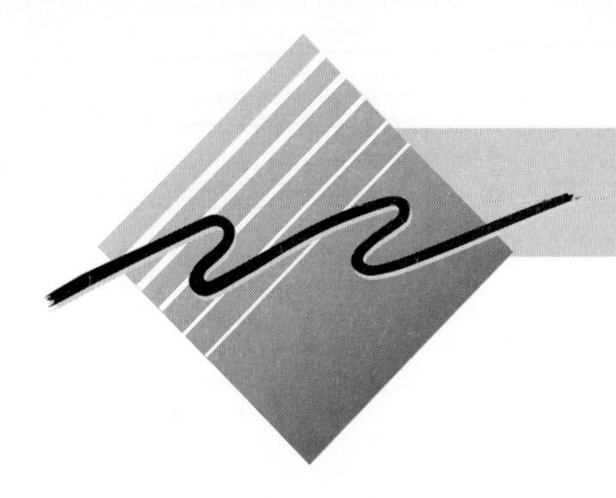

SECTION 3–18

FEEDBACK AND TIMING TOOLS

OBJECTIVES

- ❖ Write a VI that uses three LEDs as feedback devices that light when a threshold voltage is achieved in target mode or sequentially.
- ❖ Write a VI that uses a slide fill indicator and LED as a feedback device that lights and gives a message after a target voltage is achieved.
- ❖ Write a VI that demonstrates the use of LEDs using comparative functions.
- ❖ Write a VI configured as a digital timer that displays time in seconds and milliseconds.
- ❖ Write a VI configured as a countdown digital timer.

INTRODUCTION

In this chapter, several VIs will be constructed as simple ***feedback*** and ***timing*** devices that may be further modified to meet the specific demands of training sessions or experiments. In two of the three feedback devices, sensors connected directly to the computer's analog-to-digital (A-to-D) board permit real-time feedback to the user. For example, when force is applied to a transducer, the user might target on a preset threshold voltage that, when achieved, leads to sequential lighting of LEDs configured to fire at predetermined percentages of maximum values. In some cases, the threshold values or percentage of threshold values to be achieved before an LED lights were arbitrarily selected. These values are easily changed to meet specific needs. Two ***timing devices*** are described that might be used as an on-screen stopwatch and as a countdown timer.

FEEDBK1.VI

Feedbk1.vi (Figure 3–18.1) uses three ***vertically oriented*** *Round LEDs* on the front panel, which may be activated by one of two methods using a *Boolean Vertical Toggle Switch.* With the "Sequential" method, the ***bottom*** *LED* will light up when a preset threshold voltage is achieved. The ***middle*** and ***top*** *LED* will light up when 75% and 50% of the preset threshold is achieved, respectively. Using the "Target" method, when a threshold of ± "0.5" volts is achieved, the ***middle*** *LED* will light up. If ***less than*** or ***greater than*** the target value is registered, the ***lower*** or ***top*** *LED* will light up, respectively, while the ***middle*** *LED* turns off.

In the block diagram, note that a real-time voltage output by a sensor (e.g., force transducer) is acquired by the computer's A-to-D board by the *A1 Sample Channel.vi* function. The entire program is enclosed in a *While Loop* controlled by a second front panel *Vertical Toggle Switch* affording ***on/off*** control to the VI. Toggling between methods (i.e., target vs. sequential) is achieved using a *Boolean*-activated *Case Structure.*

The "Target" method toggles the *Case Structure* to the ***true*** condition, while the *In Range?* function is used to ensure that the target voltage, input via a front panel *Digital Control,* is being maintained within 0.5 volts. Build and save this VI using a convenient filename and directory. This VI may also be called up from the **CD ROM disk directory.**

FEEDBK2.VI

Feedbk2.vi (Figure 3–18.2) uses an ***enlarged*** *Vertical Fill Slide* and *Boolean Round LED* configured with a message ("Target Achieved!") as feedback devices. The size of both structures is increased by left-clicking and dragging a corner of the structure to its desired size. A "Target Value" voltage is input via a *Digital Control.* While the VI is running, the *Vertical Fill Slide* will move up or down proportional to a voltage registered by a sensor connected to the computer's A-to-D board. When the target voltage is achieved, the *Round LED* over the *Vertical Fill Slide* will switch to the ***true*** condition turning green and flashing the "Target Achieved" message.

When the *Round LED* is initially accessed from the **Controls** palette and located on the front panel, the ***false*** condition is colored ***black*** and the ***true*** condition is ***red.*** In the current VI, ***false*** is a ***light gray*** color and the ***true*** condition is ***green.*** To change the color of each condition, use the *Hand Tool* to toggle between conditions. Next, using the *Paint Brush Tool,* color the conditions accordingly. To insert the "Target Achieved!" message, first toggle to the ***true*** (green) condition. Using the *Arrow Tool,* left-click on the LED, and from the pop-up menu, choose *Show* and then *Boolean Text.* The default message that appears will be "ON." Using the *Lettering Tool,* change the message to "Target Achieved!" Toggle back to the ***false*** condition, and delete the "OFF" (default) message.

OBJECT/FUNCTION OR SUBVI LOCATOR
FEEDBK1.VI

Panel	Object/Function or SubVI	Palette/Menu or Directory
Front	*Vertical Switch* × 2	**Controls/Boolean**
	Digital Control	**Controls/Numeric**
	LED × 3	**Controls/Boolean**
Diagram	*While Loop*	**Functions/Structures**
	Case Structure	**Functions/Structures**
	AI Sample Channel.vi	**Functions/Data Acquisition/Analog Input**
	String Constant	**Functions/String**
	Numeric Constant × 5	**Functions/Numeric**
	In Range?	**Functions/Comparison**
	Greater?	**Functions/Comparison**
	Less? × 2	**Functions/Comparison**
	Greater Or Equal? × 3	**Functions/Comparison**
	Add	**Functions/Numeric**
	Subtract	**Functions/Numeric**
	Multiply × 2	**Functions/Numeric**

In the block diagram, the entire VI is enclosed in a *While Loop* that affords ***on/off*** control. Note that in addition to the front panel *LED* giving positive feedback via color change and a message, an audible ***beep*** sound is given. The sound is provided using the *Beep.vi* function enclosed in the ***true*** condition of a *Case Structure* wired to the ***output side*** of the *Greater Or Equal?* function. The ***false*** condition is ***empty.*** Build and **Save** this VI using a convenient filename and directory. This VI may also be called up from the **CD ROM disk directory.**

LEDS.VI

Leds.vi (Figure 3–18.3) uses an array of *Boolean Round LEDs* to signal when a certain condition is met compared with a randomly generated number. For example, if the random number is ***1.34,*** the ***fourth*** LED (n < 4) would light up. This type of programming logic would be useful in constructing a front panel display as a ***biofeedback*** device. This VI uses similar front panel and block diagram elements

FIGURE 3–18.1 (A) Front panel and (B) block diagram of **Feedbk1.vi.** A single channel of data is acquired from the computer's A-to-D board in real time using the *AI Sample Channel.vi* subVI in the block diagram. The signal is displayed as a feedback device in the front panel on three *LEDs.* Two display methods are provided.

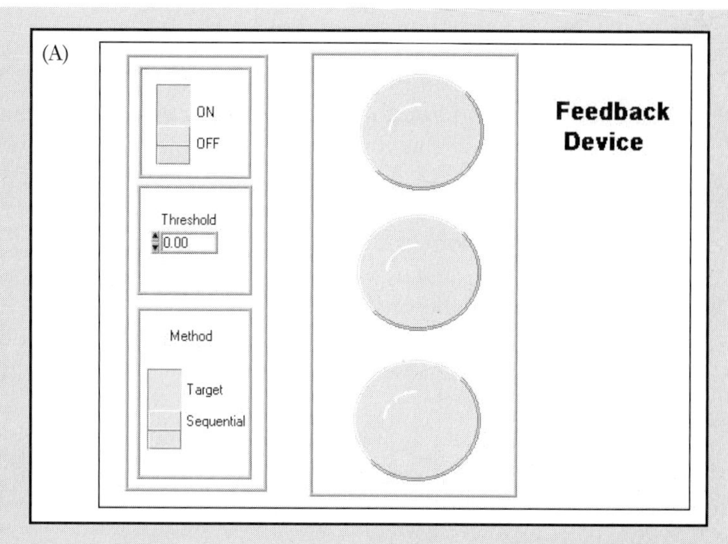

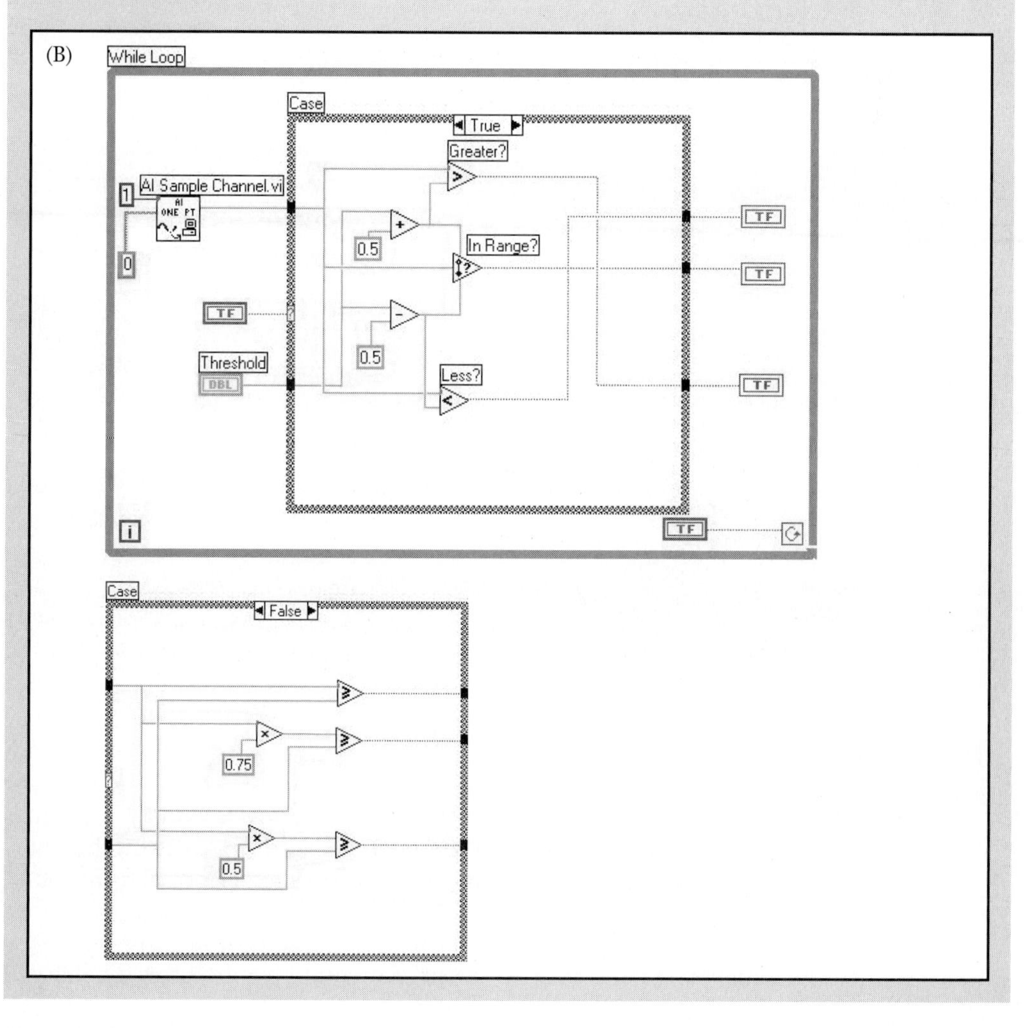

as **Feedbk1.vi** and **Feedbk2.vi.** One major difference is that the input source for this VI is produced by the **Rxcsale.vi** subVI built in Section 3–5, "Creating SubVIs." Random numbers are ***scaled*** by a factor of "10," using a *Numeric Constant,* and then compared to preset values using *Greater?* and *Less?* functions. Note also that the ***rate*** at which the random numbers are generated is controlled by *the Wait Until Next ms Multiple* function wired to a front panel *Dial,* configured as an *I32 integer* and ***scaled*** to a maximum value of "1000." The default setting is "500"; thus, a new random number is generated every 0.5 second (i.e., 500 msec). Build and **Save** this VI using a convenient filename and directory. This VI may also be called up from the **CD ROM disk directory.**

OBJECT/FUNCTION OR SUBVI LOCATOR
FEEDBK2.VI

Panel	Object/Function or SubVI	Palette/Menu or Directory
Front	*Vertical Switch*	**Controls/Boolean**
	Digital Control	**Controls/Numeric**
	Vertical Fill Slide	**Controls/Numeric**
	Round LED	**Controls/Boolean**
Diagram	*While Loop*	**Functions/Structures**
	AI Sample Channel.vi	**Functions/Data Acquisition/Analog Input**
	String Constant	**Functions/String**
	Numeric Constant	**Functions/Numeric**
	Greater Or Equal?	**Functions/Comparison**
	Case Structure	**Functions/Structures**
	Beep.vi	**Functions/Graphics & Sound/Sound**

TIMER.VI

Timer.vi (Figure 3–18.4) is a countdown timer that can be set with a front panel *Dial* to 60 seconds (default position = 10 seconds). When the VI is **Run,** the timer will countdown in ***1-second increments.*** When the timer stops, a front panel *Boolean Round LED* will light and turn red, flashing a "Finish" message. Note that the *Digital Control* associated with the *Dial* and the *LED* on the front panel has been enlarged, making them easier to see on the computer monitor. The *Round*

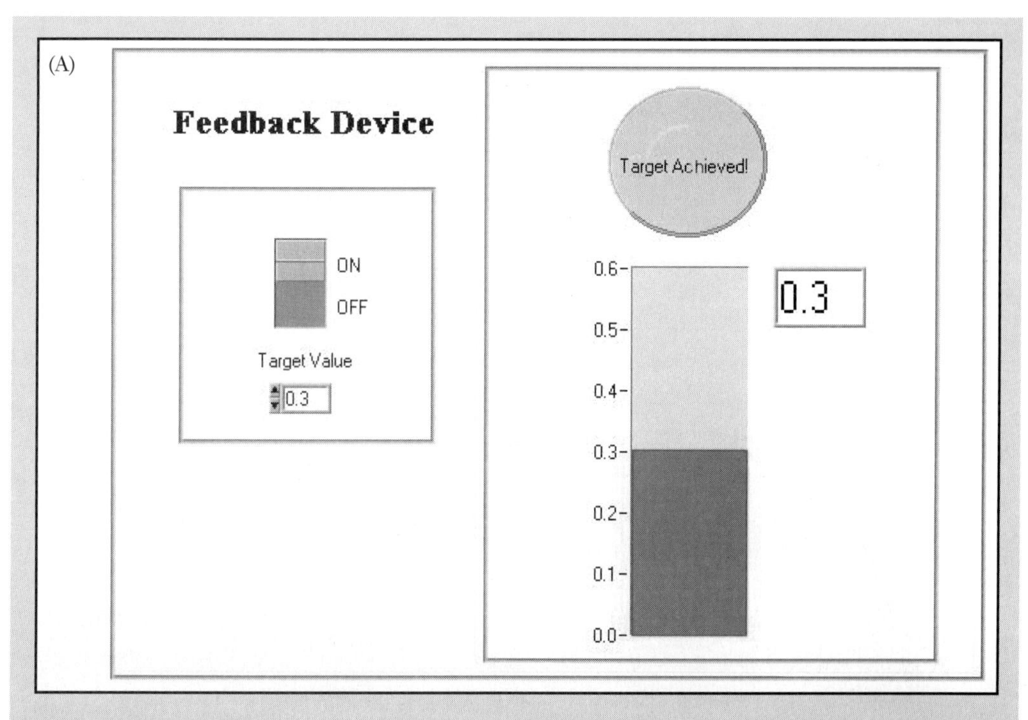

FIGURE 3–18.2
(A) Front panel and (B) block diagram of **Feedbk2.vi.** This VI also uses *the AI Sample Channel.vi* subVI in the block diagram to acquire a signal from the computer's A-to-D board in real time. A *Vertical Fill Slide* on the front panel moves upward as the signal's voltage increases. When a predetermined threshold voltage is attained, an *LED* lights and provides a feedback message. An audible signal is also given off using the *Beep.vi* subVI in the block diagram.

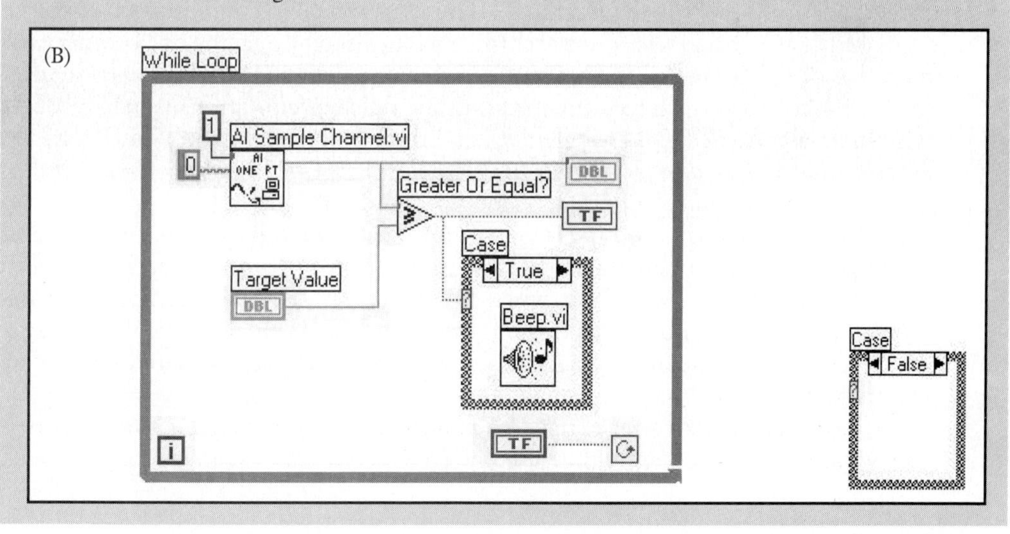

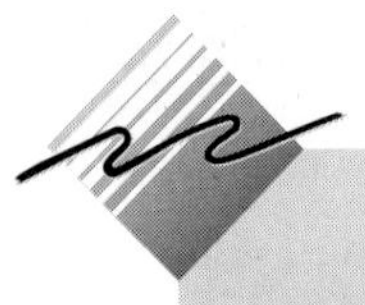

OBJECT/FUNCTION OR SUBVI LOCATOR
LEDS.VI

Panel	Object/Function or SubVI	Palette/Menu or Directory
Front	*Dial*	**Controls/Numeric**
	Labeled Oblong Button	**Controls/Boolean**
	Digital Indicator	**Controls/Numeric**
	Waveform Chart	**Controls/Graph**
	Round LED × 4	**Controls/Boolean**
Diagram	*While Loop*	**Functions/Structures**
	Rxscale.vi	**Functions/Select a VI . . . / CD ROM disk directory**
	Wait Until Next ms Multiple	**Functions/Time & Dialog**
	Greater? × 4	**Functions/Comparison**
	Less?	**Functions/Comparison**
	Numeric Constant × 5	**Functions/Numeric**

LED may be configured with color and a message in the same way as described in the previous example.

In the block diagram, the program has again been embedded in a *While Loop*, which, in this case, is controlled by a front panel *Dial* and the use of a *Shift Register* (see Section 3–3, "Block Diagram"). The *Decrement* (−1) function, wired to the right *Shift Register Element*, ***decreases*** the current time by a factor of "1" with ***each iteration*** of the *While Loop*. That value is retained in the *While Loop* and ***sequentially reduced*** until a "zero" value (i.e., timer finished condition) is achieved. At that point, the *While Loop* is toggled ***off***, and the VI stops running. The *While Loop* is ***calibrated*** to ***1 second per iteration*** using the *Wait Until Next ms Multiple* function wired on its input side with a *Numeric Constant* of "1000."

This VI uses a *Local Variable* (*Timer (secs)*—in a ***blue*** rectangular box). ***Local Variables*** are used to pass data, in this case in the form of a ***control instruction*** from the *Dial* timer to the *While Loop*, when the structures ***can't*** be wired together ***directly.*** In some cases, but not in this VI, the same *Local Variable* may appear in several places in the same block diagram. *Local Variables* may be associated with many front panel elements.

To create a *Local Variable*, right-click on the front panel element to be associated with the *Local Variable*. In this case, the *Dial* is configured as an *I32 integer*, scaled

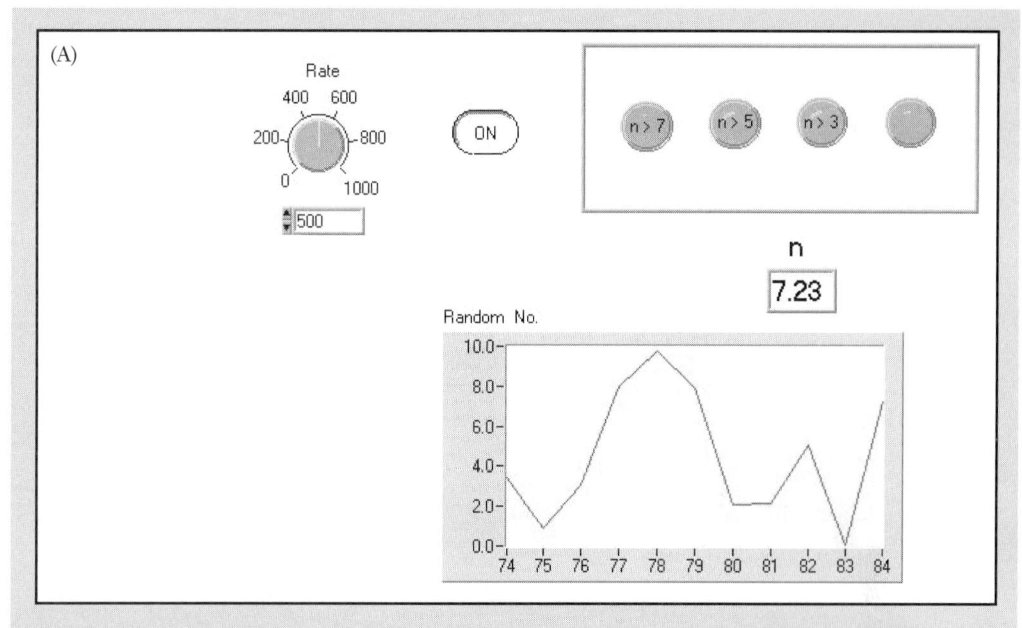

FIGURE 3–18.3
(A) Front panel and (B) block diagram of **Leds.vi** using four front panel *LEDs* to document when a random number generated by the **Rxscale.vi** subVI meets a preset condition (e.g., a number is greater than 3). When the condition is met, an *LED* lights up. The data points are also displayed on a front panel *Waveform Graph* and *Digital Indicator.*

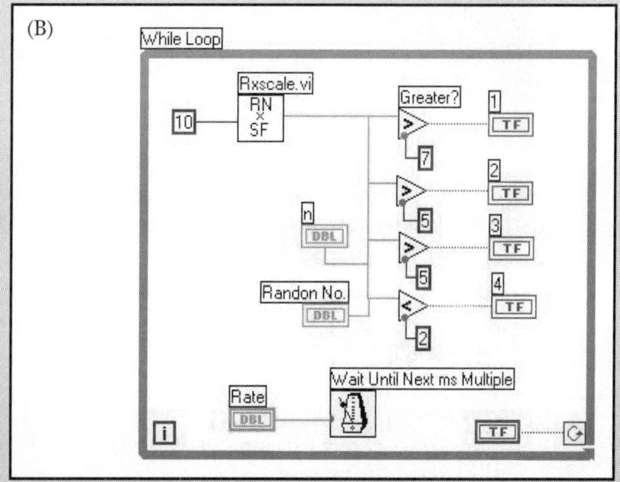

up to "60," and labeled "Timer (secs)." From the *pop-up menu,* select the *Create* option, and then left-click on *Local Variable.* This action toggles to the block diagram where a ***blue rectangular box*** (i.e., the *Local Variable*) with the inside label "Timer (secs)" appears near the *Dial* icon. At this point, the *Local Variable* is treated as any other block diagram icon and may be wired in place in the usual manner. In this VI, wire the *Local Variable* between the left side *Shift Register Element* and the *Decrement*

OBJECT/FUNCTION OR SUBVI LOCATOR
TIMER.VI

Panel	Object/Function or SubVI	Palette/Menu or Directory
Front	*Digital Control*	**Controls/Numeric**
	Dial	**Controls/Numeric**
	Round LED	**Controls/Boolean**
Diagram	*While Loop*	**Functions/Structures**
	Wait Until Next ms Multiple	**Functions/Time & Dialog**
	Numeric Constant	**Functions/Numeric**
	Not	**Functions/Boolean**
	Greater Than 0?	**Functions/Comparison**
	Decrement (−1)	**Functions/Numeric**
	Timer (sec) Local Variable	**Attached to Dial—See text**

(−1) function. Call up the remaining front panel elements, and finish wiring the VI as described in Figure 3–18.4. **Save** this VI using a convenient filename and directory. This VI may also be called up from the **CD ROM disk directory.**

DIGTIMER.VI

As its name implies, **Digtimer.vi** acts like an onscreen digital timer or stopwatch, reporting time in ***seconds*** and ***milliseconds*** (Figure 3–18.5). It has three front panel elements including a *Boolean Round Stop Button* and two *Digital Indicators:* one reading time as ***seconds*** with ***precision*** configured to ***four*** decimal places; and the other reading ***milliseconds*** with ***zero*** decimal places. A large red "Stop" button will turn off the VI.

The majority of the program in the block diagram is embedded in a *While Loop.* The timing source in this VI is the *Tick Count (ms)* function appearing both ***outside*** and ***inside*** the *While Loop.* The theory of operation is that the tick count begins when the VI is run, activating both *Tick Count (ms)* functions. The **stop_time.gbl** *Global Variable* (see following discussion), wired to the *While Loop,* freezes the tick count outside the *While Loop* while the tick counting process con-

FIGURE 3–18.4 (A) Front panel and (B) block diagram of **Timer.vi.** This VI operates like a standard timer with a maximal setting of 60 seconds defaulting to 10. When the countdown is complete, a large *LED* lights.

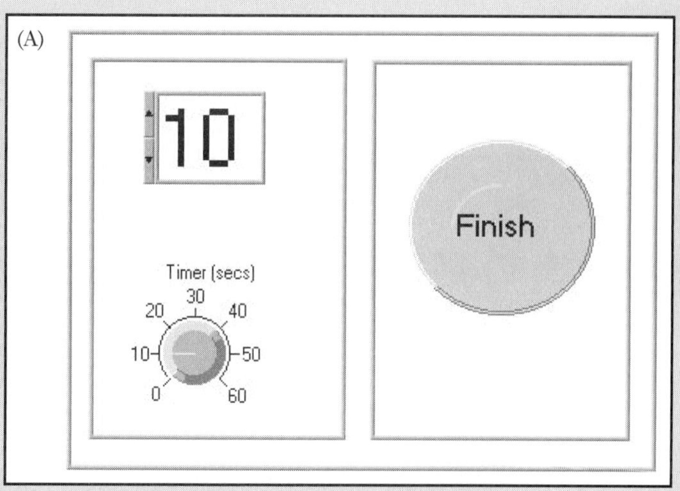

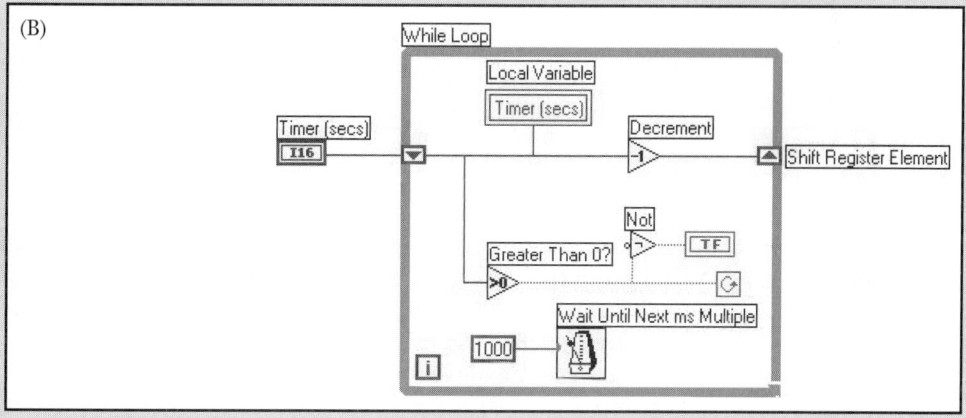

tinues inside. The ***difference*** between the ***continuous tick count*** (inside the loop) and the ***frozen tick count*** (outside the loop) is the ***elapsed time*** the VI operates. When the VI is stopped, the same *Global Variable* is used to turn ***off*** the *While Loop*, shutting down the VI.

Global Variables have a similar function to *Local Variables* (see previous example), in that the variable is associated with numerous block diagram functions. *Local Variables,* however, only function within a ***single*** VI, whereas *Global Variables* have association with elements in ***two*** or ***more*** VIs. **Digtimer.vi** demonstrates a simple use of a *Global Variable.* The fact that the *Tick Count (ms)* function resides outside and inside the *While Loop* basically defines two ***interacting*** VIs that are controlled by a ***single*** *Global Variable.* Unlike *Local Variables,* which are ***embedded***

OBJECT/FUNCTION OR SUBVI LOCATOR
DIGTIMER.VI

Panel	Object/Function or SubVI	Palette/Menu or Directory
Front	*Labeled Round Button*	**Controls/Boolean**
	Digital Indicator × 2	**Controls/Numeric**
Diagram	*Tick Count (ms)* × 2	**Functions/Time & Dialog**
	While Loop	**Functions/Structures**
	Boolean Constant	**Functions/Boolean**
	Subtract	**Functions/Numeric**
	Divide	**Functions/Numeric**
	Not	**Functions/Boolean**
	stop_time.glb	**Functions/Select a VI . . . / CD ROM disk directory**

code elements of a VI, ***Global Variables*** may be thought of as a form of subVI that is configured and saved using the **.gbl** extension.

To create a *Global Variable*, go to the block diagram, and left-click on *Global Variable* from the **Structures** palette, and place it in its approximate location. Note that in its current form, the icon appears as a small rectangle with a picture of the world in it with a ***question mark (?)*** to its right. Double-clicking on the *Global Variable* icon opens the variables front panel in which are placed front panel elements of the main VI. In this case, there are two elements: a *Boolean Round Stop Button* labeled "Stop button" and a *Digital Indicator* labeled "Time (msec)." ***Be sure each element is labeled.*** Save the *Global Variable* using the **stop_time.gbl** filename into a convenient directory.

Return to the block diagram, and make a copy of the icon by first holding down the Control (Ctrl) key and left-clicking and dragging off a copy of the icon. Right-click on one copy of the *Global Variable* icon; from the pop-up menu, choose *Select Item*, and left-click on "Stop button." Note that the ***question mark (?)*** in the variable icon changes to the word "Stop button" and the ***double-lined border*** around the icon is now ***green.*** Repeat the procedure with the second icon, but this time choose "Time (msec)" and note the ***red double-lined border.*** At this point the *Global Variable* may be used just like any subVI or other programming function.

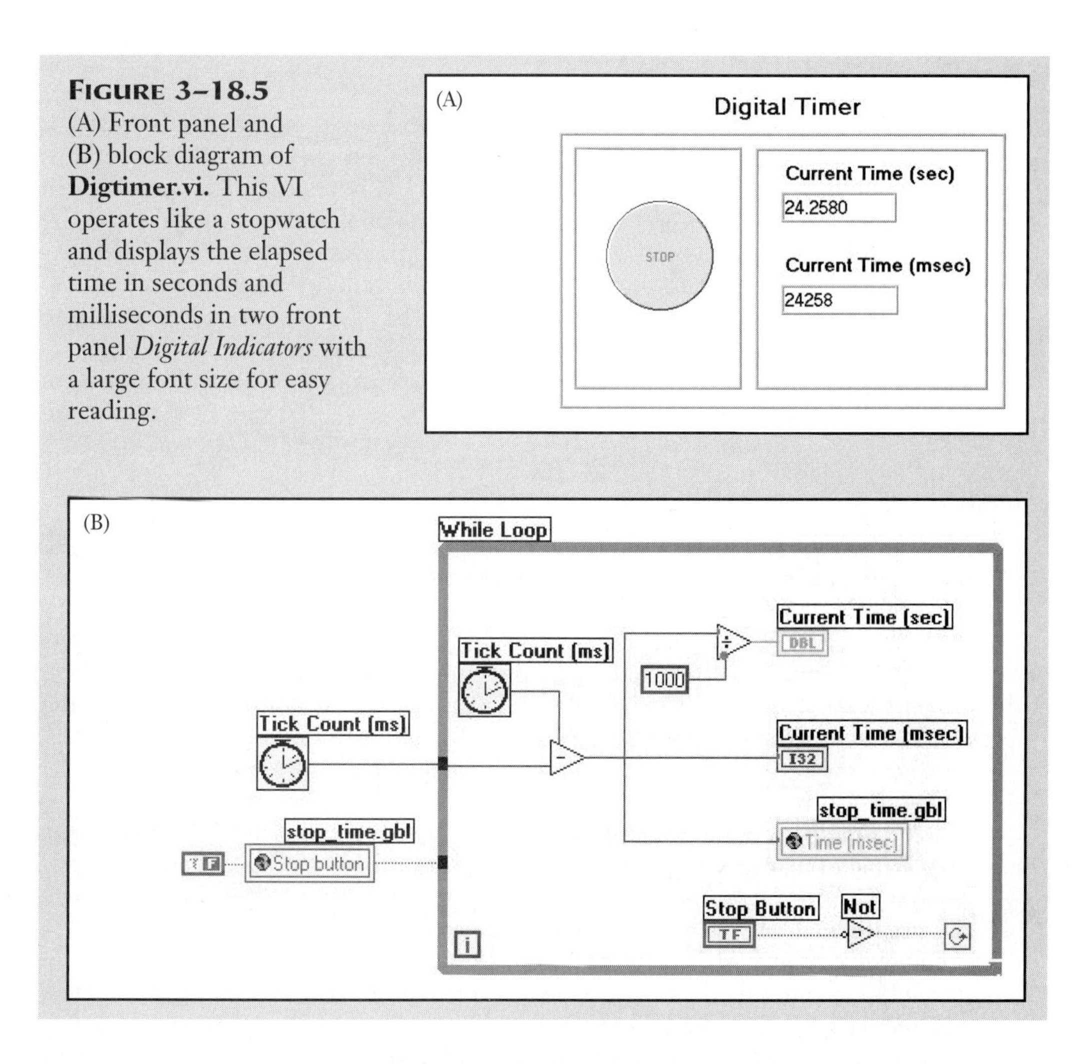

FIGURE 3–18.5
(A) Front panel and (B) block diagram of **Digtimer.vi.** This VI operates like a stopwatch and displays the elapsed time in seconds and milliseconds in two front panel *Digital Indicators* with a large font size for easy reading.

Call up and lay out the remaining front panel and block diagram elements as described in Figure 3–18.5. Move the icon labeled "Stop button" to the left side of the *While Loop*, right-click on the icon, and select *Create Constant*. Note that a *Boolean True/False Constant* pops out from the left side of the icon already wired. Keep the constant in its ***F*** (false) default position. Wire the right side of the icon to the *While Loop*. Move the icon labeled "Time (msec)" inside the While Loop, and wire it to the output side of the *Subtract* function. Complete wiring other elements, and **Save** the VI using a convenient filename and directory. This VI, including the **stop_time.gbl** *Global Variable*, may also be called up from the **CD ROM disk directory.**

SUMMARY

LabVIEW VIs used as ***feedback*** and ***timing*** devices were constructed. VIs used as ***feedback*** devices employ *LEDs*, *Digital Indicators*, and an audible ***beep*** sound as sources of visual and auditory feedback. These VIs are generally embedded in *While Loops* that afford ***on/off*** control using a front panel *Boolean* switch. Two of the VIs capture voltage signals directly from sensors connected to the computer's A-to-D board, while the third uses a random number generator as the signal source. These VIs should be thought of as prototypes whose threshold and comparative values can be changed to meet specific training and experiment needs.

Timing devices can be constructed using *Local* and *Global Variables* to control timer function.

PRACTICE EXERCISES

Modify **Feedbk1.vi** so that front panel controls may be used with the "Target" method to change the level of ***plus*** or ***minus tolerance*** used to decide whether the current voltage value is ***in range.*** Set the ***control device*** to ***default*** to "0.25" volts. Add an auditory ***beep*** signal that ***will sound*** when the ***current value*** is ***in range.*** Using the "Sequential" method, add front panel controls that permit ***varying*** the ***current scale factors*** of "0.75" and "0.50." Have the control devices default to the ***current values.*** **Save** the ***modified*** VI using the following filename: **Fd1_mod.vi.** Compare the new version with a modified version called **Fd1mod.vi** in the **CD ROM disk directory.**

In **Feedbk2.vi,** modify the VI to include a front panel control that allows the ***beep*** signal to be turned ***off*** if it's decided this additional source of feedback is not needed. ***Rescale*** the *Vertical Fill Slide* so that the ***top value*** is "0.45" volts. This will require ***decimal precision*** to be changed to ***two places.*** Change the default value in the *Digital Control* underneath the "ON/OFF" switch to "0.45" volts, and likewise change its ***decimal precision*** to ***two places.*** Finally, change the ***color*** of the *Vertical Fill Slide* to ***green*** and the LED ***target message*** to "You're There!" Save the modified version using the following filename: **Fd2_mod.vi.** Compare the new version with a modified version called **Fd2mod.vi** in the **CD ROM disk directory.**

To understand the different actions of the *Tick Count (ms)* functions in **Digtimer.vi,** call up the VI just constructed or call it up from the **CD ROM disk directory.** Switch to the block diagram, and use the ***debugging procedures*** discussed in Section 3–8, "VI Programming Errors," to understand how the VI operates. Recall that when the VI is run the *Tick Count (ms)* function outside the *While Loop* freezes while inside function continues. The ***difference*** between the two represents the ***elapsed time.*** Left-click **Highlight Execution** (light bulb), click on the **Run** arrow, and observe the values in the ***pop-up probe indicators*** inserted into the two wires leading to the *Subtract* function as the VI goes through several iterations.

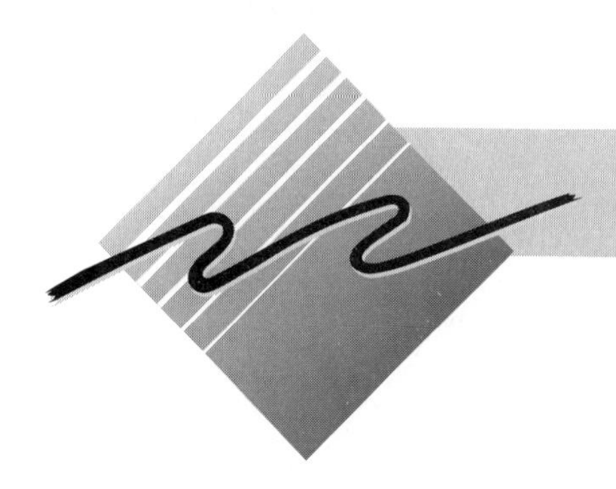

SECTION 3–19

Other Programming Functions and Tools

Objectives

- ❖ Build VIs that use additional front panel and block diagram control functions to display and analyze data.
- ❖ Build and run three VIs that demonstrate basic concepts of statistical analysis.
- ❖ Run two VIs that demonstrate the use of binary programming concepts for data acquisition and analysis.

Introduction

This chapter presents a number of VIs that demonstrate additional LabVIEW programming functions and tools that may be of use in kinesiological and biomechanical research including a demonstration of basic applications in ***statistical analysis.*** The final VIs in the "Advanced Analysis" section are quite complex and demonstrate higher level programming functions, including an introduction to data analysis using ***binary*** format data files.

Other Programming Functions

Objectives

- ❖ Build a VI that demonstrates three methods of updating *Waveform Graphs* and *Charts.*

- Build a VI that demonstrates the use of front panel *Menu* and *Text Rings*.
- Build a VI that uses an Attribute Node to automatically read x-axis (time) index positions from a *Waveform Graph* cursor display.

UPDATES.VI

Updates.vi (Figure 3–19.1) demonstrates three methods of ***displaying*** and ***updating*** data in *Waveform Graphs* and *Charts.* Build this VI, or call it up from the **CD ROM disk directory.** Three *Waveform Charts* are stacked, one on top of the other, in the front panel. Note that the same data appear on each chart when the VI is run. ***Simulated temperature*** data are generated from a National Instruments subVI called **Promon1.vi,** also found in the **CD ROM disk directory.** ***On/off*** control is afforded by embedding block diagram elements in a *While Loop* controlled by a front

OBJECT/FUNCTION OR SUBVI LOCATOR
UPDATES.VI

Panel	Object/Function or SubVI	Palette/Menu or Directory
Front	*Dial*	**Controls/Numeric**
	Vertical Switch	**Controls/Boolean**
	Waveform Graph × 3	**Controls/Graph**
Diagram	*While Loop*	**Functions/Structures**
	Promon1.vi	**Functions/Select a VI . . . / CD ROM disk directory**
	Wait Until Next ms Multiple	**Functions/**

panel *Boolean Vertical Switch.* The rate of data generation is controlled by a front panel *Dial* and by the use of the *Wait Until Next ms Multiple* function in the block diagram. The default rate has been set at "55."

The three update modes include *Strip Chart (default)*, *Scope Chart*, and *Sweep Chart.* After a *Waveform Chart* is selected, positioned, and sized on the front panel, use the *Arrow Tool*, and right-click anywhere on the graph to pop-up a menu. Left-click on *Data Operations* and again on *Update Mode.* Three chart icons will appear as described earlier. Left-click on one of the three options.

After building the VI, move the "ON/OFF" switch to the "ON" (up) position using the *Hand Tool*, **Run** the VI, and observe the ***three update modes.*** *Strip Chart* mode gives a ***continuous*** data stream that will continue uninterrupted until

part of the positioned and sized graph, and right-click. From the pop-up menu, left-click on the *Show* option, and then select *Cursor Display*. The display appears below in an inactive state and should be configured (see "Graphs and Graphing Options" in Section 3–2, "Front Panel"). The *Cursor Display* of the lower graph labeled "Rectified File" will be the one to which an *Attribute Node* will be attached. This *Cursor Display* will read predetermined start and ending points for a ***segment*** to be analyzed into *Numeric Indicators* to the right of the graph. In Figure 3–19.3, "Cursor 0" has been located at x-axis (time) point "1300," and "Cursor 1" is at "4100." These points have been designated as default settings for the *Cursor Display* by placing the *Arrow Tool* on each display and by right-clicking and choosing the *Data Operations/Make Current Value Default* option ***before*** the VI is saved.

An *Attribute Node* is associated with the *Cursor Display* by right-clicking on it directly over the phrase "Cursor 0" and by selecting the *Create* an *Attribute Node* option from the pop-up menu. In the block diagram, a rectangular icon appears, labeled "Visible." Add ***three*** more *Elements* (rectangles) to the icon by right-clicking on it and selecting *Add Element.*

At this point, the icon has four rectangular *Elements*, each one labeled "Visible." The upper two elements will be associated with Cursor 0: One will ***read*** the cursor x-axis location, and the other will ***write*** that position to a front panel *Numeric Indicator.* The next two elements will be configured in a similar way for *Cursor 1*. Right-click on the ***first*** and ***third*** elements, and from *Select Item* in the pop-up menu, choose *Active Cursor.* For the ***second*** and ***fourth*** elements, choose *Select Item*, then *Cursor Info*, and finally *Cursor Index*. Pop-up a *Numeric Constant* for the first and third elements: The first should be "0" and the other should be "1."

By default, elements have a *Write* function, as signified by a ***small arrow*** (pointing to the right) on the left side of the label "Active Cursor." Change the ***second*** and ***fourth*** elements to ***Read*** by right-clicking and selecting the *Change to Read* pop-up menu item. Note that the arrow has shifted to the right side of the label "Cursor Index." Check that the *Attribute Node* has been correctly configured in the block diagram in Figure 3–19.3. At this point, the *Attribute Node* will now ***write*** and ***read*** cursor display x-axis coordinate positions. Call up, locate, and wire the remaining functions in the block diagram, and **Save** the VI using a convenient filename and directory.

To confirm that the VI is wired correctly, run the VI; when prompted, select the data file called **Torq4.dat** from the **CD ROM disk directory,** and compare the values in the front panel *Digital Indicators* with those in Figure 3–19.3.

B_LINE.VI

During isometric torque curve analysis, it's necessary to establish a point in time when the actual torque signal ***rises*** from the ***baseline*** (see Figure 3–16.1). Once this point is determined, parameters such as ***time-to-peak-torque*** or the ***integral*** (i.e., area under the curve) of the complete torque signal may be calculated. In previous VIs, the point when the torque curve (signal) rises from the baseline

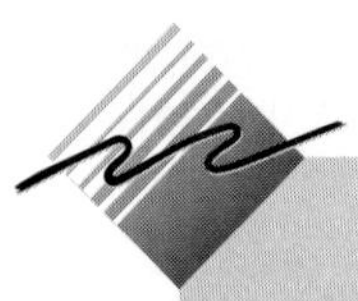

OBJECT/FUNCTION OR SUBVI LOCATOR
CURSOR.VI

Panel	Object/Function or SubVI	Palette/Menu or Directory
Front	*Waveform Graph* × 3	**Controls/Graph**
	Digital Control	**Controls/Numeric**
	Digital Indicator × 8	**Controls/Numeric**
Diagram	*Read From Spreadsheet File.vi*	**Functions/File I/O**
	Index Array	**Functions/Array**
	Array Size × 2	**Functions/Array**
	Absolute Value × 3	**Functions/Numeric**
	Attribute Node	**Attached to Cursor Display—see Text**
	Subtract	**Functions/Numeric**
	Array Subset	**Functions/Array**
	Mean.vi	**Functions/Mathematics/ Probability and Statistics**
	SDsam.vi	**Functions/Select a VI . . . / CD ROM disk directory**
	Array Max & Min	**Functions/Array**
	Add	**Functions/Numeric**

(noise) has been determined using the segment of code described in the block diagram of Figure 3–19.4. Key elements of this routine include the *Array Subset* and *Threshold Peak Detector.vi* functions. The maximal amplitude of a predetermined, rectified, and filtered segment of baseline noise (default = 500) is identified. This segment is referenced using an *Array Subset* function where a *Numeric Control* variable or *Constant* (default = 500) is wired to the "length" terminal (lower left terminal). A small voltage (default = 0.001 volts) is added to the maximal amplitude determined using an *Array Max & Min* function. This represents the ***differentiation point*** between baseline ***noise*** and the ***true torque signal*** arising from baseline. An alternate method would be to add 2 ***standard deviations*** from the mean baseline amplitude. Either value is used to ***index*** the *Threshold Peak Detector.vi* function, which in turn, passes on the signal to determine the minimum index point using a second *Array Max & Min* function. This point represents the ***torque signal rise point*** from the baseline.

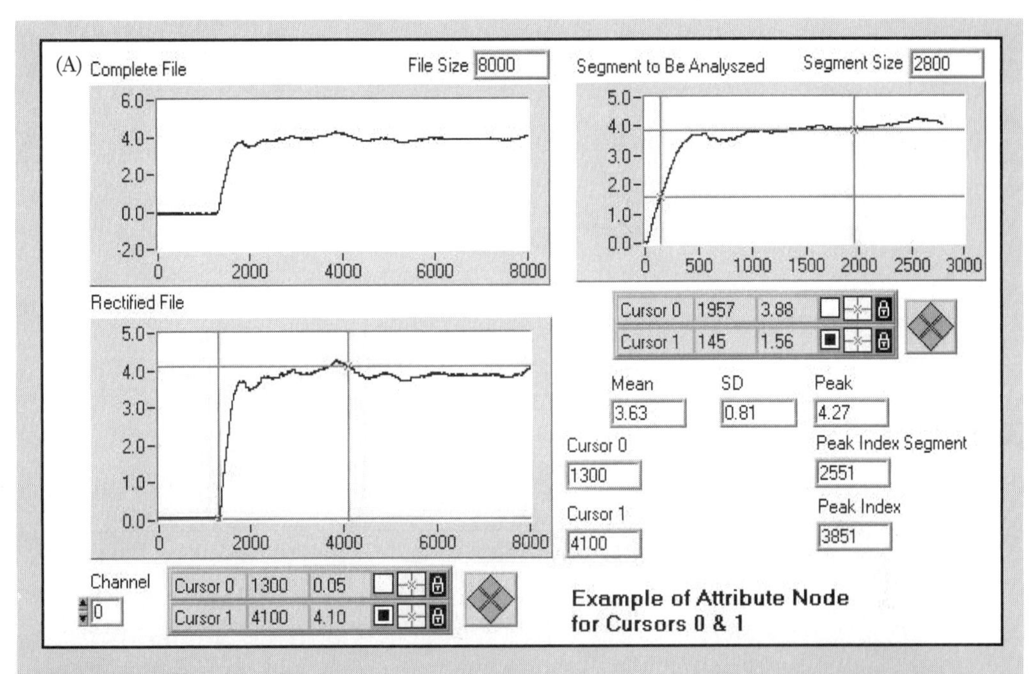

FIGURE 3–19.3
(A) Front panel and (B) block diagram of **Cursor.vi.** An *Attribute Node* is used to identify the start and ending points of a segment of data to be analyzed. After the VI is run for the first time, the cursors of the lower *Waveform Graph* in the front panel are positioned over the segment to be analyzed. The second time the VI is run, the selected segment will be displayed in the upper right *Waveform Graph.*

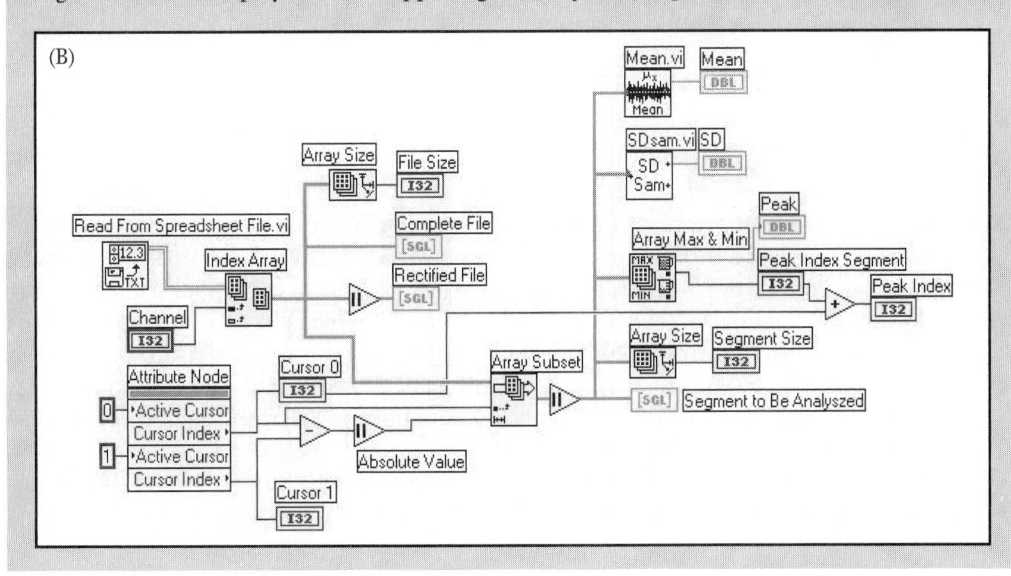

B_line.vi is a subVI that incorporates the program code described in Figure 3–19.4. As discussed in Section 3–5, "Creating SubVIs," there are two methods for constructing a subVI. The first is to call up, lay out, and wire all block diagram elements described in Figure 3–19.4. A second, easier method, is to ***capture*** this segment of code from a previously written VI such as **Torque.vi** (see Figure 3–16.1) or **Tor&ang2.vi** (see Figure 3–16.5), ***create an icon face***, and save the subVI with a unique filename for future use.

OBJECT/FUNCTION OR SUBVI LOCATOR
B_LINE.VI

Panel	Object/Function or SubVI	Palette/Menu or Directory
Front	*Array*	**Controls/Array & Cluster**
	Digital Control × 2	**Controls/Numeric**
	Digital Indicator	**Controls/Numeric**
Diagram	*Array Subset*	**Functions/Array**
	Numeric Constant × 3	**Functions/Numeric**
	Array Max & Min × 2	**Functions/Array**
	Add	**Functions/Numeric**
	Threshold Peak Detector.vi	**Functions/Signal Processing/Measurement**

In the front panel of Figure 3–19.4, a "Data Input" array (*Array* + *Digital Control*) is used to input data to the *Array Subset* function. A *Numeric Control* with a default setting of "500" establishes the length of the baseline that will be used to determine maximal baseline amplitude. A *Numeric Indicator* labeled "Start of Rise from Baseline" identifies the point where the torque signal rises from the baseline.

Use the previously constructed VI called **Torque.vi** from Section 3–16, "Torque and Velocity Measurements," or call up this VI from the **CD ROM disk directory.** Using the ***capture method*** described in Section 3–5, "Creating SubVIs," create this subVI and an identifying icon face, and **Save** it with the **B_line.vi** filename into the directory of subVIs.

DATA DISPLAY AND ANALYSIS

OBJECTIVES

- ❖ Build a VI that emulates a simple one-channel oscilloscope.
- ❖ Build a VI that computes the slope and Y-intercept of a line fitted to a preselected segment of data.
- ❖ Build a VI that automatically determines the amplitude of a force transducer signal at the point where an event marker is activated.

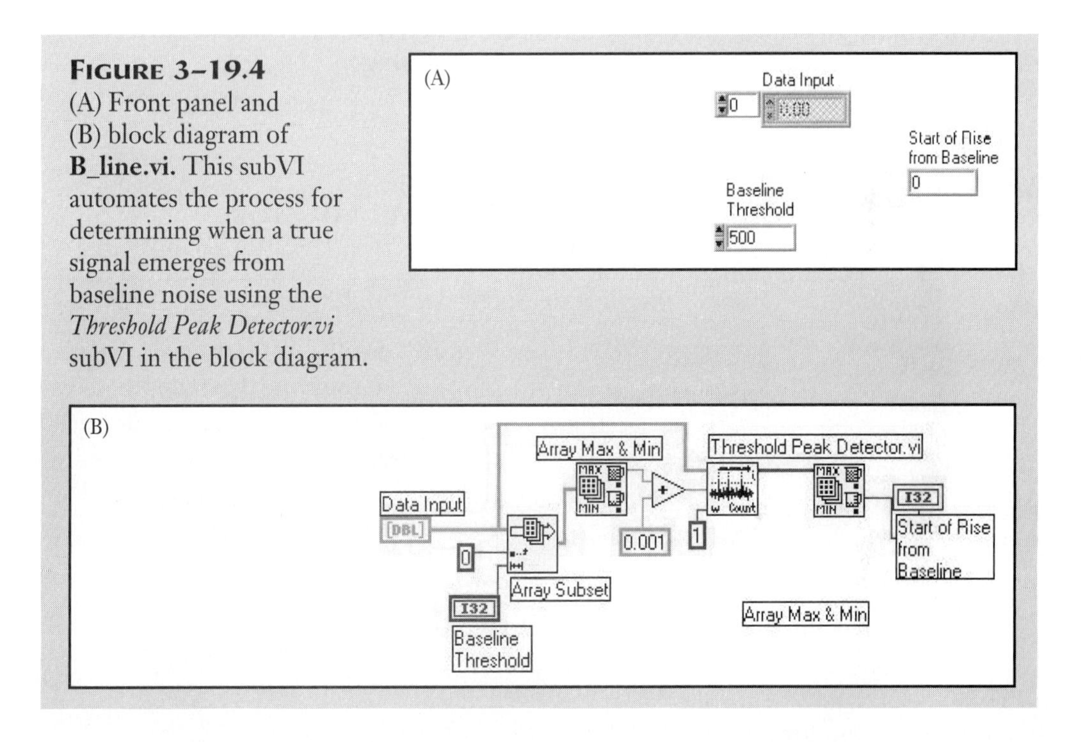

FIGURE 3–19.4 (A) Front panel and (B) block diagram of **B_line.vi.** This subVI automates the process for determining when a true signal emerges from baseline noise using the *Threshold Peak Detector.vi* subVI in the block diagram.

SCOPE1.VI

Scope1.vi (Figure 3–19.5) is a one-channel VI that displays a ***real-time*** signal acquired from the computer's analog-to-digital (A-to-D) board ***emulating*** an oscilloscope. Build this VI, or call it up from the **CD ROM disk directory.**

Four elements are required for the front panel. A *Waveform Chart*—calibrated to display a signal of ± 2.0 volts with a ***black*** (default) ***background*** and ***green gridlines***—displays the real-time signal from, for example, an EMG amplifier. Grid lines may be selected by right-clicking anywhere on the *Waveform Chart* and by selecting either *X Scale* or *Y Scale* from the pop-up menu and choosing the *Formatting* option. Left-click on the *Grid Options* icon, and choose the ***far-right*** icon. A ***green*** (or other color) gridline is selected by left-clicking on the box directly to the right of the *Grid Options* icons and by selecting a color from the palette. *Auto-Y scaling* permits the vertical axis to automatically ***rescale*** itself as the input voltage fluctuates by left-clicking on the *Waveform Chart* and selecting the *Y Scale* and then *AutoScale Y* option. A *Dial*—configured as an *I32 integer* and scaled to "3"—permits access to one of four channels defined by a *String Control* in the lower right corner.

A *Boolean Rectangular Stop Button* controls the VI that is embedded in a *While Loop* in the block diagram. The signal is acquired by an *AI Sample Channels.vi* function that acquires the signal from the A-to-D board configured as "Device No. 1" (*Numeric Constant* = "1"). **Save** the VI using a convenient filename and directory. The VI may be tested only if the computer has an A-to-D board.

OBJECT/FUNCTION OR SUBVI LOCATOR
SCOPE1.VI

Panel	Object/Function or SubVI	Palette/Menu or Directory
Front	*Waveform Chart*	**Controls/Graph**
	Labeled Oblong Button	**Controls/Boolean**
	Dial	**Controls/Numeric**
	String Control	**Controls/String**
Diagram	*While Loop*	**Functions/Structures**
	AI Sample Channels.vi	**Functions/Data Acquisition/Analog Input**
	Index Array	**Functions/Array**

FITLINE2.VI

Fitline2.vi (Figure 3–19.6) ***fits a line*** and computes the ***slope, Y-intercept, and mean*** and ***standard deviation*** of a ***segment*** of isometric torque data selected from a complete data file. This VI might be used to look at the slope characteristics of torque curves during their initial phase as the signal begins to rise from the baseline before it plateaus. Build this VI, or call it up from the **CD ROM disk directory.**

On the front panel, a *Waveform Graph* with a *Cursor Display* is used to display the complete data file during a first pass. A ***segment*** of the data is selected for analysis using the **Segment.vi** subVI constructed in Section 3–6, "More SubVIs." As with the previous VIs that used a segment analyzer, cursors are used to determine the "*Begin(ning)*" and "*End(ing)*" points of the segment of interest. X-axis (time) coordinates are input into two *Digital Controls*, and the VI is run again with the ***segment analyzer*** turned "ON." The data are filtered using the **Filters.vi** subVI. An *XY Graph* is used to plot the segment to be analyzed, and a line is fit to that segment using the *Linear Fit.vi* function in the block diagram. To its left are five *Digital Indicators* that report the fitted line's "Slope," (Y) "Intercept," "Mean," "SD"(standard deviation), and the number of data points analyzed ("n").

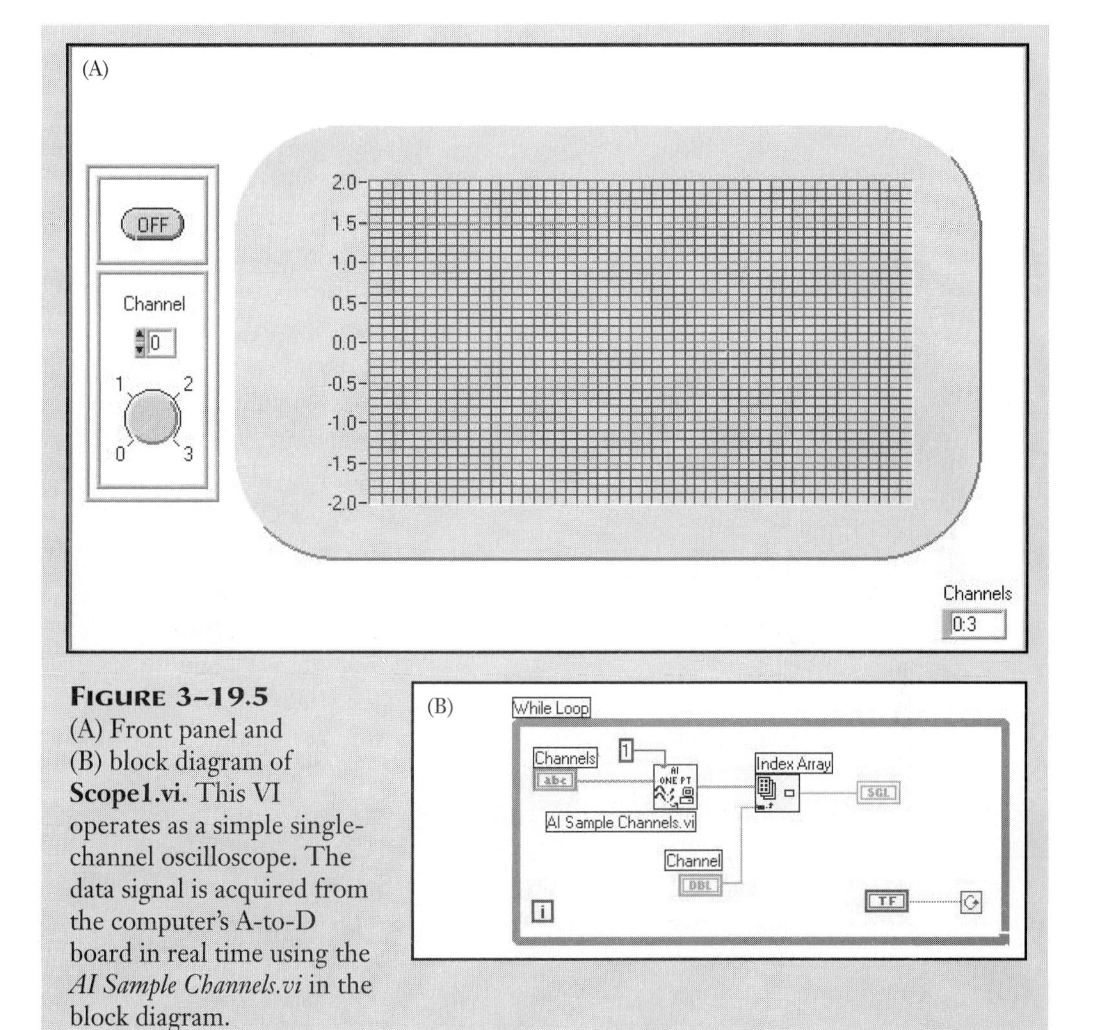

FIGURE 3–19.5 (A) Front panel and (B) block diagram of **Scope1.vi.** This VI operates as a simple single-channel oscilloscope. The data signal is acquired from the computer's A-to-D board in real time using the *AI Sample Channels.vi* in the block diagram.

In the block diagram, file reading, indexing, filtering, and segment selection are handled in a similar manner to previous VIs that were constructed in Section 3–16, "Torque and Velocity Measurements" (see Figure 3–16.1, for example). The *Linear Fit.vi* function requires x and y coordinates to ultimately plot the fitted line

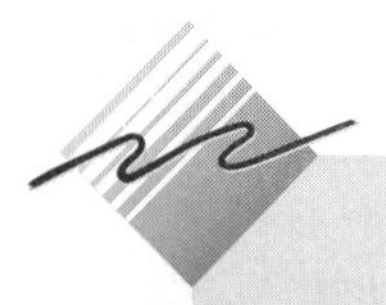

OBJECT/FUNCTION OR SUBVI LOCATOR
FITLINE2.VI

Panel	Object/Function or SubVI	Palette/Menu or Directory
Front	*Labeled Oblong Button* × 2	**Controls/Boolean**
	Dial	**Controls/Numeric**
	Digital Control × 6	**Controls/Numeric**
	Digital Indicator × 8	**Controls/Numeric**
	Array × 2	**Controls/Array & Cluster**
	Waveform Graph	**Functions/Graph**
Diagram	*Read From Spreadsheet File.vi*	**Functions/File I/O**
	Positive Infinity	**Functions/Numeric/ Additional Numeric Constants**
	Index Array	**Functions/Array**
	Multiply	**Functions/Numeric**
	Filters.vi	**Functions/Select a VI . . . / CD ROM disk directory**
	Segment.vi	**Functions/Select a VI . . . / CD ROM disk directory**
	Subtract	**Functions/Numeric**
	Mean.vi	**Functions/Mathematics/ Probability and Statistics**
	SDsam.vi	**Functions/Select a VI . . . / CD ROM disk directory**
	Linear Fit.vi	**Functions/Mathematics/ Curve Fitting**
	Bundle × 2	**Functions/Cluster**
	Build Array	**Functions/Array**
	For Loop	**Functions/Structures**
	Increment (+1)	**Functions/Numeric**

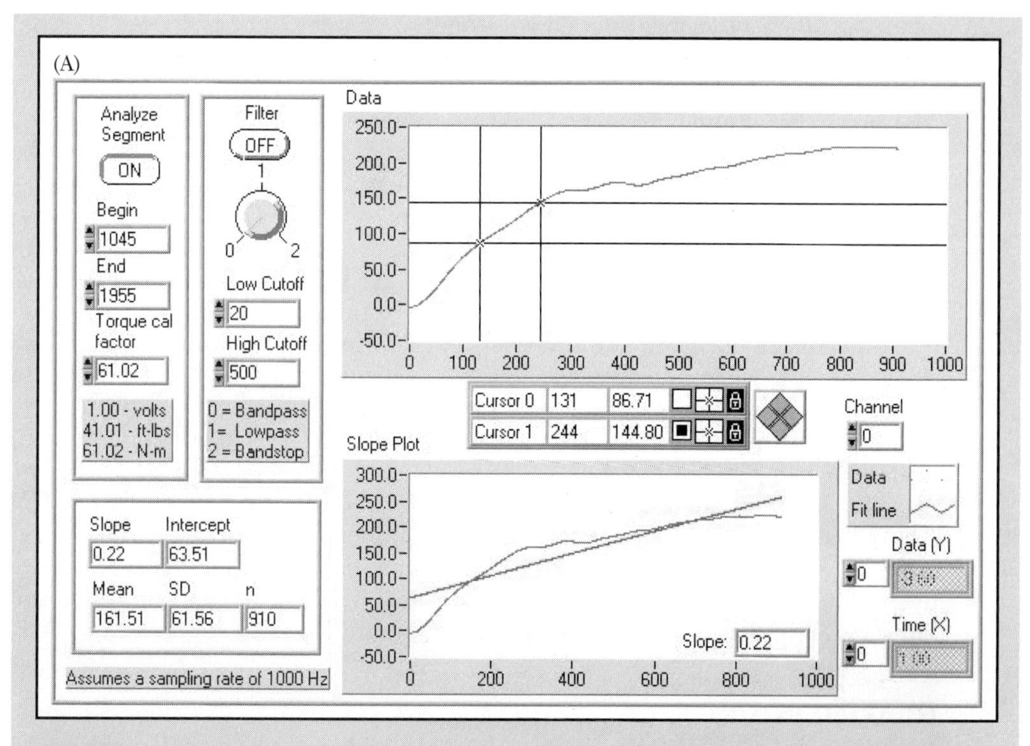

FIGURE 3–19.6
(A) Front panel and (B) block diagram of **Fitline2.vi.** This VI reads a previously saved data file and fits and plots a line on a *Waveform Graph* of a segment of the signal. Slope, Y-axis intercept, and mean value are calculated and displayed in *Digital Indicators* on the front panel. Line fitting is provided by the **Linear Fit.vi** subVI in the block diagram, and a *For Loop* is used to generate X-axis values.

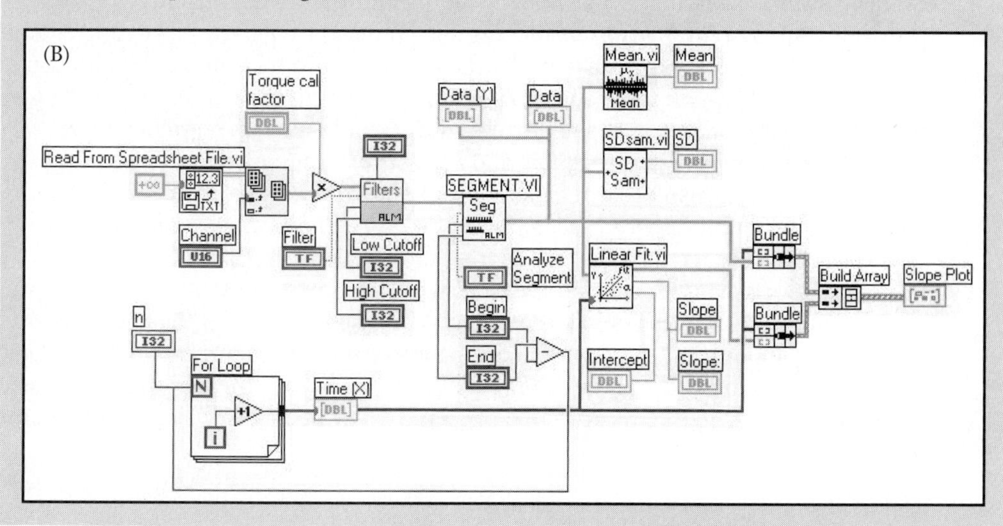

on an *XY Graph*. ***Y coordinates*** derive from the data file. The array of data from the output side of the **Segment.vi** subVI is wired to the "Y" terminal on the upper left corner of the *Linear Fit.vi* function. ***X coordinate*** data, against which the y coordinates are plotted, are generated by a *For Loop* whose "N" terminal is wired to the *Digital Indicator* that reports the number of data points analyzed. That is, the *For Loop* will cycle for *n* iterations. Two *Bundle* functions are used to construct a *Build Array* function that outputs its coordinates to the *XY Graph*. The ***top*** *Bundle* input terminals are wired to the data file from the output terminal of the **Segment.vi** subVI and the ***x data*** from the *For Loop*, respectively. The ***lower*** *Bundle* input terminals are wired to the "Best Linear Fit" terminal of the *Linear Fit.vi* function (upper right corner) and the ***x data*** from the *For Loop*, respectively. The *Build Array* function, when called up, defaults to a ***one-input terminal*** configuration. In this case, a second terminal is added by left-clicking on the lower right corner with the *Arrow Tool* and dragging down a second terminal. **Save** this VI using a convenient filename and directory.

To confirm that the VI is operating correctly, run the data file in the **CD ROM disk directory** called **Torq2.dat** with the segment analyzer turned "ON" and the "Start" and "End" points of the segment at "1045" and "1955," respectively. The "Filter" in this case has been turned "OFF." Compare the slope and other values in the VI just built with those in Figure 3–19.6.

READTRAN.VI

Readtran.vi (Figure 3–19.7) is a two-channel VI intended to read the output of a Piezo electric ***force transducer*** and an ***event marker*** that documents a point in time along the x-axis. Build this VI, or call it up from the **CD ROM disk directory.**

The VI automatically reads the x-axis (time) coordinate when the event marker (lower graph) is switched on and uses this coordinate to ***index*** the force curve in a *Waveform Graph* described earlier. For example, in Figure 3–19.7, the event marker is switched on at point "2006," and the force output is 3.40 kg. In previous testing, a ***calibration factor*** was determined (1 volt = 6.25 kg) and is multiplied, as a block diagram constant, by the transducer input voltage. In addition to the indexed force, ***peak force*** and its ***index*** are calculated in several formats and reported in *Digital Indicators* at the bottom of the front panel. A ***segment analyzer*** is included. A bandpass filter, with ***low*** and ***high cutoff*** frequencies of "20" and "500" Hz, respectively, is also provided using a *Butterworth Filter* in a *Case Structure* toggled by a front panel *Labeled Oblong Button*. A *Vertical Toggle Switch* provides the option to rectify the signal.

The block diagram is organized and wired in much the same way as the previous example. Note that the **B_line.vi** subVI, described earlier, has been used to document the point on the x-axis when the ***event marker*** is turned on. The ***index*** value is used to index the *Array Subset* function to identify the transducer force at the time the event marker is switched on. **Save** this VI using a convenient filename and directory.

To confirm that the VI is operating properly, run it using the data file called **Trans4.dat** in the **CD ROM disk directory**, and compare the values in the *Digital Indicators* of the VI just built with those in Figure 3–19.7. Note that the ***segment analyzer*** is turned "OFF," and the ***bandpass filter*** is turned "ON."

STATISTICAL ANALYSIS

OBJECTIVES

- ❖ Build a VI that plots a running histogram of data points generated from two simulated function generators.
- ❖ Build a subVI that calculates the Pearson product moment correlation coefficient.
- ❖ Build a VI that performs a one-way analysis of variance on three data sets.

HISTGRM.VI

Histgrm.vi (Figure 3–19.8) uses the *Uniform White Noise.vi* and *Periodic Random Noise.vi* simulated ***function generator*** subVIs to plot a ***histogram*** and calculate the ***mean***, ***standard deviation***, and ***mode*** of the data points generated. Build this VI, or call it up from the **CD ROM disk directory.**

On the front panel, an *XY Graph* plots the histogram, which is updated after a ***predetermined*** number of "Samples" (default = 120) are generated. Simultaneously, individual data points are displayed in real time on a *Waveform Chart.* A *Boolean Vertical Switch* is used to toggle between the two data point generators. ***Descriptive statistics*** are reported in three *Digital Indicators.* Both *Vertical Switches* have been ***enlarged*** for easy viewing and access.

In the block diagram, the entire VI is embedded in a *While Loop* that is switched "On" and "Off" with a front panel *Vertical Switch.* The "Rate" at which data points are generated is controlled by the *Wait Until Next ms Multiple* function controlled by a front panel *Vertical Slide* that defaults to a rate of "686" and is scaled to a maximal value of "1000." The number of "Samples" generated per iteration of the *While Loop* and the "Interval" spacing of the data points on the x-axis of the *Waveform Chart* are controlled by two front panel *Digital Controls.* A *Case Structure*, toggled by a front panel *Vertical Switch*, with two labeled choices ("Uniform" and "Random"), permits the selection of the simulated function generator. Note the setup instructions in the lower left corner of the *While Loop:*

Waveform graph set line interpolation to "none"
XY graph set line interpolation to "step"

Interpolation functions are set up as follows: With the *Arrow Tool*, right-click anywhere on the graph, and left-click on *Show* and then *Legend* from the pop-up menu. A *Legend* will appear near the upper right corner of the graph. Right-click

OBJECT/FUNCTION OR SUBVI LOCATOR
READTRAN.VI

Panel	Object/Function or SubVI	Palette/Menu or Directory
Front	*Labeled Oblong Button* × 2	**Controls/Boolean**
	Digital Control × 6	**Controls/Numeric**
	Digital Indicator × 10	**Controls/Numeric**
	Vertical Toggle Switch	**Controls/Boolean**
	Waveform Graph × 2	**Controls/Graph**
	File Path Indicator	**Controls/Path & Refnum**
Diagram	*Read From Spreadsheet File.vi*	**Functions/File I/O**
	Positive Infinity	**Functions/Numeric/ Additional Numeric Constants**
	Index Array × 2	**Functions/Array**
	Case Structure × 3	**Functions/Structures**
	Butterworth Filter.vi × 2	**Functions/Signal Processing/Filters**
	Numeric Constants × 9	**Functions/Numeric**
	Segment.vi × 2	**Functions/Select a VI . . . / CD ROM disk directory**
	B_line.vi	**Functions/Select a VI . . . / CD ROM disk directory**
	Subset Array	**Functions/Array**
	Mean.vi	**Functions/Mathematics/ Probability and Statistics**
	Multiply **× 6**	**Functions/Numeric**
	Absolute Value	**Functions/Numeric**
	Array Max & Min	**Functions/Array**
	Array size **× 2**	**Functions/Array**

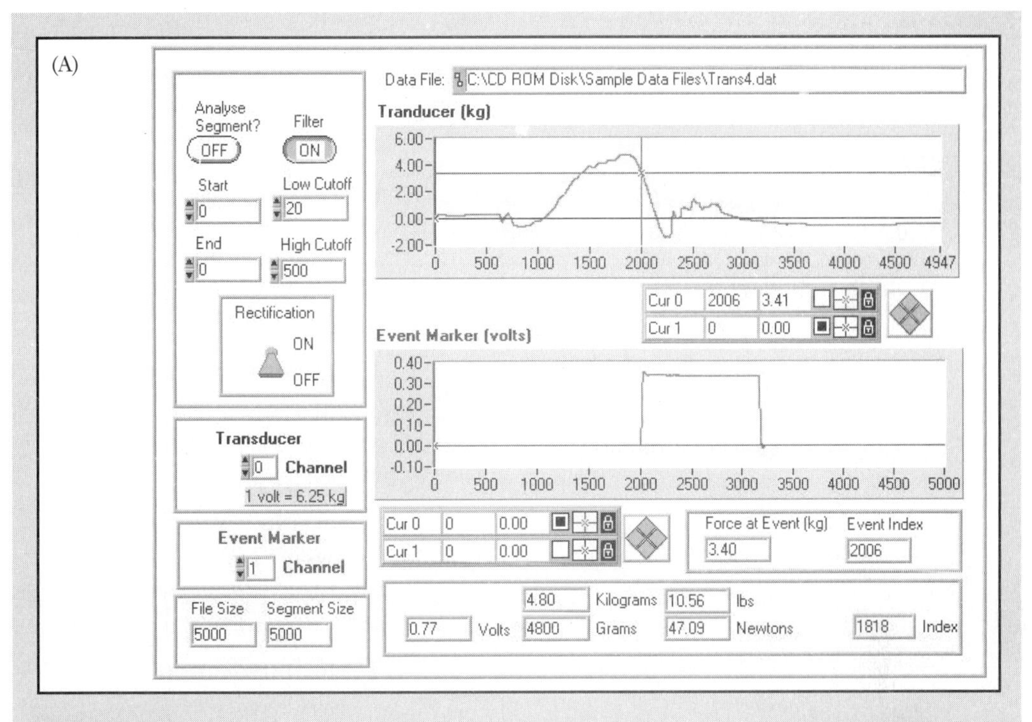

FIGURE 3–19.7
(A) Front panel and (B) block diagram of **Readtran.vi.** This VI calculates force applied to a transducer at the point at which an event marker rises from the baseline of a previously saved data file. The transducer and event marker signals are displayed in two *Waveform Graphs* in the front panel.

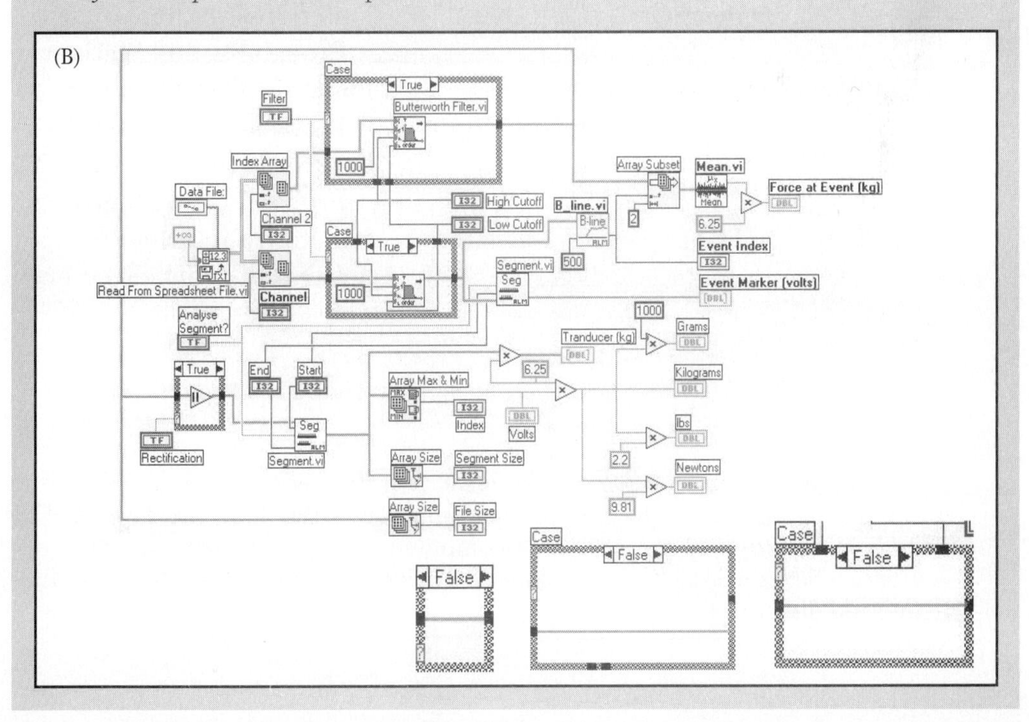

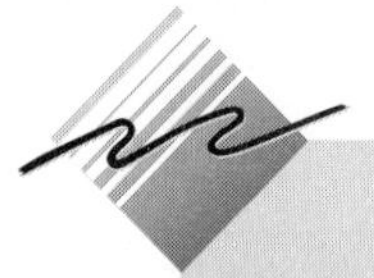

OBJECT/FUNCTION OR SUBVI LOCATOR
HISTGRM.VI

Panel	Object/Function or SubVI	Palette/Menu or Directory
Front	*Vertical Slide Switch* × 2	**Controls/Boolean**
	XY Graph	**Controls/Graph**
	Waveform Chart	**Controls/Graph**
	Digital Control × 2	**Controls/Numeric**
	Vertical Slide	**Controls/Numeric**
	Digital Indicators × 3	**Controls/Numeric**
Diagram	*While Loop*	**Functions/Structures**
	Case Structure	**Functions/Structures**
	Wait Until Next ms Multiple	**Functions/Time & Dialog**
	Uniform White Noise.vi	**Functions/Signal Processing/Signal Generation**
	Periodic Random Noise.vi	**Functions/Signal Processing/Signal Generation**
	Histgrm.vi	**Functions/Mathematics/ Probability and Statistics**
	Mode.vi	**Functions/Mathematics/ Probability and Statistics**
	Mean.vi	**Functions/Mathematics/ Probability and Statistics**
	SDsam.vi	**Functions/Select a VI . . . / CD ROM disk directory**

on the *Legend*, select *Interpolation* from the pop-up menu, and then choose the desired function. After the *Interpolation* function is set, hide the *Legend.* The ***standard deviation of the sample*** is computed using the **SDsam.vi** subVI described in Section 3–5, "Creating SubVIs." **Save** this VI using a convenient filename and directory.

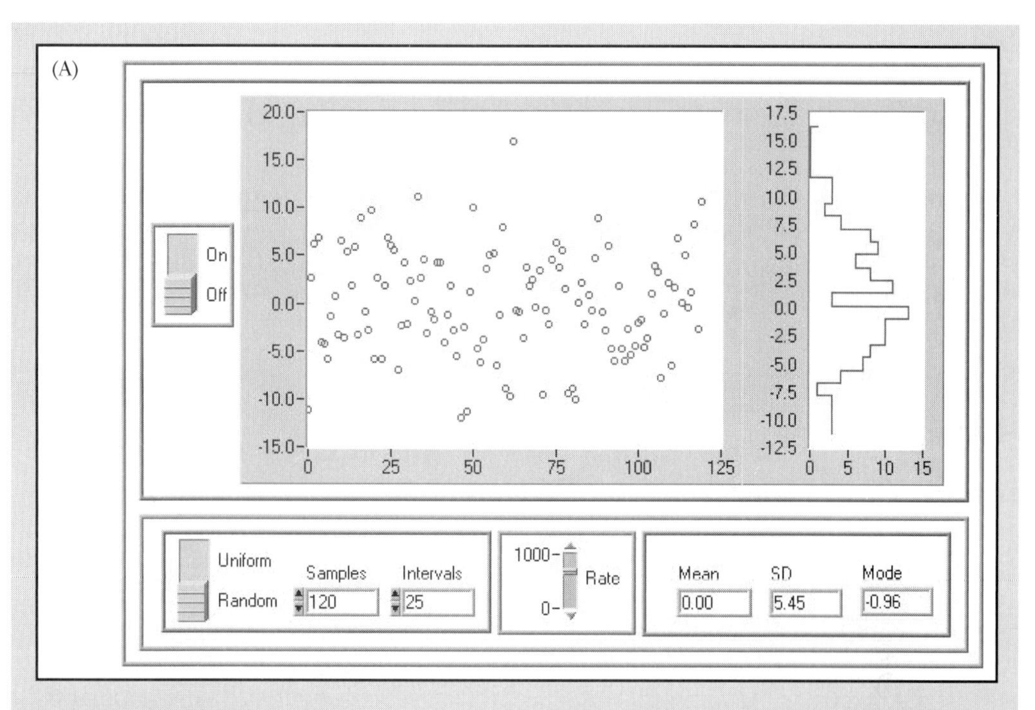

Figure 3–19.8
(A) Front panel and (B) block diagram of **Histgrm.vi.** This VI uses a front panel *XY Graph* to generate a scatter plot and histogram of the frequency of data points from a predetermined number of samples from two sources. Descriptive statistics are calculated and displayed in front panel *Digital Indicators.*

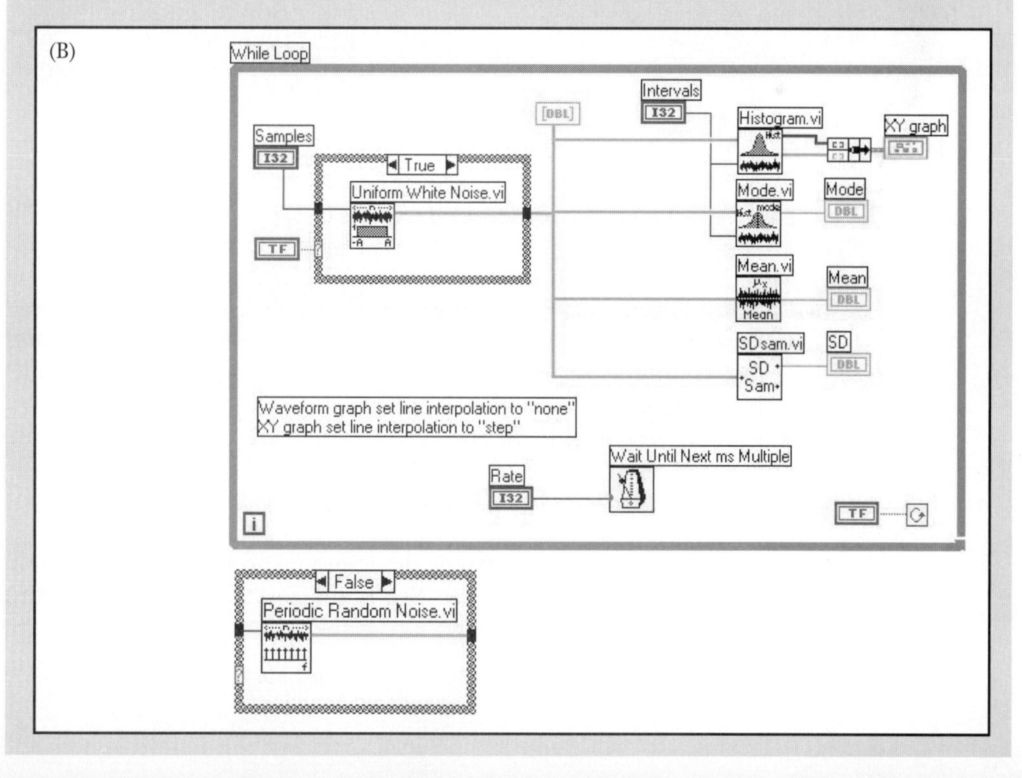

PEARSN_R.VI

The ***Pearson product moment correlation coefficient (r)*** is computed from two data sets previously saved in a two-column spreadsheet as a text (**.txt**) file by the **Pearsn_r.vi** SubVI (Figure 3–19.9). While this program is intended as an ***embeddable*** subVI, it could also ***stand alone*** (see following discussion). Build this VI, or call it up from the **CD ROM disk directory.**

OBJECT/FUNCTION OR SUBVI LOCATOR
PEARSN_R.VI

Panel	Object/Function or SubVI	Palette/Menu or Directory
Front	*Array* × 2	**Controls/String & Table**
	Digital Control × 2	**Controls/Numeric**
	Digital Indicator × 2	**Controls/Numeric**
Diagram	*Mean.vi*	**Functions/Mathematics/ Probability and Statistics**
	Subtract × 2	**Functions/Numeric**
	Multiply × 4	**Functions/Numeric**
	Add Array Elements × 3	**Functions/Numeric**
	Square Root	**Functions/Numeric**
	Array Size	**Functions/Array**

The front panel includes two *Arrays of Digital Controls* to input "X" and "Y Data." Note that in Figure 3–19.9, the *Arrays* have been expanded so that 15 cells have been exposed. If this program is used as a subVI, the *Arrays* need not be expanded. Two *Digital Indicators* are used to report the "Pearson r" coefficient and "No. of Comparisons," respectively. The upper indicator is set to ***two decimal points of precision,*** while the lower one is configured as an *I32 integer.* Both indicators have been ***enlarged*** for easier visualization.

In the block diagram, means for the two data sets are calculated using the *Mean.vi* function and a series of arithmetic functions. Note that the *Add Array Elements function* provides the "sum of . . ." function signified by the traditional use of a ***Sigma*** (Σ).

Move back to the front panel, and edit the icon face in the upper right corner of the monitor screen, as discussed in Section 3–5, "Creating SubVIs," to uniquely identify it. ***Four terminals*** should next be wired: ***two*** for ***inputs*** for the

"X" and "Y Data" *Arrays* and ***two*** for ***outputs*** for the "Pearson r" coefficient and the "No. of Comparisons" *Digital Indicators.* **Save** this subVI using a convenient filename and in subVI directory.

To confirm that the subVI operates properly, use it as a ***stand-alone*** VI. Using the *Lettering Tool,* insert the values that appear in Figure 3–19.9 and **Run** the (sub)VI. The "Pearson r" correlation coefficient should read "0.96."

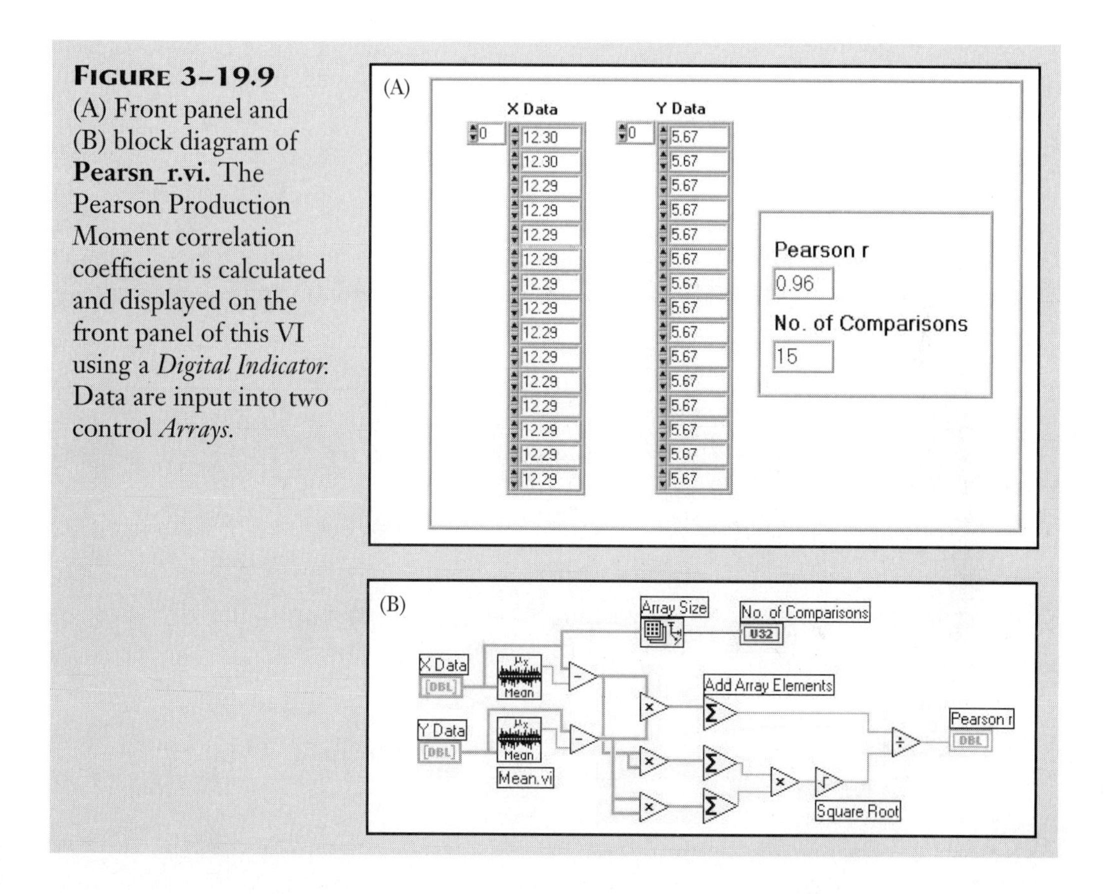

FIGURE 3–19.9
(A) Front panel and (B) block diagram of **Pearsn_r.vi.** The Pearson Production Moment correlation coefficient is calculated and displayed on the front panel of this VI using a *Digital Indicator.* Data are input into two control *Arrays.*

1WANOVA.VI

LabVIEW provides a number of statistical functions that allow pairwise (e.g., *t*-tests) and multiple data sets comparisons including one-, two-, and three-way analysis of variance (ANOVA). **1Wanova.vi** (Figure 3–19.10) performs a one-way ANOVA on three dependent variables and reports the results using a conventional ANOVA table in the front panel. Build this VI, or call it up from the **CD ROM disk directory.**

In the front panel, two *Arrays* of *Digital Controls* are used to input "X" (dependent variables) and "Grouping Factor" variables. A *Digital Control* identifies the "No. of Groups" being studied. In this case, the number is "3." An "ANOVA Table" has been set up using 10 *Digital Indicators* and appropriate labels using the *Lettering Tool.*

The main component of the VI in the block diagram is the *1D ANOVA.vi* subVI to which are wired the ***inputs*** and ***outputs*** represented in the front panel. Since a number of terminals are associated with this function, it may be useful to turn on the **Help** window to assist in wiring. Note that all of the *Digital Indicator* icons are labeled, but only some of these labels are displayed in the front panel. To turn off a label in the block diagram so that is does not appear in the front panel, right-click on the icon, and then left-click the *Show* and then *Label* options from the pop-up menu. **Save** this VI using a convenient filename and directory.

OBJECT/FUNCTION OR SUBVI LOCATOR
1WANOVA.VI

Panel	Object/Function or SubVI	Palette/Menu or Directory
Front	*Array* × 2	**Controls/Array & Cluster**
	Digital Control × 3	**Controls/Numeric**
	Digital Indicator × 9	**Controls/Numeric**
Diagram	*1D ANOVA.vi*	**Functions/Mathematics/ Probability and Statistics/Analysis of Variance**
	Array Size	**Functions/Array**
	Decrement (−1)	**Functions/Numeric**
	Subtract × 2	**Functions/Numeric**

To confirm that the VI is working properly, ***expand*** the two *Control Arrays* to expose at least 15 cells and input the values that appear in Figure 3–19.10. Input the "No. of Groups" (i.e., "3") in the *Digital Control,* and **Run** the VI, comparing the "ANOVA Table" results with the VI just constructed and those in the figure. Figure 3–19.11 is an ANOVA table from the SPSS™ statistical software package. Confirm that the results of both ANOVA tables are the same (within decimal error).

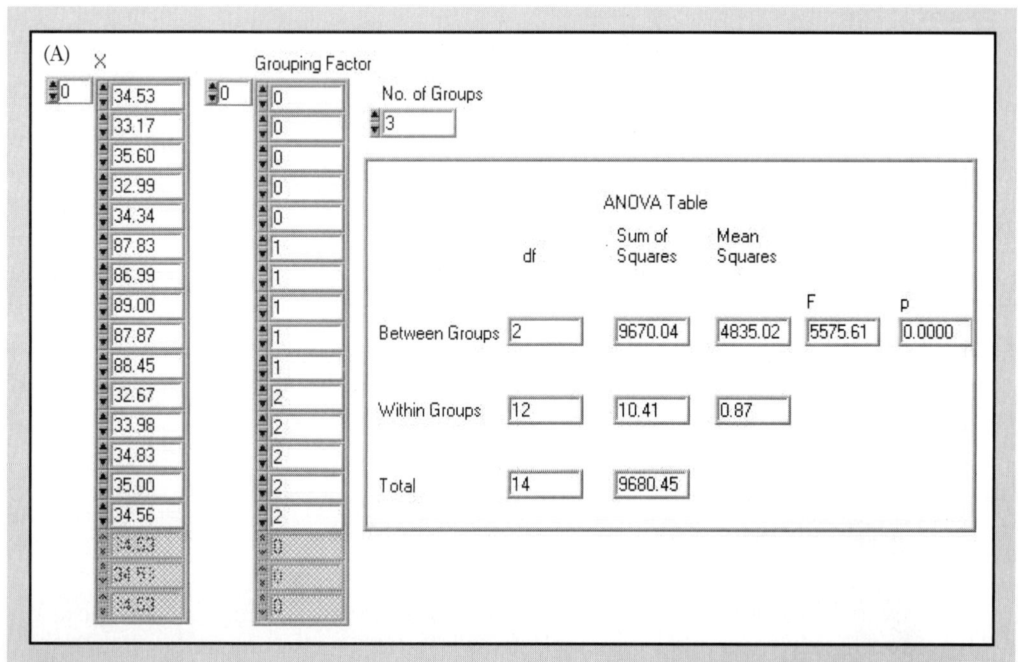

FIGURE 3–19.10
(A) Front panel and (B) block diagram of *1Wanova.vi.* This VI performs a one-way analysis of variance (ANOVA) from groups of variables input into two control *Arrays* on the front panel. A standard ANOVA table is configured in the front panel using *Digital Indicators.*

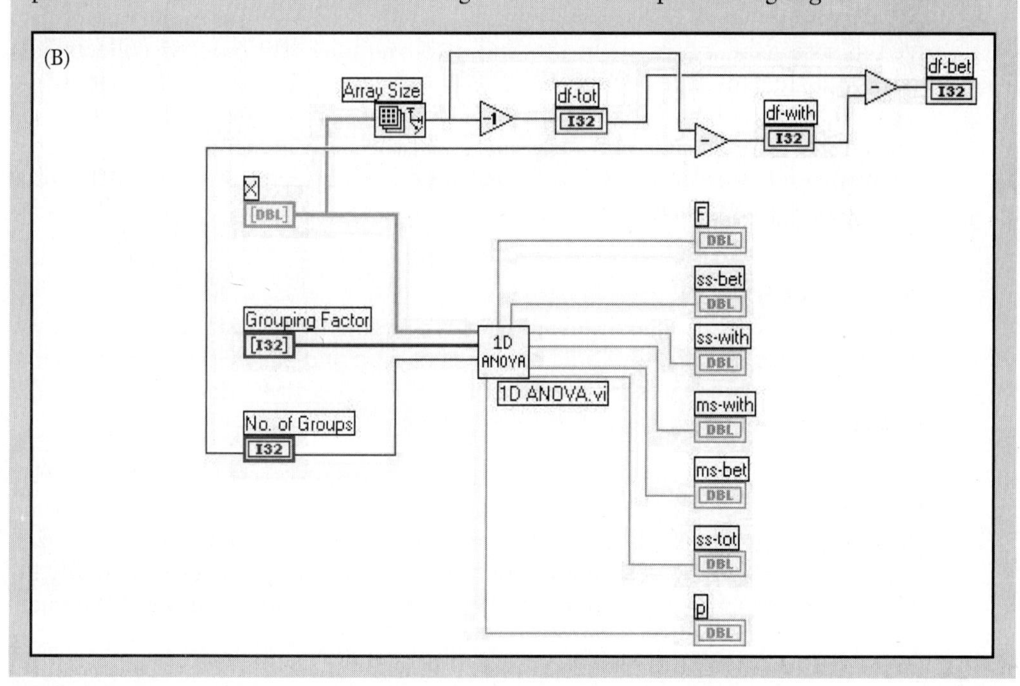

ANOVA

	Sum of Squares	df	Mean Square	F	Sig.
Between Groups	9670.41	2	4835.021	5575.610	.000
Within Groups	10.46	12	.867		
Total	9680.447	14			

FIGURE 3–19.11
An ANOVA table generated by the SPSS™ statistical package using the same data described in Figure 3–19.10.

ADVANCED TOOLS

Three VIs in this final part of this section are presented. All three are advanced VIs requiring advanced programming skills. The latter two acquire and process signals using ***binary*** format files. Binary processing is inherently more efficient and uses less hard drive storage space, especially when memory is at a premium. Experiments requiring long data collection periods (e.g., 1 minute or longer) may be handled more efficiently using VI written in binary format. Data saved to disk in ***binary format*** require VIs that ***save, read,*** and ***analyze*** files, just as in the case of data saved in spreadsheet format. In the final two examples, **Bincolct.vi** collects data from an analog-to-digital (A-to-D) board and saves it in binary format, while **Hread.vi** reads and analyzes a ***binary*** file. Since it is not expected that these VIs will be used as basic programming exercises, the descriptions that follow focus principally on the front panel of each and describe VI operations. Each VI is provided in the **CD ROM disk directory.**

OBJECTIVES

- ❖ Use a generic VI that analyzes and saves a segment of a data file "on-the-fly."
- ❖ Use a VI that acquires multiple channels of data and saves it in binary format.
- ❖ Use a VI that measures a single channel of H-reflex EMG data previously saved in binary format.

ANALYZE.VI

In previous discussions, VIs that were used to analyze data were run ***twice:*** the ***first*** time to view the ***entire*** file and a ***second*** time to partition a ***segment*** of the file for further analysis. **Analyze.vi** (Figure 3–19.12) is a generic data analysis VI that permits partitioning of a segment of data ***on-the-fly*** without having to run and rerun the program numerous times. Once the segment of interest is selected using cursors, that segment may be saved to disk in spreadsheet format. The same ***filtering*** and ***voltage/unit conversion*** functions developed in previous chapters have been incorporated into this VI. For example, a front panel *Dial* permits selection of a bandpass (default), lowpass, or bandstop "Filter" after a *Boolean Square Labeled Button* is pushed "ON." Another button switches unit "Calibration" from "Volts" (default) to microvolts and millivolts, foot-pounds, or Newton-meters using a *Vertical Slide* control. A third button permits rectification ("Rectify") of the signal, while a fourth allows the current data set to be appended ("Append") to a previously saved data file. The *Waveform Graph* to the left displays the ***entire*** data file. A *Cursor Display* for this graph is linked to an *Attribute Node* that ***automatically*** reads the ***start*** and ***end*** coordinates on the x-axis. These points are used to display the ***segment of interest*** in the *Waveform Graph* to the right when the "Analyze Selected Subset" button is pushed. Between the two graphs are a *Cluster* of *Simple Digital Indicators* and an *Array Indicator* that computes ***descriptive statistics*** and ***index coordinates.***

(A)

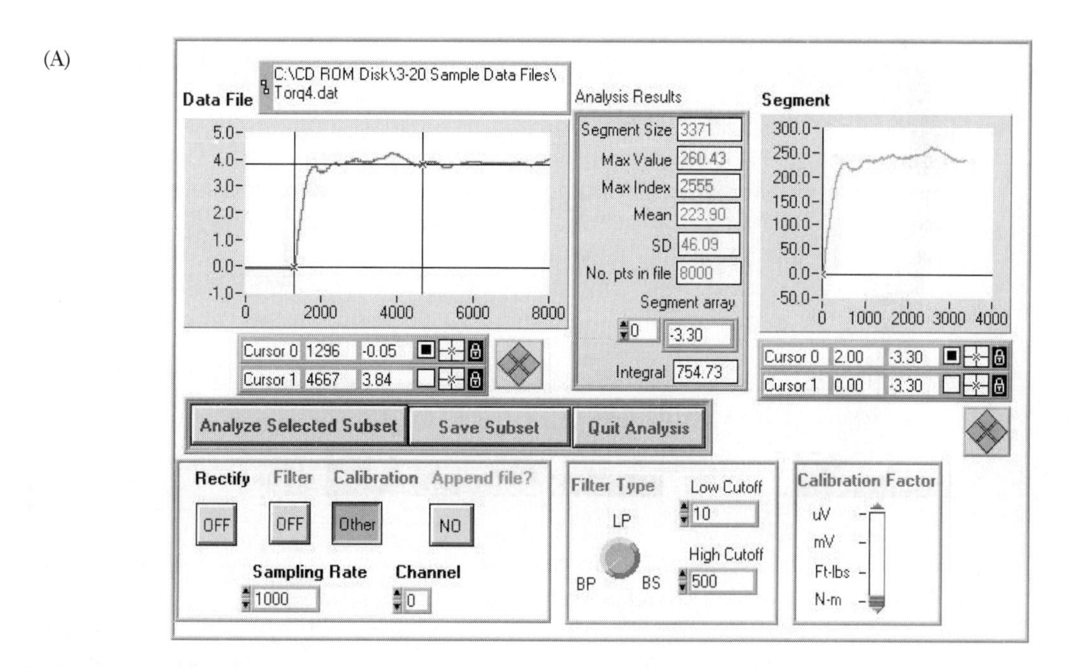

FIGURE 3–19.12
(A) Front panel and (B) block diagram of **Analyze.vi.** This VI is a generic data analysis program that calculates and displays descriptive statistics from a segment of a presaved data file in a data *Cluster* on the front panel. This VI has the ability to make calculations "on-the-fly" without having to run and rerun the program several times.

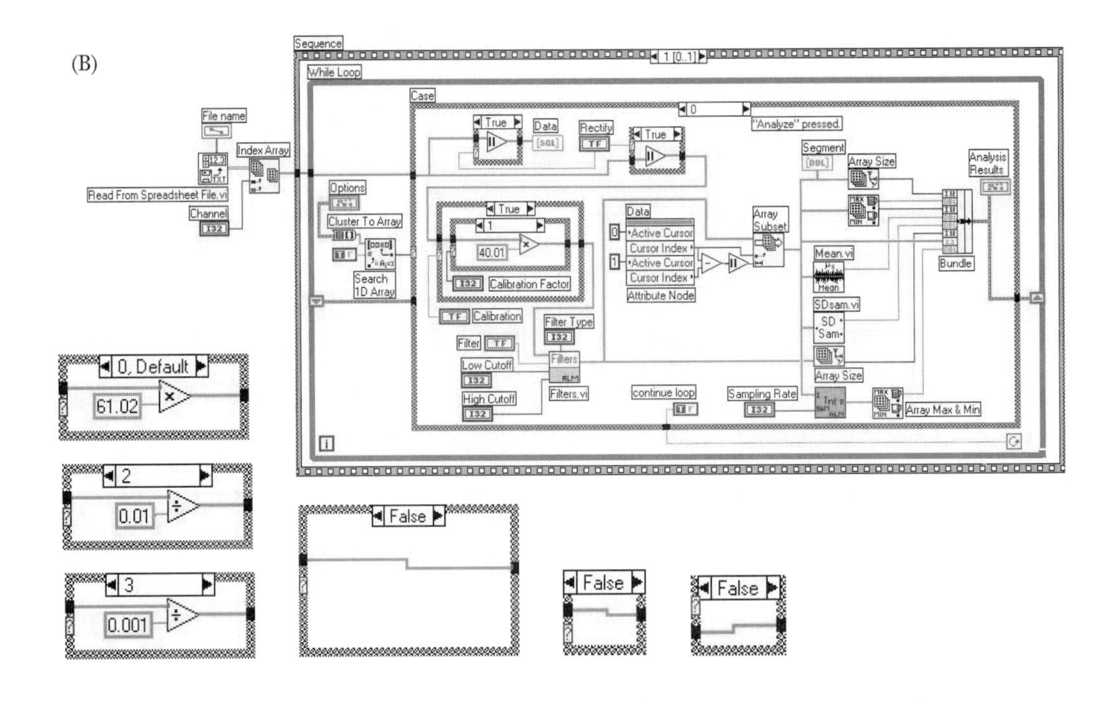

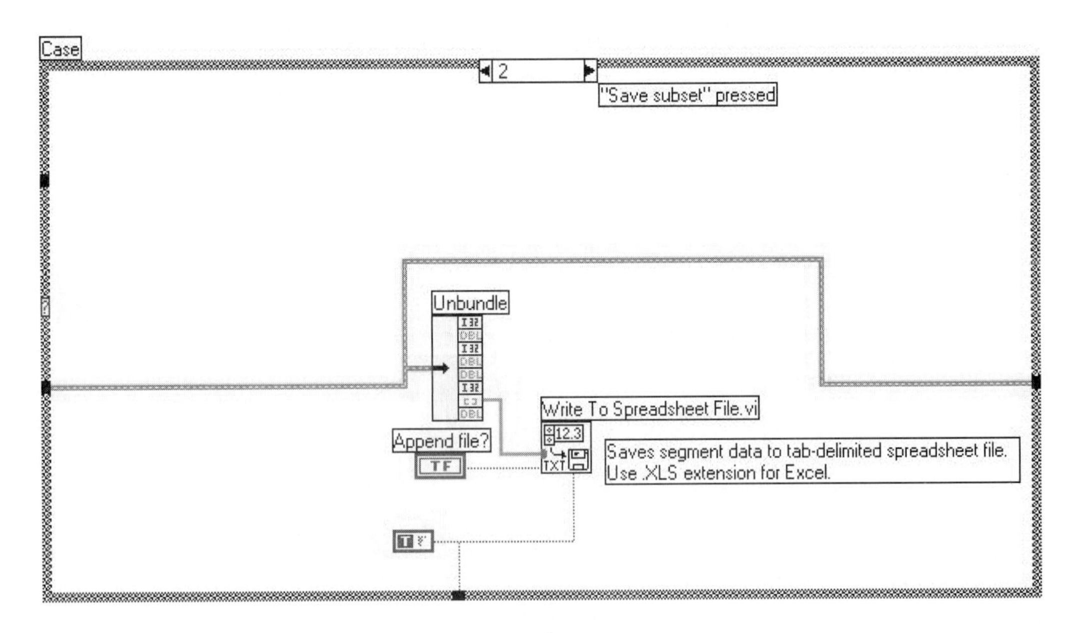

FIGURE 3–19.12
Continued.

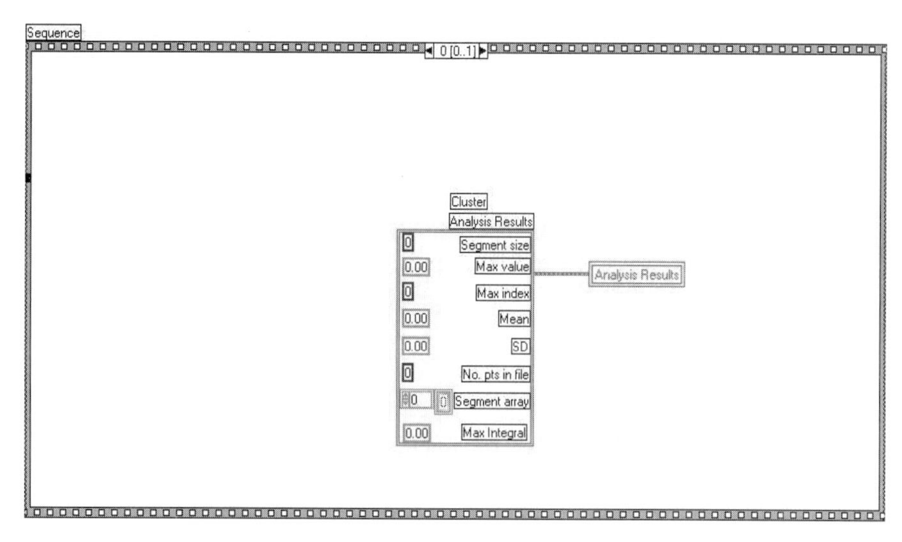
Sequence
0 [0..1]
Cluster
Analysis Results
Segment size
Max value
Max index
Mean
SD
No. pts in file
Segment array
Max Integral
Analysis Results

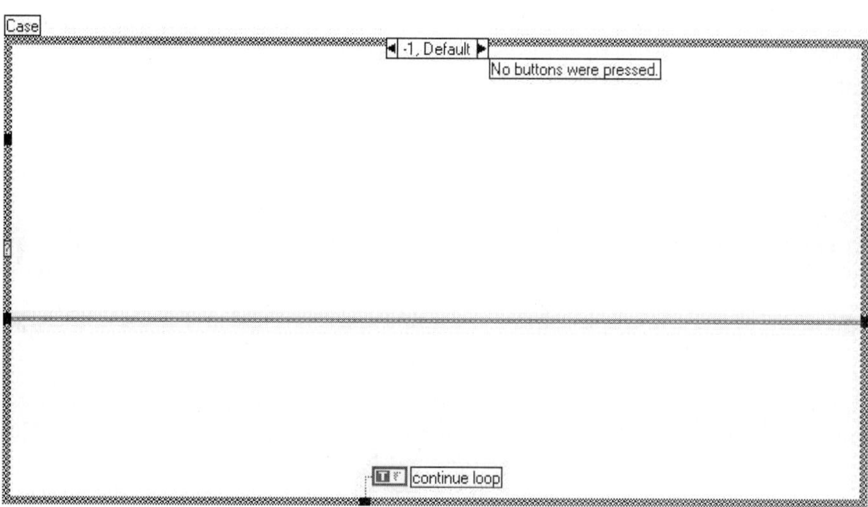
Case
-1, Default
No buttons were pressed.
continue loop

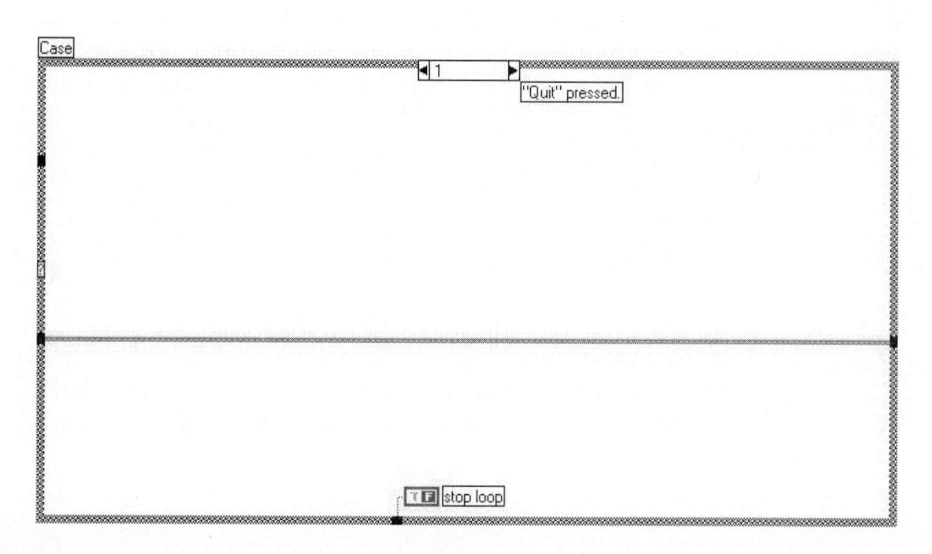
Case
1
"Quit" pressed.
stop loop

Call up this VI from the **CD ROM disk directory,** and note in the block diagram that the ***on-the-fly*** capability of this VI is achieved using a series of ***nested*** *Sequence* and *Case Structures* and *While Loops.* Three subVIs including **Filters.vi, SDsam.vi** and **Intgrl2.vi** have been used to provide their respective functions.

To understand how this VI operates, **Run** it, and when prompted, use the ***isometric torque*** data file called **Torq4.dat.** Press the "Calibration" button to the "Other" position, and move the *Cursors* in the left *Waveform Graph* with the *Hand Tool,* so that "Cursor 0" is on x-axis data point "1296," and "Cursor 1" is on "4667." Using the *Hand Tool* again, press the "Analyze Selected Subset" button, and note that the *Cluster* data ***between*** the graphs are the same as displayed in Figure 3–19.12. Note also the ***segment*** of the torque curve in the right *Waveform Graph* labeled "Segment."

BINCOLCT.VI

Bincolct.vi (Figure 3–19.13) acquires multiple channels of data from an A-to-D board of a computer and saves the data in ***binary*** format. This VI is a stand-alone and modified version of the *AI Continuous Scan.vi* function that was resaved using the **Bincolct.vi** filename. **Bincolct.vi** is available from the **CD ROM disk directory.**

Open a **New** blank VI from the **File** option on the task bar, and move to the block diagram. Call up *AI Continuous Scan.vi* from the **Functions** palette, and select the **Data Acquisition/Analog Input/Utilities** menus. Position the subVI in any convenient spot. Using the *Arrow Tool,* left double-click on the icon face opening up to the front panel. Compare the front panel with Figure 3–19.13, noting the similarities of the front panel elements. When finished, close out of the subVI ***without saving*** the VI.

Before running **Bincolct.vi,** a *String Control* is used as a "User Supplied Header" for identifying information about the subject. Note that the VI, by default, will scan the first ***four*** "Channels" ("0:3") of the A-to-D board. This parameter may be modified using the *Lettering Tool.* The "Max(imum) No. of Scan to Write to File" is likewise input by the user. Note in the "Scan Functions" panel the default settings for "Scan Rate," "Buffer Size," and "Min(imum) No. of Scans to Write at a Time." These may also be modified to meet the needs of a specific experiment.

HREAD.VI

In the previous VI, multiple channels of data were acquired from the computer's A-to-D board and saved in ***binary*** format. **Hread.vi** (Figure 3–19.14) is a VI intended to ***read*** and ***analyze H-reflex*** files saved in ***binary*** format. This VI is a modified version of one of National Instruments' **Example** VIs.

H-reflexes are elicited after a muscle is stimulated with a galvanic stimulator and are used as an index of ***alpha motorneuron excitability*** at the spinal cord level. Recordings are made using surface EMG electrodes applied to the skin overlying

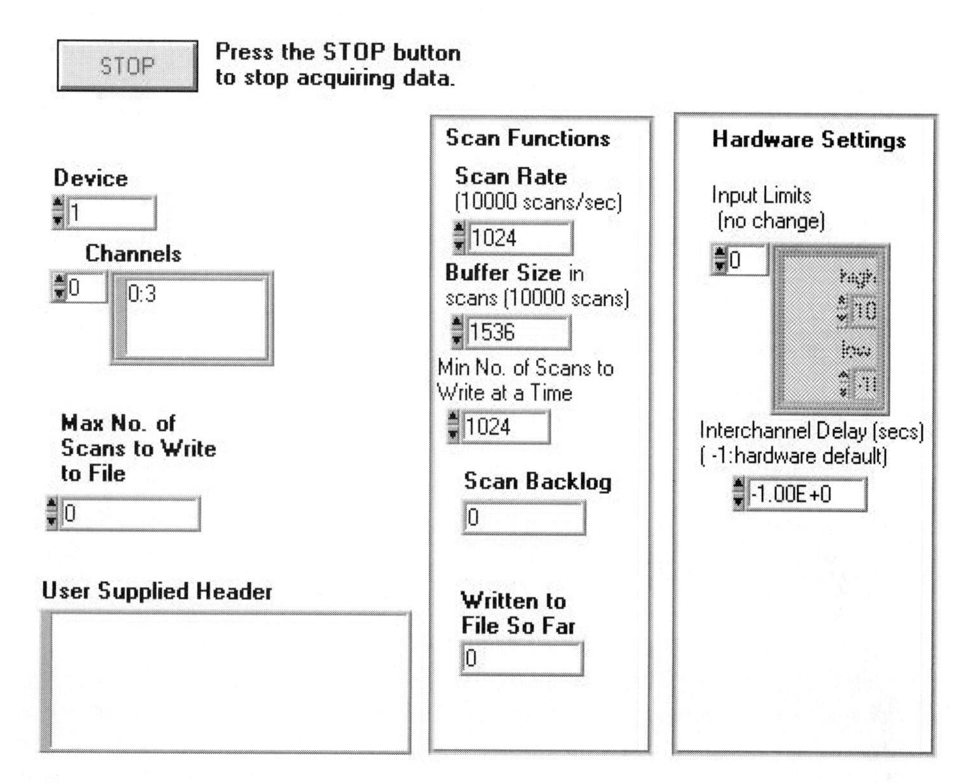

FIGURE 3–19.13
Front panel of **Bincolct.vi.** This VI collects multiple channels of data and saves them in binary format.

the muscle. H-reflexes may be thought of as an ***evoked*** form of ***deep tendon reflex.*** Three waveforms (Figure 3–19.14) are generated during the procedure to evoke an H-reflex. The ***first*** electrical spike is the ***stimulus artifact*** (upward deflection located at x-axis point "695"), the point where electrical stimulation begins. The ***second*** waveform is the ***M-wave*** (point "712"), the muscle's direct response to electrical stimulation, and the ***third*** waveform is the ***H-reflex*** (point "720").

Waveforms are displayed on the front panel on a *Waveform Graph* with a *Cursor Display.* A *String Indicator* displays "User Header" information about the subject that was originally input when the data were saved using the **Bincolct.vi** VI (see preceding discussion). The "Numbers of Scans Read at a Time" is controlled by a *Digital Control* and defaults to "1000." Other indicators identify "Maximum" and "Minimum (signal) Amplitudes," a "Channel List from File," and the "No. of Scans from File" that have been read. Physiological waveforms are quite variable and may be displayed in an ***inverted*** form. A "Scale Factor" *Digital Control,* defaulting to

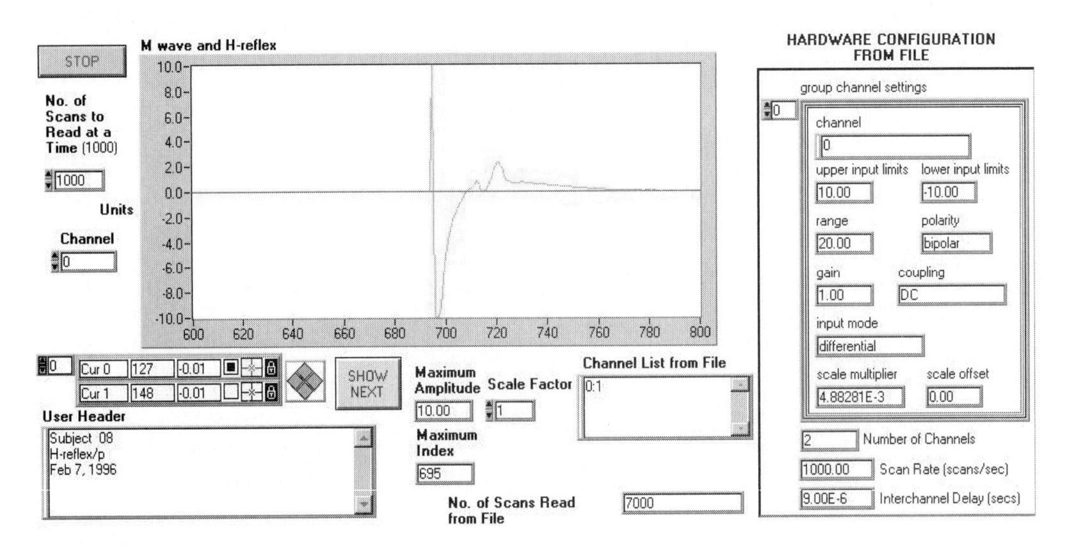

FIGURE 3–19.14
Front panel of **Hread.vi.** This VI reads and displays binary files in a front panel *Waveform Graph.* This VI was configured to display H-reflexes processing 1000 data points (default value) at a time. In this example, the stimulus artifact, M-wave, and H-reflex are displayed, respectively.

"+1," will ***invert the signal.*** As the VI begins running, a ***prompt window*** appears asking for a ***data filename.*** After the file is selected, the *Waveform Graph* displays the signal "1000" points at one time by pressing the "SHOW NEXT" button. The VI will shut down after the last data scan has occurred or if the "STOP" button is pushed using the *Hand Tool.*

To understand how this VI works and to review the block diagram, call this VI up from the **CD ROM disk directory. Run** the VI, and when prompted, select the data file called **Hreflex.bin** (binary file). Note that a nonspecific EMG interference pattern is first apparent. Press the "SHOW NEXT" button, using the *Hand Tool,* ***six times*** until the waveforms displayed in Figure 3–19.14 appear. ***Stop*** the VI at this point. Note that the three waveforms described previously will be located slightly off-center and to the right. They will also appear ***horizontally compressed*** and located approximately between x-axis points "695" and "775." To ***center*** the waveforms and ***horizontally stretch*** them out for easier identification, change the "0" x-axis point to "600," and change the "999" point to "800" by ***swiping over*** the numbers with the *Lettering Tool* and inputting the new numbers when each x-axis number is highlighted. Note that this has the effect of ***zooming-in*** on the waveforms. ***Zoom-in*** even further using the same procedure again with a narrower range of x-axis values. The y-axis (***signal amplitude***) may be controlled in a similar way.

SUMMARY

Additional front panel and block diagram display, data collection, and analysis functions were discussed. Most of the VIs described may be reconfigured to meet specific application needs. The final two VIs in this section, modified from existing National Instruments' **Example** VIs, introduced ***binary*** programming functions.

PRACTICE EXERCISES

To practice using ***Rings,*** open the **Rings.vi** VI created earlier in this chapter, or call it up from the **CD ROM disk directory.** Modify the VI in the following way. First, change the *Text Ring* to a *Menu Ring,* and label it "Option 1." Second, change the label of the original "Menu Ring" to "Option 2." Third, add another entry to this *Menu Ring* that creates a beep sound and displays the message: "THIS IS THE LAST ENTRY FOR THIS OPTION" in a dialog window. Fourth, bundle the two *Menu Rings* with a frame to create a control panel area. **Save** the modified VI using the filename **2_Options.vi** into a convenient directory. Compare the new version just created with the VI called **2Options.vi** in the **CD ROM disk directory.**

To practice using an *Attribute Node,* build a simple VI that **will read a force transducer data file** with the following elements and functions. Include two *Waveform Graphs,* the first of which will use a *Cursor Display* to determine the ***start*** and ***end*** points of a ***segment*** of an entire data file. Associate an *Attribute Node* with the *Cursor Display* that will read the segment ***start*** and ***end*** points, and use this information to display the segment on a second *Waveform Graph* after the VI is **Run** a second time. Compute the ***mean force*** and ***standard deviation*** of the sample ***for the segment*** that is selected, and display these two values on the front panel in two *Digital Indicators.* Use two other *Digital Indicators* to display the ***start*** and ***end*** points of the segment. Use the following ***conversion factor*** to display the graph and *Digital Indicator* data in kilograms: 1 volt = 6.25 kg. Configure the VI such that Channel "0" is the transducer channel. ***Lowpass filter*** the signal with a ***low-frequency cutoff*** of "20 Hz" using the **Filters.vi** SubVI.

To test that the VI is working properly, **Run** it using the ***transducer data*** with the **Trans3.dat** filename, which may be found in the **CD ROM disk directory.** For the segment that ***starts*** with an x-axis coordinate of "1525" and ***ends*** at "3000," the "Mean Force" should be "2.60 kg" with a "Standard Deviation" of "0.65." After the VI is built, **Save** it to a convenient directory using the **Trans_1.vi** filename. Compare the version just built with the VI in the **CD ROM disk directory** called **Trans1.vi.**

In this chapter, the subVI **B_line.vi** was created to identify the point on the x-axis (time) where a ***torque curve*** began to ***rise from the baseline.*** In the VI called **Torque.vi** (see Figure 3–16.1), in Section 3–16, "Torque and Velocity

Measurements," this function was handled using icons wired together to achieve the same function.

Open the **Torque.vi** VI created previously, or call it up from the **CD ROM disk directory.** In the block diagram, identify the area of the program where the ***rise from baseline*** function is handled, and ***substitute*** the **B_line.vi** subVI for the comparable code. **Save** the modified version using the filename **Tor_mod.vi.** Compare the new version just created with the VI called **Tormod.vi** in the **CD ROM disk directory.** To ensure that the VI correctly identifies the ***rise from baseline*** x-axis coordinate, use the same data file (**Torq3.dat**) recommended to test the original **Torque.vi** VI in the **CD ROM disk directory.** The *Digital Indictor* labeled "Start of Rise from Baseline (msec)," with the ***segment analyzer*** and ***filter*** options both turned "OFF," should read "1014."

Open the **Scope1.vi** VI (see Figure 3–19.5), or call it up from the **CD ROM disk directory.** Add a ***second*** channel display capability to the front panel. Label the upper chart "Channel 0" and the lower chart "Channel 1." Also, add a front panel control that will permit the two signals to be scaled by factors of "1x," "2x," and "3x," and label them accordingly. The ***default setting*** for this control should be "1x." **Save** the modified version of this VI using the filename **Scope_2.vi** into a convenient directory. Compare the new version just created with the VI called **Scope2.vi** in the **CD ROM disk directory.**

Using a spreadsheet software package such as Excel™ or Quattro Pro™, create a ***two-column spreadsheet*** data file with the following values. Do ***NOT*** use headers in the columns:

56.3	23.6
55.4	22.6
53.7	24.7
58.0	22.3
58.9	26.4
55.5	30.0
56.9	24.5
58.1	22.9
56.2	25.8
59.0	25.6
58.1	29.3
56.8	22.7

Save the spreadsheet as a ***tab-delimited (text)*** file using the filename **Testdat.dat.** Build a simple VI that will ***read*** the **Testdat.dat** file just created, and insert the

Pearsn_r.vi subVI, created in this chapter, into the block diagram. Include two *Digital Indicators* in the front panel labeled "Pearson r Correlation Coefficient" and "No. of Comparisons," respectively. **Run** the VI with the data file just created, and confirm that the "Pearson r Correlation Coefficient" is "0.04" and that the "No. of Comparisons" is "12." Compare the VI just created with the VI called **Pear_r.vi** in the **CD ROM disk directory.**

The **1Wanova.vi** VI created in this chapter was designed as a ***stand-alone*** VI. Open this VI, or call it up from the **CD ROM disk directory.** Configure and **Save** it as a subVI, providing ***output terminals*** for three parameters including the "F" statistic, "Degrees of Freedom," and "p" probability value. Label them accordingly. Edit the ***icon face*** of this subVI with the label "1Way," and **Save** the subVI with the filename **1_Way.vi** into your subVI directory. Review Section 3–5, "Creating SubVIs," concerning terminal wiring and editing the icon face.

Next, create a ***two-column spreadsheet data file*** using the ***same*** values that appear in the "X" and "Grouping Factor" *Arrays* in Figure 3–19.10. **Save** the spreadsheet as a ***tab-delimited (text)*** file using the filename **1Waydat.dat.** Finally, create a simple VI, using the **1_Way.vi** subVI in the block diagram, that will ***read*** the data file just created. Construct it so that it will compute and display "F," "Degrees of Freedom," and "p" values in front panel *Digital Indicators.* **Run** the VI using the **1Waydat.dat** data file, and compare the values noted previously with those in Figure 3–19.10. Compare the versions of the subVI and VI just created with the subVI called **1Way.vi** and the VI called **Anova.vi** in the **CD ROM disk directory.**

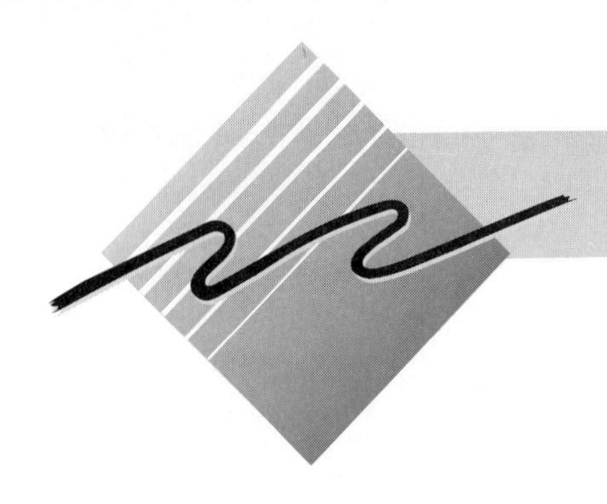

SECTION 3–20

Sample Data Files

To help the user confirm that VIs and subVIs have been constructed and are working properly, a series of ***sample data files*** have been included on the accompanying **CD ROM disk.** Various types of instruments were used to acquire these data including EMG, dynamometers providing torque and angular displacement and velocity measures, events markers, and force transducers. In some cases, data were collected simultaneously from ***several*** instruments (e.g., EMG and an isokinetic dynamometer).

These files may be especially useful if an analog-to-digital (A-to-D) board is not immediately available to take real-time measurements. Even if a converter board is available, it is still a good idea to run some sample data files through VIs that have been constructed, because specific measurements are often referred to as a means of checking program accuracy.

The following chart identifies the data ***filename*** and describes the ***source*** of the signal, ***channels,*** and the ***elapsed time*** the data were collected. Most data files have been saved in a ***tab-delimited (ASCII)*** spreadsheet format and usually have a **.dat** extension appended. The file with a **.bin** extension was saved in ***bin*ary** format and is described in detail in Section 3–19, "Other Programming Functions and Tools."

Sample Data Files

Filename	Description
EMGx11S.dat	Single channel of EMG data for 1 second.
EMGx12s.dat	Single channel of EMG data for 2 seconds.
EMGx14s.dat	Single channel of EMG data for 4 seconds.
EMGx21s.dat	Two channels of EMG data for 1 second.
EMGx22s.dat	Two channels of EMG data for 2 seconds.
EMGx24s.dat	Two channels of EMG data for 4 seconds.
Torq1.dat	Single channel of isometric torque data for 8 seconds.
Torq2.dat	Single channel of isometric torque data for 8 seconds.
Torq3.dat	Single channel of isometric torque data for 8 seconds.
Torq4.dat	Single channel of isometric torque data for 8 seconds.
3Chn.dat	Isometric torque data on channel 0, and EMG data on channels 1 and 2 for 8 seconds.
Hreflex.bin	Single channel of H-reflex EMG data for 60 seconds in binary format.
TorqEMG1.dat	Isometric torque data on channel 0, and EMG data on channels 1 and 2 for 8 seconds.
TorqEMG2.dat	Isometric torque data on channel 0, and EMG data on channels 1 and 2 for 8 seconds.
TorqEMG3.dat	Isometric torque data on channel 0, and EMG data on channels 1, 2, and 3 for 8 seconds.
Powspec1.dat	Single channel of EMG data for 5 seconds.
Powspec2.dat	Single channel of EMG data for 5 seconds.
Torqang1.dat	Isokinetic (concentric) torque data on channel 0, and joint angle data on channel 1.
Torqang2.dat	Isokinetic (concentric) torque data on channel 0, and joint angle data on channel 1.
Trans1.dat	Force transducer data on channel 0, and event marker data on channel 1 for 5 seconds.
Trans2.dat	Force transducer data on channel 0, and event marker data on channel 1 for 5 seconds.
Trans3.dat	Force transducer data on channel 0, and event marker data on channel 1 for 5 seconds.
Trans4.dat	Force transducer data on channel 0, and event marker data on channel 1 for 5 seconds.
1Waydat.dat	Two-column tab-delimited (text) spreadsheet file; the first column is for dependent variables, and the second for group factors.

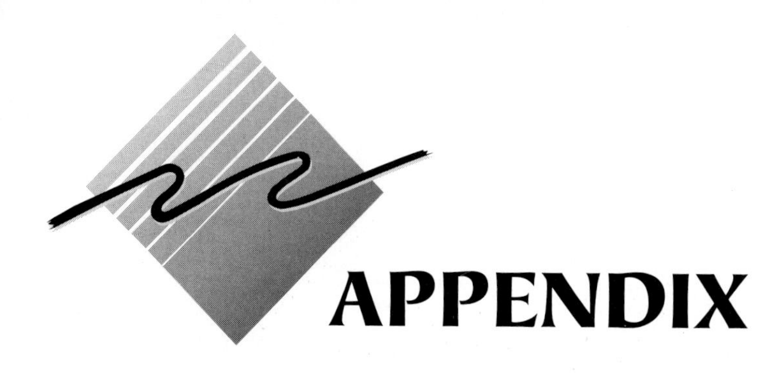

APPENDIX

CD ROM Disk Directory with VI and SubVI Descriptions

Directory	Filename	Description
3–1 Basics	None	
3–2 Front Panel	**Readtran.vi**	VI that reads a force transducer file and displays the signal in a *Waveform Graphs.* A second graph displays an event marker that is used to automatically calculate a force (in kg) at the time the event marker is triggered.
	Index.vi	VI that demonstrates indexing.
	Front.vi	Sample front panel elements for a Practice Exercise.
	Front2.vi	Modified version of **Front.vi.**
3–3 Block Diagram	**Block.vi**	Simple VI that uses several mathematical functions to calculate a numerical value.
3–4 Build and Run Two Simple VIs		
	Percent.vi	Computes and displays a percentage score.
	Random.vi	Generates scaled random numbers and plots them on a *Waveform Chart.*
3–5 Creating SubVIs		
	Rxscale.vi	SubVI that generates and scales random numbers.

Directory	Filename	Description
	2Random.vi	Simple VI that incorporates **Rxscale.vi** subVI.
	Descrip.vi	VI that computes descriptive statistics including mean, standard deviation of a population and sample and n.
	SDsam.vi	SubVI that computes the standard deviation of a sample.
3–6 More SubVIs		
	EmptyVI.vi	VI with unopened subVI demonstrating the *Replace* function.
	Disvolts.vi	SubVI that permits signal to be displayed as volts, millivolts, or microvolts using a *Case Structure*.
	Torque.vi	VI that measures torque parameters from an isokinetic dynamometer demonstrating the use of several subVIs.
	Segment.vi	SubVI that permits the analysis of a selected segment of a data file.
	Integrl2.vi	SubVI that computes and displays the integral of a signal.
	Bpass.vi	Bandpass filter subVI with low and high cutoffs of 20 and 500 Hz, respectively.
	Filters.vi	SubVI that provides, bandpass, lowpass, or bandstop digital filtering using a Butterworth filter.
	Filtered.vi	VI that displays raw and filtered data using the Filters.vi and Disvolts.vi subVIs.
3–7 Loops and Structures		
	Forloop.vi	VI that demonstrates the use of *For Loops*.
	Shifreg.vi	VI that demonstrates the use of *Shift Registers* in a *While Loop*.
	Casebool.vi	VI that demonstrates the use of Boolean-configured *Case Structure*.
	Casenum.vi	VI that demonstrates the use of a numeric-configured *Case Structure*.

Directory	Filename	Description
	Seqlocal.vi	VI that demonstrates the use of a *Sequence Local* in a *Sequence Structure.*
	Formod.vi	Modified version of **Forloops.vi.**
	Shiftmod.vi	Modified version of **Shifreg.vi.**
	Casebmod.vi	Modified version of **Casebool.vi.**
	Casenmod.vi	Modified version of **Casenum.vi.**
	Seqmod.vi	Modified version of **Seqlocal.vi.**
3–8 VI Programming Errors		
	Debug.vi	Simple VI to demonstrate debugging techniques.
	Broke.vi	Simple VI with errors to practice debugging.
	Fixed.vi	Debugged and operating version of **Broke.vi.**
3–9 Strings		
	Strings1.vi	VI that demonstrates the use of string variables including the *Concatenate strings* function.
	Strings2.vi	VI that integrates string and numeric variables to generate and display random numbers indicating the date and time each iterated random number is generated.
	Strings3.vi	Modified version of **Strings2.vi** that compares the current random number to a threshold value and saves the data to a spreadsheet.
3–10 Indexing		
	Index.vi	VI that demonstrates indexing.
3–11 Formula Nodes		
	Formula.vi	VI that demonstrates the use of a *Formula Node.*
	Square.vi	VI that demonstrates the use of multiple *Formula Nodes.*
	Formnode.vi	VI that demonstrates the computation of a number using a *Formula Node* and standard LabVIEW arithmetic functions.

Directory	Filename	Description
3–12 Tables		
	Gen3col.vi	VI that generates a three-column table on the front panel using an *Attribute Node*. Data are also saved to a spreadsheet. Headers in the spreadsheet are optional.
	Gen5col.vi	A five-column version of **Gen3col.vi.**
3–13 Data Acquisition		None
3–14 Writing and Reading Data		
	Write2ch.vi	VI that writes (saves) two channels of data collected from an A-to-D board to disk using a spreadsheet format. Sample rate and the number of samples collected are variably controlled.
	Read2ch.vi	VI that reads and displays two channels of data saved using a spreadsheet format.
	Read3ch.vi	Three-channel version of **Read2ch.vi** with filtering voltage display options.
3–15 Electromyography		
	4Chanemg.vi	VI that acquires and displays four channels of EMG data and saves the data to disk using a spreadsheet format. Sample rate and the number of samples collected are variably controlled.
	Filt&int.vi	VI that reads and displays a single channel of raw and filtered data and computes and displays the maximal integral. Analysis of a segment of the data file using the **Segment.vi** subVI.
	IEMGx2.vi	VI that reads and displays two channels of EMG raw and conditioned data. The data are bandpass filtered and rectified, and the maximal integral for each muscle is computed.
	Normalx2.vi	VI that computes the maximal integral of two channels of EMG data during a submaximal contraction and normalizes same to a maximal effort.

Directory	Filename	Description
	Spec.vi	VI that reads and displays a single channel of data. Data are displayed as raw, rectified, and filtered. The power spectrum and the integration of the spectrum are displayed using a Fast Fourier Transform, and the median and mean power frequencies are computed.
	Pspecx2.vi	VI that reads and displays two channels of data. The power spectra are displayed using a Fast Fourier Transform, and the median and mean power frequencies are computed.
	Iemg_mod.vi	Modified version of **Iemgx2.vi** with segment analysis capabilities included.
	Nor_mod.vi	Modified version of **Normalx2.vi** with segment analysis capabilities included.
3–16 Torque and Velocity Measurements		
	Torque.vi	VI that measures various torque parameters from an isokinetic dynamometer. Filtering and segment analysis are options.
	Tor&seg.vi	Modified version of **Torque.vi** that displays the complete torque signal on one *Waveform Graph* and a segment of the signal to be analyzed on another.
	Mntorq.vi	VI that computes mean torque of a single channel of data. The entire signal and a segment of the signal to be analyzed are displayed on two *Waveform Graphs.* Data may be displayed as volts, ft-lbs, or Newton-meters.
	Tor&ang2.vi	VI that computes and displays on two *Waveform Graphs* various torque and angular data from an isokinetic dynamometer. Segment analysis and filtering options are provided.

Directory	Filename	Description
	Torx3.vi	VI that creates an overlay plot of three channels of torque data using a *Sequence Structure*. The point at which the signal rises from the baseline must be specified to ensure all three signals start at the same relative point. The rise point is determined using another VI such as **Torque.vi.**
	Mtormod.vi	Modified version of **Mntorq.vi** that calculates peak torque, time to peak torque, and the start of rise from the baseline.
	Torx4.vi	Modified version of **Torx3.vi** that permits four torque curves to be simultaneously plotted.
3–17 Torque and EMG Measurements		
	Tor&emg2.vi	VI intended to simultaneously acquire and display, on *Waveform Graphs*, one channel of torque from an isokinetic dynamometer and two channels of EMG.
	Tor&iemg.vi	VI that reads a spreadsheet format data file and displays a raw and mean torque signal for 500 data points from the point of peak torque and integrates two channels of EMG. The data are first bandpass filtered.
	Tor&iemg_ mod.vi	Modified version of **Tor&iemg.vi** that integrates three channels of EMG.
3–18 Feedback and Timing Tools		
	Feedbk1.vi	VI feedback tool using three vertically oriented LEDs that are serially lighted as predetermined target threshold values are attained. The signal is acquired in real time via a sensor connected to an A-to-D board.
	Feedbk2.bk	VI feedback device using a slide indicator and top-mounted LED that lights when a target threshold value is achieved. The signal is acquired in real time via sensor connected to an A-to-D board.

Directory	Filename	Description
	Leds.vi	VI with four LEDs that are variably lighted as scaled random numbers are compared using greater than or equal to and less than or equal to statements. The random numbers are graphed on a *Waveform Chart* as the LEDs are lighted. A timing control is added using a *While Loop.*
	Timer.vi	VI that functions as a count-down timer. When the zero point is reached, a red LED lights up with the word "Finish."
	Digtimer.vi	VI that functions as a digital timer stating the time in seconds and milliseconds.
	stop_time.gbl	A global variable used in **Digtimer.vi.**
	Fdbk1mod.vi	A modified version of **Feedbk1.vi.**
	Fdbk2mod.vi	A modified version of **Feedbk2.vi.**
3–19 Other Programming Functions and Tools		
Other Programming Functions	**Updates.vi**	VI that demonstrates three ways to update a signal displayed on a *Waveform chart.*
	Rings.vi	VI that demonstrates the use of *Text* and *Menu Ring* controls.
	Cursor.vi	VI using a cursor *Attribute Node* to read the x (time) coordinates of a single data file to determine a segment of a file to be analyzed. The mean, standard deviation of the sample, peak value, and peak value index are read and displayed in digital indicators from the selected segment.
	B_line.vi	SubVI that indexes the point in time when a signal rises from the baseline.
Data Display and Analysis	**Scope1.vi**	VI that functions as a simple real-time single-channel oscilloscope acquiring the signal from an A-to-D board.
	Fitline2.vi	VI that fits a line to a segment of a data file and determines its slope and slope intercept. The full data file and segment to be analyzed are displayed on two *Waveform Graphs.* A digital filter is provided.

Directory	Filename	Description
	Readtran.vi	VI that reads a force transducer file and displays the signal in a *Waveform Graphs.* A second graph displays an event marker that is used to automatically calculate a force (in kg) at the time the event marker is triggered.
Statistical Analysis	**Histgrm.vi**	VI that plots a running histogram of data points. A front panel slide switch is used to select between a uniform white noise or random noise pattern. The mean, mode, and standard deviation of the sample are calculated.
	Pearsn_r.vi	A SubVI that calculates the Pearson product moment correlation coefficient between two arrays of data.
	1Wanova.vi	VI that performs a one-way ANOVA on three arrays of data.
Advanced Tools	**Analyze.vi**	VI that calculates various measurement parameters in real time. Cursor control *Attribute Nodes* are used to select a segment of a signal to be analyzed. The segment analyzed may be optionally saved to disk in a spreadsheet format.
	Bincolct.vi	VI that acquires a single channel of data from the computer's A-to-D board and saves the data in binary format.
	Hread.vi	VI that reads binary format files and displays H-reflexes. Cursor controls are used to measured signal amplitudes and x-coordinate time values.
Practice Exercises	**2Options.vi**	A modified version of **Rings.vi.**
	Iemgx1.vi	A modified version of **Iemgx2.vi** that demonstrates the use of an *Attribute Node* associates with the *Cursor Display* of a *Waveform Graph.*

Directory	Filename	Description
	Tormod.vi	A modified version of **Torque.vi** that uses the **B_line.vi** subVI to replace a segment of code that determines when a torque curve rises from the baseline.
	Scope2.vi	A modified version of **Scope1.vi** to which has been added a second display channel.
	Pear_r.vi	A simple VI using the **Pearsn_r.vi** subVI to compute a Pearson product moment correlation coefficient.
	1Way.vi	SubVI created from the **1Wanova.vi** VI that computes the F statistic, degrees of freedom, and *p* value.
	Anova.vi	VI that uses the **1Way.vi** subVI to compute the F statistic, degrees of freedom, and *p* value.
3–20 Sample Data Files		
	EMGx11S.dat	Single channel of EMG data for 1 second.
	EMGx12s.dat	Single channel of EMG data for 2 seconds.
	EMGx14s.dat	Single channel of EMG data for 4 seconds.
	EMGx21s.dat	Two channels of EMG data for 1 second.
	EMGx22s.dat	Two channels of EMG data for 2 seconds.
	EMGx24s.dat	Two channels of EMG data for 4 seconds.
	Torq1.dat	Single channel of isometric torque data for 8 seconds.
	Torq2.dat	Single channel of isometric torque data for 8 seconds.
	Torq3.dat	Single channel of isometric torque data for 8 seconds.
	Torq4.dat	Single channel of isometric torque data for 8 seconds.
	3Chn.dat	Isometric torque data on channel 0 and EMG data on channels 1 and 2 for 8 seconds.
	Hreflex.bin	Single channel of H-reflex EMG data for 60 seconds in binary format.
	Torq EMG1.dat	Isometric torque data on channel 0 and EMG data on channels 1 and 2 for 8 seconds.

Directory	Filename	Description
	TorqEMG2.dat	Isometric torque data on channel 0 and EMG data on channels 1 and 2 for 8 seconds.
	TorqEMG3.dat	Isometric torque data on channel 0 and EMG data on channels 1, 2, and 3 for 8 seconds.
	Powspec1.dat	Single channel of EMG data for 5 seconds.
	Powspec2.dat	Single channel of EMG data for 5 seconds.
	Torqang1.dat	Isokinetic (concentric) torque data on channel 0 and joint angle data on channel 1.
	Torqang2.dat	Isokinetic (concentric) torque data on channel 0 and joint angle data on channel 1.
	Trans1.dat	Force transducer data on channel 0 and event marker data on channel 1 for 5 seconds.
	Trans2.dat	Force transducer data on channel 0 and event marker data on channel 1 for 5 seconds.
	Trans3.dat	Force transducer data on channel 0 and event marker data on channel 1 for 5 seconds.
	Trans4.dat	Force transducer data on channel 0 and event marker data on channel 1 for 5 seconds.
	1Waydat.dat	Two-column tab-delimited (text) spreadsheet file; the first column is for dependent variables and the second for group factors.

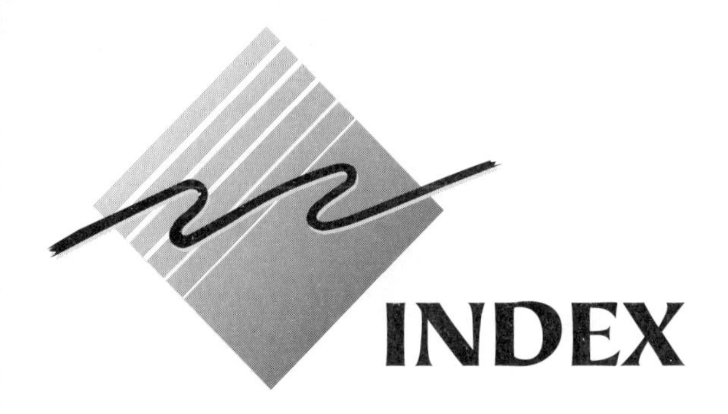

INDEX

P

R

S

T